Family Nursing

Theory & Assessment

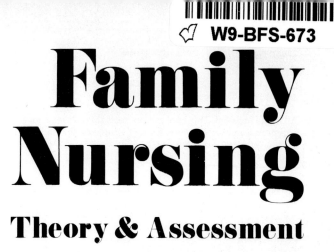

Marilyn M. Friedman
R.N., M.S.

Professor , Department of Nursing
California State University, Los Angeles
Los Angeles, California

Appleton-Century-Crofts/New York

To my family of past and present

81 82 83 84 85 / 10 9 8 7 6 5 4 3

Prentice-Hall International, Inc., London
Prentice-Hall of Australia, Pty. Ltd., Sydney
Prentice-Hall of India Private Limited, New Delhi
Prentice-Hall of Japan, Inc., Tokyo
Prentice-Hall of Southeast Asia (Pte.) Ltd., Singapore
Whitehall Books Ltd., Wellington, New Zealand

Library of Congress Cataloging in Publication Data

Friedman, Marilyn M
　　Family nursing, theory and assessment.

　　Includes bibliographical references and index.
　　1. Nursing—Social aspects.   2. Family—
Health and hygiene.   3. Community health nursing.
I. Title.
RT86.5.F75　　　610.73　　　80-13796
ISBN 0-8385-2532-6

Text and cover design: Dana Kasarsky
Production: Philip Alkana

PRINTED IN THE UNITED STATES OF AMERICA

Contributors

BARBARA E. BAILEY, R.N., M.S.
Assistant Professor
Department of Nursing
California State University, Los Angeles;
Private Practice in Mental Health
Los Angeles, California

MAXENE JOHNSTON, R.N., M.A.
Director of Nursing
Ambulatory Services
Children's Hospital of Los Angeles
Los Angeles, California

DE ANN M. YOUNG, R.N., M.S.
Associate Professor
Department of Nursing
California State University, Los Angeles
Los Angeles, California

Contents

Preface

Within the last ten to fifteen years there have been numerous texts and articles written for nurses and other health professionals about family health care. In reviewing these writings one can readily see that there is no consensus of what family health care, family nursing, family-centered nursing, or family-centered community nursing mean or involve.*

Since my initiation into community health nursing and later into teaching, I have been struck by the contrast between what has been promulgated in nursing literature (in particular community health nursing) and by the American Nurses Association (ANA) and National League for Nursing (NLN), and what actually exists in practice. The family-centered approach is a stated ideal rather than prevailing practice—not only in the primary care settings, but also in the community health settings, where for years community health nurses have been proselytizing the concept that the "family is the patient and focus of our services."

To discharge a stroke patient with thorough instructions on how to transfer from wheelchair to toilet, and then find that the wheelchair does not fit through the small doorway at home is an illustration of the common problems we run into when family and home are not considered. Furthermore, the return into the family network of a family member who has been removed due to illness changes the person's participation in the family and frequently requires serious professional help. Mauksch states:

> It does not matter whether those issues ought to be the concern of the physician, the nurse, the social worker, or any other member in the galaxy of health functionaries. What does matter is that the family as a target of health care and as a conceptual autonomous unit requires professional perspectives which go far beyond the commonly observed approaches to problems and complaints.[1]

Unfortunately, our practice and specialty areas in community health nursing health care delivery patterns belie this approach. Maternal–child health, occupational health, school health, and geriatrics all show the emphasis to be on the individual rather than the family unit. Our health care delivery patterns, particularly the convenient working hours, also make it impossible to provide services to families. As early as 1955 Johnson and Hardin showed that patients, not families, were the primary targets of a community health nurse's service.[2]

My ardent belief is that health professionals who work with families, regardless of the setting, for the purpose of providing effective service must broaden

---

* These terms seem to be used interchangeably in nursing and health literature, with one possible exception—family health care is seen in some texts as a broader term denoting care delivered by more than one health profession.

their commitment so that they serve families as units, as well as individual family members. One of the primary obstacles to providing family health care is a lack of substantive knowledge. Vast amounts of literature are available on the family—in the fields of sociology (family sociology), social psychology, anthropology (cross-cultural family studies), psychiatry, social work, and nursing. But how much and what really do we teach in nursing that actually enables a nurse to work with families, such as knowledge and skill in taking family health assessments, making family diagnoses, and planning and implementing family care plans? I would suggest that very few nursing schools include adequate family theory to provide the necessary foundation for family-centered practice in their curriculum. In all the health professions, such as nursing, medicine, and social work, there is an enormous concentration of curricular focus on the individual client or patient, with little focus on the family system. No one would negate the importance of studying the client comprehensively, but because the family is greater and different from the sum of its parts, both the familial and individual level of assessment and intervention must be the focus when working with families. Sweeney expresses a similar conviction:

> The difference between philosophy and practice in public health nursing will be reconciled only when the public health nurse internalizes family concepts in relation to the needs of individuals and the needs of the family as a whole.[3]

Not only is there a paucity of knowledge provided in nursing and other health curricula, but in nursing literature there also is a serious lack of systematic, comprehensive family assessment tools. Several community health texts have included a family data collection instrument as part of their book (notably Tinkham and Voorhies, Freeman, and Leahy et al.[4–6]) but there have been little related theory or in-depth descriptions of the family structural and functional dimensions.

A comprehensive family assessment tool, based upon a structural–functional theoretical framework, is presented in Part II, which elaborates upon each facet of the tool from both a theoretical and applied perspective. Although several chapters are devoted to other major theoretical frameworks used for family analysis, the structural–functional approach has been selected because of my belief that this approach provides an umbrella framework, sufficient to cover the many relevant concepts and areas needed for assessment. The family assessment tool becomes the basis for the selection of family content and the organizing framework for the book. The family assessment process and much of the family theory

presented in this textbook represent the product of my teaching in community health nursing for 13 years. I started with a very rudimentary tool. Gradually, as the result of insights gained from usage and student and faculty feedback, the family health assessment tool grew into a series of self-learning modules incorporating much of the content within this book. The learning objectives and study questions have been retained from these original modules to assist students with their learning. The study questions (evaluation) at the end of the chapter test the objectives, and upon successful completion of the study questions (all correct) the learner will have mastered the chapter objectives.

The assessment process presented in the following chapters has proved to be a valuable teaching–learning tool in the several schools that use it. One obvious limitation to its usage in its pure form is that it is quite detailed and elaborate, precluding use in every day practice. I believe, however, that a detailed approach is initially necessary to learn family nursing meaningfully. Once the content and skills are grasped, a more practical, attenuated assessment process may be initiated.

I have heard students say that all this information about families is just common sense. It is true that studying the family in one's own society is different from studying many other subjects like mathematics, science, or history due to our personal familiarity with families. This familiarity and expertise in family relations can be both a help and a hindrance: a help because we have some understanding of what goes on in families, how important they are, and some reference from which to tie theory; a hindrance because our own experiences with family life are constricted and biased. Our very familiarity may stand in our way of attempting to step back and assess families objectively and from a broader perspective.

Another observation I have made is that most of us have the natural tendency to assume that the way one's own family does things is, if not the only way, certainly the best way (a brand of ethnocentrism). This, of course, constricts and biases our observations and assessments.

Reiss believes that the study of family theory and research should help students increase their understanding of human interaction since "the reality of human social interaction is a complex phenomenon, and simple truisms and common sense will not be sufficient to understand it."[7] Robischon and Smith[8] strongly emphasize the need for nurses to become skilled in family assessment as a requisite for family nursing. With the increasing emphasis in nursing on the nursing process and with assessment being the foundation for practice, I believe that family health assessment will grow in importance as has the recent interest in nursing assessment of individuals. This is not to suggest that assessment alone provides sufficient knowledge and skill for family health care. Education in family nursing must include discussion of and practice in the other components of the nursing process—diagnosis, planning, intervention, and evaluation.

This book is subdivided into three broad areas. Part I includes four introductory chapters that discuss the family's importance and family definitions; family nursing goals and roles; nursing process; and the basic approaches used in family analysis. The chapter on family-centered roles covers the new thrust of health care—health promotion, wellness training, and prevention of illness and dysfunction. As I am sure most of you are aware, this positive approach to health care is not new. Community health and nursing have been advocating its primacy for a number of years. But because of the present recognition that life style and the environment are the major determinants of disease and illness, and because of the rising costs of crisis-oriented medical care, health promotion and preventive modalities are receiving renewed enthusiasm from both health providers and consumers (albeit limited primarily to the middle and upper classes).

Part II introduces the reader to the actual family assessment model (tool), which forms the core of this text. A modified structural–functional approach has been used as the tool's guiding theoretical framework. I have integrated pertinent theory and content within each of the assessment chapters. The four large areas of assessment are: identifying data, environmental data, family structure, and family functions. Family structural dimensions are crucial to family assessment since they cover family dynamics consisting of power structure, role structure, communication patterns, and value system. The affective function, socialization function, health care function, and family coping function are four essential family functions discussed under family functions. Chapter 17 explains cultural differences and contains family descriptions of the two largest ethnic groups in the United States, the black and Chicano cultures.

The appendixes contain the complete family assessment tool, a family case, and an analysis of the family to give students an opportunity to retest themselves on all the significant areas of family assessment by applying their knowledge to a hypothetical family situation.

Throughout the book I have used the word client rather than patient because of its broader meaning and applicability. Client covers all recipients of our services—individuals, family groups, and even communities, regardless of the recipient's health status.

I wish to extend my thanks to Chris Barnett and Krista Barrett, who diligently typed the manuscript, my family, who encouraged this endeavor and tolerated all the inconveniences associated with having a partially absent mother, and Leslie Boyer, Nursing Editor at Appleton-Century-Crofts who provided not only support but also superb guidance and direction throughout the book's writing.

REFERENCES

1. Mauksch H: A social science basis for conceptualizing family health. Social Science and Medicine 8:525, 1974
2. Johnson WL, Hardin CA: Content and Dynamics of Home Visits of the Public Health Nurse, Part I. New York, American Nurses Foundation, 1955
3. Sweeney BT: Family-centered care in public health nursing. Nursing Forum 9:2: 170, 1970
4. Tinkham C, Voorhies E: Community Health Nursing: Evolution and Process. New York, Appleton, 1972
5. Freeman R: Community Health Nursing Practice. Philadelphia, Saunders, 1970
6. Leahy K, Cobb M, Jones M: Community Health Nursing. New York, McGraw-Hill, 1977
7. Reiss I: Family Systems in America, Second Edition. Hinsdale, Illinois, Dryden Press, 1976, p 399
8. Robischon P, Smith, JA: Family assessment. In Reinhardt A, Quinn M (eds): Current Practice in Family-Centered Community Nursing. St. Louis, Mosby, 1977

I

INTRODUCTORY CONCEPTS AND APPROACHES

INTRODUCTION

One of the most important aspects of pediatric, maternity, community health, and mental health nursing is the emphasis placed on the family unit. Empirically we realize that the quality of family life is closely related to the health of family members. Nevertheless, remarkably little attention has been paid to the family as an object of systematic study in nursing curricula. Apart from simple evaluative labeling of families with terms such as "good," "problem," "multiproblem," or "disorganized," nurses are generally unable to describe objectively the families they see. Furthermore, too little research has been devoted to examining the relationships between the family—its structure and functions—and the health and development of its individual members.

This chapter will attempt to set the stage for a systematic study of the family by describing basic purposes of the family, basic family definitions, how the society and family mutually influence each other, and, most importantly, the salient interrelationship between the health status of family and the health status of its individual members.

Because the family forms the basic unit of our society, it is the social institution which has the most marked effect on its members. This basic unit so strongly influences the development of an individual that it may determine the success or failure of that person's life.

The family serves as the critical intervening variable (or as some authors term it, "buffer" or "bargaining agent") between society and the individual. In other words, the basic purpose of the family is *mediation*—taking the basic societal expectations and obligations and molding and modifying them to some extent to fit the needs and interests of its individual family members. At the same time the family provides new "recruits" and prepares them for assuming roles in society.[1]

Each family member has basic physical, personal, and social needs. The family must serve to mediate the demands and wishes of all the individuals within the unit. A family is expected to be concerned with the needs and demands of parent(s) as well as children, making it a difficult task to assign priorities to diverse individual needs at any particular time. On the other hand, society expects each member to fulfill certain obligations and demands. The family has to mediate the needs and demands of the family member with those of society.

A number of groups have a mediating function, but the family is important in that it is *the* primary group for the individual. Each family member belongs to a number of groups, but usually only the family is concerned with the total individual and all facets of his or her life. The highest priority of the family is usually the welfare of its family members. Other groups such

1

Introduction to the Family

LEARNING OBJECTIVES

1. Describe the basic purposes the family serves for society, the individual family member, and the health care provider.
2. Define:
   a. family
   b. nuclear (conjugal) family
   c. extended family
   d. family of orientation or origin
3. Describe how family and society mutually affect each other.
4. Give examples of how the family influences the health status of its members and how the family is influenced by illness or injury of one or more of its members.
5. Define variant family forms and give examples of several types of traditional and nontraditional (experimental) family forms.
6. Identify several stressors commonly found in single-parent families.

as co-workers, church, school, and friends do not have this concern for the complete individual, but usually limit themselves to one facet of the individual's life; for example, cooperation and friendliness at work, sincerity and involvement in church affairs, or productivity and achievement in school. This is not to say that other groups cannot serve as, or even replace, the family. In communes, monasteries, custodial hospitals, kibbutzim, or various rooming situations, nonfamily primary groups may provide the critical mediating function. The main difference between these primary groups and the family is that the family still retains the replacement or reproduction responsibility. The other primary groups do not generate new members in order to guarantee the survival of the group.

To restate the family's role, the family unit occupies a position between the individual and society, and its functions are twofold: (1) to meet the needs of the individuals in it and (2) to meet the needs of the society of which it is a part. These functions, which are fundamental to human adaptation, cannot be fulfilled separately. They must be joined in the family.

For society, the family functions to fill a vital need through its procreation and socialization of new members. It forms a grouping of individuals that society treats as an entity; it creates a network of kinship systems that help stabilize a society, even in its industrialized state; and it provides status, incentives, and roles for its members within the larger social system.[2]

As mentioned above, the family also functions to meet the needs of its members. For the spouse or adult members it serves to stabilize their lives—meeting their affectional, socioeconomic, and sexual needs. For the children, the family provides physical and emotional care, and concomitantly directs their personality development. The family system is the main learning context for an individual's behavior, thoughts, and feelings. The family's mediating function also protects individuals from direct contact with society.

Parents are the primary "teachers," since parents interpret the world and society to children.* The environment—outside forces—is important mainly as it affects parents, since the parents are the ones who are translating to the children the major meanings these outside forces will have on the family.

The family has a crucial influence on the formation of an individual's identity and feelings of self-esteem.

---

*The interpretation parents give of the world and society is naturally based on their experiences and their "reality." If they have been discriminated against or lived in a crime-ridden community, they may see the world as being "dangerous," "hostile," a place to avoid, and thereby impart these perceptions to their children. If, on the other hand, the world has provided stability and security for them, this perspective will be transmitted to their children.

An individual is the repository of group (especially primary group or family) experience. His or her identity is both individual (intrapersonal experiences) and social (interpersonal experiences). A person's intrapsychic experiences are largely developed from his or her interpersonal experiences, e.g., as through the parent–child relationship. It has been repeatedly found that a meaningful conception of an individual's mental health status can be achieved only as we relate the functioning of the individual to the human relation patterns of that person's primary group or family.

Why Work with the Family?

In the preface it was noted that family-centered practice has been promulgated by community health nursing for quite some time. Why has there been the emphasis on working with families? The family provides the critical resource for delivering efficacious health services to people. Tinkham and Voorhies refer to the family as being the community health nurse's "patient," with the major focus being family health needs and their resolution.[3]

The following are the most cogent reasons why the family unit needs to be focused on:

1. There is the belief that in a family unit, any dysfunction (illness, injury, separation) which affects one or more family members may, and frequently will, in some way affect other members and the unity as a whole. The family is a closely knit, interdependent network where the problems of an individual "seep in" and affect the other family members and the whole system. If a nurse assesses only the individual and not the family, she or he may be missing the gestalt needed to gain a holistic assessment. One of the important tenets of family therapy is that the symptoms of the identified patient (the family member with the overt behavioral problems or psychosomatic illness) are indices of family pathology.
2. There is such a strong interrelationship between family and the health status of its members that the role of the family is crucial during every facet of health care, from preventive strategies through the rehabilitative phase; thus assessing and rendering family health care is critical for assisting each family member to achieve an optimum level of wellness.
3. Through family health care that focuses on health promotion, "self-care," health education, and family counseling, significant inroads can be made to curtail risks which life style and environmental indiscretions create. The goal is to raise the level of wellness of the whole family,

which should then significantly raise the wellness level of each of its members.

4. Case finding is another good reason for providing family health care. Disease in one member may lead to discovery of disease or risk factors in others, as is common with many of the communicable and chronic diseases. The family-centered nurse works through the family to reach individuals.

5. One can achieve a clear perspective of the individual and his or her functioning only when the person's family is also assessed. This enables the nurse to view the individual in his or her primary social context.

THE FAMILY-SOCIETY INTERFACE

As the basic unit in society, the family shapes and is shaped by the external forces (community, large social systems) surrounding it. Most sociologists would agree that the influence of society on the family is greater than that of the family on society, although the family exerts an effect on the society also. In spite of the greater impact society exerts on the family, the family should not be considered a passive, reactionary agent in the process of social change. Through history the family has demonstrated its tremendous resiliency and adaptiveness, just as political, educational, and other societal institutions have shown their ability to change as need dictates. Moreover, the forces operating in society and in the family are continually intervening, interacting, and changing.

Tinkham and Voorhies point out that tacit sanction by society of the communal form of group living, for instance, has modified socialization patterns of the family. The adulation of youth by society has completely altered the function of the family relative to its role in assisting parents and grandparents.[4] Society, with its beliefs, values, and customs pervades every facet of family life such as the age at which children may go to work and the age at which they are legally given adult status. Society also sanctions illness definitions, sick role behaviors, and the appropriateness of treatments.

On the other hand, the family influences society, which in turn may alter societal norms. Tinkham and Voorhies again cite a case in point by explaining that when families socialize their children to settle disputes and conflicts by nonviolent means, the use of war as a means for handling disputes becomes a less acceptable strategy. Also the egalitarian roles which women have assumed in family life have made drastic changes in the way society now views women and their roles and capacities.[5]

The controversies over family planning services and, later, abortion laws exemplify the way in which the family exerts pressure on society to change. In order for parents to be liberated and maintain an acceptable living standard, families are urging society to make birth control services accessible.

The great forces of a modern industrial nation, with its emphasis on individual achievement and autonomy, have been effective in shaping family patterns in such a way that the atomistic nuclear family has emerged. Its organization is geared to the needs of a complex, urban, industrialized society. In contrast, the organization of the extended family consisting of parents, grandparents, children, aunts, uncles, and cousins is more tailored to a rural, agricultural society, which is rapidly disappearing in the United States. Goode summarizes this process in the following statement:

> Because of its emphasis on performance, such a system (industrialization) requires that a person be permitted to rise or fall, and to move about wherever the job market is best. A lesser emphasis on land ownership also increases the ease of mobility. The conjugal family is neo-local (each couple sets up its own household), and its kinship network is not strong, thus putting fewer barriers than other family systems in the way of class or geographic mobility. In these ways the conjugal family system "fits" the needs of industrialization.[6]

Without the extended family's great involvement, nuclear family relationships become more intensified and continuous. There is little cushioning of the negative impact which some family members have on others and few relatives available to participate in child rearing, i.e., babysitting or giving counsel and support to parents.

HEALTH STATUS OF FAMILY AND FAMILY MEMBERS

Health and illness behavior are learned, and the family is the primary source for health education. In one way or another, the family tends to be involved in the decision making and therapeutic process at every stage of a family member's health and illness, from the state of being well (when promotion of health and preventive strategies are taught) to diagnosis, treatment, and recuperation. The process of becoming a "patient" and receiving health services encompasses a series of decisions and events involving the interaction of a number of persons, including family, friends, and professional providers of care. Generally speaking, the role the family plays in the process varies over time depending on an individual's health, the type of health problem, i.e., whether it is acute, chronic, severe, etc., and the degree of familial concern and involvement. Six stages of health/illness* will be presented to further illustrate the family's major involvement.

Prevention of Illness and Promotion of Health

The family can play a vital role in all forms of health promotion and prevention. Modern medical science has produced vaccines and suggested preventive behavioral measures such that many forms of illness can be avoided. Vaccines for poliomyelitis, measles, mumps, smallpox, and diphtheria are among the more common vaccines available to the public for preventive purposes. Smoking, lack of exercise, poor diet, high blood pressure, prolonged stress, and obesity have been well documented as factors influencing the occurrence of coronary heart disease and other major diseases, and preventive behaviors have been recommended to reduce their deleterious effects. Many other examples of recommended preventive practices could be cited, but these few suffice to make the point that many forms of health promotion and prevention exist. Whether a child gets a particular vaccine, whether a father is encouraged to get more exercise and eat less, or whether a mother receives proper prenatal care, all involve family decisions and participation to a great degree. *Public health begins in the family.* Wellness strategies usually require improvements in the life style of an entire family, and varying degrees of conflict may ensue because of the wider impact on the family. Moreover, an individual's body image and self-view—as either healthy and active or sickly and frail—are learned largely within the family context.

Symptom Experience Stage

The symptom experience stage begins when symptoms are (1) recognized, (2) interpreted as to their seriousness, possible cause, and importance or meaning, and (3) related to with varying degrees of concern.

The family serves as the basic point of reference for assessing health behavior and provides basic definitions of health and illness, thus influencing the individual's perceptions. In the American family, the mother is frequently the major determiner of the health behavior in the family. Litman reported in family studies he conducted that the mother acted as health decision maker 67.7 percent of the time, while the father acted in this capacity only 15.7 percent.[8]

Disease and socioeconomic status are interrelated. In general, there exists an inverse relationship between prevalence rates and socioeconomic status, resulting from the greater susceptibility of lower income groups

to disease. This inverse relationship also reflects the fact that members of lower income groups are slower to respond to initial symptoms or may not recognize symptoms as signs of disease or as needing medical attention.[9] The family exposes its members to health hazards to a varying degree and provides the basic interpretations of symptoms.

Families not only influence recognition and interpretation of symptoms of illness, but they may be the *genesis* of illness among family members. Family social disorganization often has negative health consequences for family members. A variety of specific health problems have been found more frequently in "socially disorganized families," among them tuberculosis,[10] arthritis,[11] mental disorders,[12] hypertension,[13] coronary heart disease,[14] and stroke fatalities.[15] The classic Newcastle-upon-Tyne studies[16] showed the pervasive influence of family on health. When deprivation, deficiency of care, and dependence on community were all present within a family, there was a higher incidence of infections, enuresis, short stature of children at age three, convulsions, and strabismus. This study also showed a higher incidence of streptococcal infections and childhood accidents following an acute family crisis.

The Care-Seeking Stage

The care-seeking stage begins when the family decides that the ailing member is really sick and needs help. The ill person and family start to seek alleviation, information, advice, and professional validation from extended family, friends, neighbors, and other nonprofessionals (the lay referral structure). The decision as to whether a member's illness should be treated at home or medical clinic or hospital tends to be negotiated within the family. For example, Richardson, in a study of low-income, urban households, found that about one-half of those with illnesses reported consulting another family member concerning what they should do about the situation.[17] Knapp also found that the family was the most frequently mentioned source of information concerning home remedies and self-medication.[18]

Not only does the family provide the basic definitions of health, but family members may press the individual into this stage if they believe he is failing to react favorably. This process is extremely difficult for the family, particularly when a psychiatric disorder is the major problem, because it may mean that the family must label the person as mentally ill and isolate him and/or acknowledge their own feelings of guilt and shame. The problem is compounded when the affected person denies the disorder or blames the family.[19]

---

*The following six stages represent an adaptation of Suchman's five stages of illness and medical care.[7]

The Medical Contact Stage

This stage commences when contact is made with the health services. Studies have clearly shown that the family is again instrumental during this stage. The family (usually the mother-wife) will refer a family member to whatever type of service is felt appropriate. The family, serving in this capacity, is referred to as "the primary health referral agent."[20]

In the 1950s Koos noted that while families may consult a different physician in special circumstances, the family doctor remains the one to whom they turn for all the family's ordinary medical needs.[21] This pattern probably still exists among many inner-city, poor families due to the lack of availability of specialists. Most health data, however, show that emergency rooms are fast becoming the poor family's most common resource for initial medical care. Among working and middle-class families, there has been a growth in the number of families making use of group practice arrangements and medical clinics.[22]

The type of health care sought varies tremendously. The folk practitioner, the unorthodox "healer," the holistic health practitioner (using sometimes esoteric modalities such as hair analysis and iridology), the superspecialist (such as a neurosurgeon), the independent nurse practitioner, and the primary care physician should all be considered as possible sources of health care (thus broadening antiquated definitions of medical care).

We know that families with higher income, families with children present in the home, and families who have resided in the community for some time usually have a regular physician or source of health care and that the reverse is often true—families not possessing one or more of the above characteristics do not routinely make use of the same care source.[23]

How do families decide what clinic or health provider to contact? While such variables as acceptability, appropriateness, perceived adequacy of service, and seriousness of condition are important, the proximity to a primary care facility seems to be a prime determinant of whom families contact. In other words, the closer the facility, the greater the usage factor.[24]

The Dependent-Patient Role Stage

As the patient accepts care of health practitioners, he or she surrenders certain prerogatives and decisions, and is expected to assume the patient role, characterized by a dependence on the health professional's advice, the willingness to comply with medical advice, and a striving to recover. How this role is further defined and enacted at home will be individually determined within each family. Some families exclude the sick member from all responsibilities and "serve and assist" to the fullest extent. Other families expect little change in the ill member's behavior, hoping that he or she can carry on as usual; this way of handling is seen frequently when it is the mother who is sick. Litman explains the difficulty mothers often have when sick:

> In view of both her rather pervasive and pivotal role as an agent of cure and care within the family setting, the mother may find it not only extremely difficult to fulfill her obligations to all the members of the household when one or more is ill, but she may experience considerable difficulty in maintaining her normal role and responsibility when she herself is the one who is ill.[25]

Hence, mothers generally have a great deal of reluctance in accepting a patient role.

Thus the family unit plays a pivotal role in determining the sick member's patient role behaviors. The family is also instrumental in deciding where the treatment should be given—hospital, home, clinic, etc. Efforts to treat illness and promote good health may often conflict with family values and attitudinal patterns, making medical compliance problematic.

The Rehabilitation Stage

The presence of a serious, chronic illness in one family member usually has a profound impact on the family system, especially to its role structure and to the carrying out of family functions. The disruptive effect may, in turn, negatively affect the outcome of rehabilitation efforts. Can the patient reassume his or her prior (preillness) role responsibilities or is he or she able to establish a new, "workable" role in the family? The way in which this question is solved usually has to do with two factors: (1) the seriousness of the disability and (2) the "centrality" of the patient within the family unit.[26] When either the nature of the person's condition is serious (greatly disabling or progressively deteriorating) or the family member is a pivotal, crucial person to the family's functioning, the impact on family is much more pronounced.

Families play an important supportive role during the course of a client's convalescence or rehabilitation, and, in the absence of this support, the success of convalescence/rehabilitation decreases significantly.

In summarizing the six stages, Haggerty highlighted the ways in which families influence the health of their members as being (1) a cause or the source of illness, (2) a factor affecting the outcome of illness once present, (3) a locus for spread of illness from one family member to another, and (4) a determinant of who is brought to the doctor and when.[27]

FAMILY DEFINITIONS

The family has been defined in various ways. These definitions of the family differ depending on the theoretical orientation of the "definer," that is, by the kind of explanation the writer seeks to make concerning the family. For instance, writers who follow the interactionist theoretical orientation of the family see the family as an arena of interacting personalities, thus emphasizing the dynamic transactional characteristics.

Burgess identifies the following characteristics as being common to families and distinguishing them from other social groups:

1. The family is composed of persons joined together by bonds of marriage, blood, or adoption.
2. The members of a family usually live together in a single household; or, if they live separately, consider the household their home.
3. Family members interact and communicate with each other in family social roles such as husband and wife, mother and father, son and daughter, brother and sister.
4. The family shares a common culture which is derived primarily from societal culture containing some unique features of its own.[28]

This definition is commonly used and certainly covers a large majority of families. It negates, however, the relevance of the extended family, whose members may live in two or more households, and precludes the communal types of families where there are no legal or hereditary ties. Also in some families there are tremendous value differences especially between the generations, so that the maintenance of common culture cannot be narrowly defined. For the purposes of this text, I will define "family" in its broadest sense to allow sufficient flexibility in assessing this social unit:

Family—A family is composed of people (two or more) who are emotionally involved with each other and live in close geographical proximity.*

The following additional family definitions connoting general family types are presented to facilitate our understanding of the family.

---

*Emotional involvement means that there is a perception of reciprocal obligations, a sense of commonness, and a sharing of certain obligations, coupled with a caring and commitment to each other. Because this definition is purposefully broad, it will then cover the type of relationships formally excluded by definition. For example, two members of the same sex linked through homosexual attachment and living together would fit, or two friends living together for a sustained period of time would be subsumed under this definition. The single parent with young children living near her parents and relating on a close, continual basis would also be considered a family.

Nuclear (conjugal) family—This is the family of marriage, parenthood, or procreation; it is composed of a husband, wife, and their immediate children—natural, adopted, or both.
Family of orientation (family of origin)—The family unit into which a person is born.
Extended family—The nuclear family and other related (by blood) persons, who are most commonly members of the family of orientation of one of the nuclear family mates. These are "kin"—grandparents, aunts, uncles, and cousins. The traditional extended family was one in which the couple shared household arrangements and expenses with parents, siblings, or other close relatives. The children were then reared by several generations and had a choice of models on which to pattern their behavior. This type is still frequent in working-class families and immigrant milieus, and is often cohesive and effective.

Advances in transportation and communication have made the extended family ties possible in spite of geographic distance, and thus extended family ties among the middle class are more widespread today. The nuclear American family is not as isolated as it superficially appears. The many ways in which such families rely on one another create an extended family context that has been verified in several important studies. The frequently repeated myth that the nuclear family is isolated from family supports is not borne out by this research, the evidence showing that a modified extended family usually exists within a rich network of generational interaction.[29] Parents and siblings of spouses form the most important network of extended kinship relations. The common modified extended family of today differs from the isolated nuclear family in that it provides significant support and continuing assistance to other nuclear families within the extended family network. This type of extended family is set up on an egalitarian basis and is composed of a series of nuclear families who equally value these extended family bonds.[30]

VARIANT FAMILY FORMS

Families using health services come from all walks of life and represent all types of life styles. Many, if not most, of our clients are not part of the idealized nuclear family. Thus it is imperative for health professionals to understand and appreciate the wide varieties of family forms, as well as some of the reasons for their existence.

One of the primary reasons for the growing number of variant family forms is our affluent and truly pluralistic society, which is to say one that is highly differentiated and specialized. Never in recorded history has a society been composed of a greater multiplicity of attitudes, values, behaviors, or life styles. These social, behavioral, and cultural differences are reflected in a variety of family forms.

According to some social scientists, the basic structure of the family is related to the dominant value orientation of the culture or subculture. For example, the white middle-class orientation is toward small nuclear families, relatively isolated from extended family. With the weakening of the Protestant ethic and the greater acceptability of divergent values, the nuclear family form has lost ground. Yet it has been noted that tying family structure to the dominant value orientations of society may be too simplistic an explanation. Billingsley discusses the reasons for various family forms among black families by stating that

> In every Negro neighborhood of any size in the country, a wide variety of family structures will be represented. This range and variety does not suggest, as some commentaries hold, that the Negro family is falling apart, but rather that these families are fully capable of surviving by adapting to the historical and contemporary social and economic conditions facing the Negro people. How does a people survive in the face of oppression and sharply restricted economic and social support? There are, of course, numerous ways. But surely one of them is to adapt the most basic of its institutions, the family, to meet the often conflicting demands placed on it. In this context, then, the Negro family has proved to be an amazingly resilient institution.[31]

Diversity is based on the right of individuals to live in any form they feel will be beneficial to them in achieving their desired quality of life. A pluralistic society such as ours must realize that any of the currently existing family forms may be suited to certain individuals in their search for fulfillment. It is true that certain of these forms are probably more suitable for fulfilling certain basic functions than other forms. To date, however, we have little objective knowledge about the outcomes or superiority of one family form over another.[32]

Before proceeding further, it is important to explain how the term "variant family form" is used. This term includes all deviations from the traditional nuclear family, which is characterized by households of husband, wife, and children living apart from both sets of parents with the male as the breadwinner and wife as the homemaker.[33] Thus people are getting more "various" in their family behavior. "What was defined a decade ago as 'deviant,'" observes Rossi, "is today labelled 'variant' in order to suggest that there is a healthy experimental quality to current social explorations beyond monogamy and the nuclear family."[34]

The term "variant" is used in an attempt to avoid negative connotations toward any existing type of family and to recognize the diversity of the number and types of options available to people and families.

As can be seen from the listing of the variations in the family (Table 1.1), a multitude of forms exist. Nevertheless, when one thinks of family, a model of a parent team—mother and father—is conjured up. As biological and social parents they carry out the parental functions of child rearing, providing economic support, and meeting their own and their children's needs. Today this is an ideal which is not accessible or does not operate in many American families (only 36 percent of our nuclear families meet this ideal norm of father–mother–children today).[35] Because of their significance for family nursing, several types of family forms will be described.

Single-Parent Family

Single parents include "parents without partners" (usually divorced or separated women), widows or widowers with children, unmarried mothers, adoptive parents, step-parents, and, finally, foster parents. The most common single-parent type in our society is the mother rearing her children alone. At least 17 percent of United States households in 1978 were single-parent families, most often headed by women.[36] The woman who is divorced, separated, deserted, widowed, and unmarried falls into the single-parent family type. Because these women do not have the usual economic and emotional resources and because single-parent families are so numerous today, an exploration of some of the generic features of single-parent families and their special problems and needs follows.

Generic Features of Single-Parent Family

Poverty. Although households headed by women comprised only about 17 percent of all United States households in 1978, they constituted a large percentage of those on welfare. Goode, in a study of women divorcees, found financial problems to be a major complaint of divorced women. Approximately 40 percent of the divorced husbands in this study were delinquent in their support payments.[37]

Poverty is extremely relative, as is deprivation. In practically all cases of divorce, there is a reduction in the standard of living, reflecting the costs of maintaining two households on the same financial resources.[38]

Role Conflicts. Single-parent women tend to be either overloaded with roles or in conflict over their various role commitments, since they were forced to add the father role to their parental responsibilities. With a spouse to depend on, there is role flexibility—

TABLE 1.1
Types and Percentages of Different Family Forms in the United States.*

Traditional Variant Family Forms

The most prominent traditional types of variant family forms now existing are:

1. Nuclear family—dual career, husband, wife, and children living in same household (16%)
2. Nuclear dyad—husband and wife alone: childless, or no children living at home (10%)
   a. Single career
   b. Dual career
      1. Wife's career continuous
      2. Wife's career interrupted
3. Single-parent family—one head, as a consequence of divorce, abandonment, or separation (with financial aid rarely coming from the second parent), and usually including preschool and/or school age children (16%)
   a. Career
   b. Noncareer
4. Single adult living alone (20%)
5. Three generation family—may characterize any variant of family forms 1, 2, or 3 living in a common household (5%)
6. Middle-aged or elderly couple—husband as provider, wife at home (children have been launched into college, career, or marriage) (13%)
7. Kin network—nuclear households or unmarried members living in close geographical proximity and operating within a reciprocal system of exchange of goods and services.
8. "Second career" family—the wife enters the work force when the children are in school or have left the parental home.

Nontraditional, Experimental Variant Family Forms

Emerging (experimental) variant family forms (4%) include:

1. Commune family
   a. Household of more than one monogamous couple with children, sharing common facilities, resources, and experiences; socialization of the child is a group activity.
   b. Household of adults and offspring—a "group marriage," where all individuals are "married" to each other and all are parents to the children. Usually there is a charismatic leader.
2. Unmarried parent and child family—usually mother and child, where marriage is not desired or possible.
3. Unmarried couple and child family—usually a common-law type of marriage with the child their biological issue or informally adopted.
4. Cohabiting couple—unmarried couple living together.
5. Homosexual unions—persons of same sex living together as "marital partners."

---

* Adapted from: Sussman MB: Family systems in the 1970s: Analysis, policies and programs in volume no. 396 of THE ANNALS of The American Academy of Political and Social Science. © 1971 by The American Academy of Political and Social Science.

---

someone to help with chauffeuring, filling in when mother is sick, etc. But for the single parent, her working hours often conflict with child-care hours. Even though there is no wife role to be involved with, dating and courtship often enter in and create demands on the mother's time.[39]

Role Shifts. Eighty to ninety percent of the mothers who are single parents will eventually remarry, necessitating another role change—first taking over the father's role and then relinquishing it and forming new marital and parental roles on remarriage.[40]

Social Stigma. Single parents face some degree of social stigma (less certainly for the widowed than for the divorced or separated, and they less than the unmarried). This should be qualified, however, by emphasizing that the extent to which this is true depends on the single parent's subculture or reference group. In poor communities, for example, an unmarried woman living with children is not as stigmatized by the community as she would be if she were living in a middle-class community.

The divorced or separated mother has several advantages over the deserted mother, who appears more traumatized by the unilateral decision of her husband to leave and her unresolved legal status (support payments and marital status). The divorcee at least has legal recourse through the domestic relations court and is free to associate with other men and remarry, in addition to not having to share the parental decisions with a partner, with whom she probably could not agree in the past.

The divorced father also encounters some major difficulties. He often hates to be separated from his children. He still has financial responsibility of a father but few of the joys of parenthood. These fathers often voice their frustration and concern about their relationships with their children.

The Unmarried Mother. This mother quite obviously has all the problems of the other single parents and a few more (financial, perhaps a disadvantaged background, greater social stigma).[41] It is well known that the mother–child family is prevalent among the poor of all racial and ethnic backgrounds. As Billingsley suggests, these families need not be deviant or distorted family forms, since they may be the only viable and appropriate form for the particular setting in which they exist. Keller points out that "its defects may stem more from adverse social judgments than from intrinsic failings. Deficient in cultural resources and status, it may nevertheless provide a humane and spirited setting for its members, particularly if some sense of stability and continuity has been achieved."[42]

LeMasters addresses a related question, "Is the one-parent family pathological?", by citing studies conducted in this area that report no conclusive research data to prove the two-parent family is any better than the one-parent family. He goes on to say that he believes "one good parent is enough to rear children adequately or better in our society ... enough prominent Americans have been reared by widows or other solo parents to prove the point."[43]

A careful review of the effects of fatherless families on children concludes that there is little convincing evidence that the mere absence of a father produces serious distortions in the child's intellectual and emotional development or sexual identity. The manner in which the mother functions with her children in such a family, along with the adequacy of child-care arrangements made if the mother works, is far more significant than the presence of both parents.[44]

Single Adult Living Alone

As seen in the list of variant family forms, the solitary person is included as a variant family form. Many community health clients, especially the chronically ill, disabled, and older individuals are single persons living alone. Although these "solitary people" do not fit into the definition of "family," they do have a family of the past to consider. Most solitary people are also part of a loosely formed family network. They may have no relatives, but share a family-type relationship with others such as those residing in the same rooming house, nursing home, or neighborhood or relate closely with pets. There are also people who are truly "loners." They have a greater need for health service, since they have no support system. Helping them achieve socialization through provision of a supportive, affective relationship (albeit limited in time and scope) may be a significant service.

Experimental Variant Family Forms

Experimental variant family forms cover a wide gamut of family forms which are very different from one another in structure and dynamics, although probably more similar in goals and values than vis-à-vis the traditional nuclear family. Specific family forms referred to as "experimental" include open marriages, communes, cohabiting couples, group marriages, and ho-

mosexual unions. Cogswell reports that one theme implicit in the literature related to experimental family forms is the rejection of the myth of the idealized traditional nuclear family. Advocates of experimental-type families see the nuclear family as restrictive, since no one person (mate) can meet all of another person's needs, and deleterious, because of distorted myths about child rearing (such as total parental responsibility for child-rearing outcomes) and male superiority. There is the implicit assumption that the orientation of the traditional nuclear family is based primarily on the value system of the dominant culture (white Anglo-Saxon Protestant culture) and that individuals living in experimental families have rejected some of these basic values and selected an alternative culture.[45]

It is the affluent, bourgeois, middle-class family with its Protestant work ethic from which these experimentalists of the alternate culture are usually trying to escape. In contrast, their values and goals consist of self-actualization, independence, gender equality, intimacy in a variety of interpersonal relationships (not marital exclusively), openness in communication, and sexual variety. There is an emphasis on enjoying the present rather than postponing satisfaction to the future. From this array of values each particular experimental family form selects and stresses different priorities.[46]

Many of those involved in the new family forms are college-educated people who have been indoctrinated into the philosophy of choice and freedom. The delay of marriage, the delay of parenthood, the reduction of family size, and the high divorce rates are all evidences that other options besides marriage and family are present for both sexes.[47]

Keller sums up the anticipated future for the American family in the following:

> Thus if we dare to speculate further about the future of the family we will be on safe ground with the following anticipations: (1) a trend towards greater, legitimate variety in sexual and marital experience; (2) a decrease in the negative emotions—exclusiveness, possessiveness, fear and jealousy—associated with these; (3) greater room for personal choice in the kind, extent, and duration of intimate relationships; ... (4) entirely new forms of communal living arrangements in which several couples will share the tasks of childrearing and economic support as well as relaxation pleasures; (5) multi-stage marriages geared to the changing life cycle and the presence or absence of dependent children.[48]

FAMILY NURSING IMPLICATIONS

This illustrates the broad range of structures prevalent in families today. There is no "right," "wrong," "proper," or "improper" form of family. Families must be understood for themselves. Labels and types serve only as a reference to family structural form. Every effort must be made to understand the uniqueness of each particular family. Society places conflicting demands on people; hence the need for a range of family forms to coexist. Persons serving families must be tolerant of existing family forms and should abandon the traditional model of the "ideal" family.

REFERENCES

1. Williams JI, Leaman T: Family structure and function. In Conn H, Rakel R (eds): Family Practice. Philadelphia, Saunders, 1973, p 5
2. Lidz T: The Family and Human Adaptation. New York, International University Press, 1963, p 45
3. Tinkham C, Voorhies E: Community Health Nursing—Evolution and Process. New York, Appleton, 1977, p 118
4. *Ibid.*
5. *Ibid.*
6. Goode WJ: The Family. Glencoe, Ill, The Free Press, 1964, p 108
7. Suchman EA: Stages of illness and medical care. J Health Human Behav 6(3):114, 1965
8. Litman TJ: The family as a basic unit in health and medical care—A social behavioral overview. Social Sci Med 8:502, 1974
9. Koos E: The Health of Regionville. New York, Columbia University Press, 1954
10. Holmes T: Multidiscipline studies of tuberculosis. In Spacer P (ed): Personality Stress of Tuberculosis. New York, International University Press, 1956
11. Scotch N, Greiger J: The epidemiology of rheumatoid arthritis—A review with special attention to social factors. J Chronic Dis 15:1037, 1962
12. Leighton D, Harding JS, Macklin DB, et al: The Character of Danger. New York, Basic Books, 1963
13. Harburg E, et al: Stress and heredity in black-white blood pressure differences. Progress Report to National Institutes of Health, Ann Arbor, 1971
14. Syme S, Hyman M, Enterline P: Some social and cultural factors associated with the occurrence of coronary heart disease. J Chronic Dis 17:277, 1964
15. Neser W: Fragmentation of black families and stroke susceptibility. In Kaplan B, Cassel J: Family and Health: An Epidemiological Approach. Chapel Hill, NC, Institute for Research in Social Science, 1975
16. Spence JC: A Thousand Families in Newcastle-upon-Tyne: An Approach to the Study of Health and Illness in Children. London, Oxford University Press, 1954
17. Richardson W: Measuring the urban poor's use of physicians' services in response to illness episodes. Med Care 8:132, 1970
18. Knapp DA, Knapp DE, Engle J: The public, the pharmacist and self-medication. J Am Pharmacol Assoc 56:460, 1966
19. Vincent CE: Mental health and the family. In Glasser PH, Glasser LN (eds): Families in Crisis. New York, Harper & Row, 1970
20. Williams JI, Leaman T: Family structure and function. In Conn H, Rakel R (eds): Family Practice. Philadelphia, Saunders, 1973, p 6
21. Koos E: The Health of Regionville. New York, Columbia University Press, 1954
22. Litman TJ: Health care and the family—A three generational study. Med Care 9:67, 1971
23. Wolfe S, Badgley RF: Patients and their families (part 2 of The family doctor). Millbank Mem Fund Bull 50:73, 1972
24. Abernathy WJ, Schrems EL: Distance and health services—issues of utilization and facility choice for demographic strata. Research Paper No. 19, Stanford University Graduate School of Business, Palo Alto, California, 1971
25. Litman TJ: The family as a basic unit in health and medical care—A social behavioral overview. Social Sci Med 8:505, 1974
26. Sussman MG, Slater SB: Reappraisal of urban kin networks—Empirical evidence. Paper presented at the Annual Meeting of the American Sociological Association, Los Angeles, August 28, 1963
27. Haggerty RC: Health and the family. Paper presented at the Annual Symposium of the American Academy of Pediatrics, Chicago, 1963
28. Burgess EW, Locke, HJ, Thomas MM: The Family, 3rd ed. New York, American Book, 1963, p 1
29. Hill R: Interdependence among the generations. Family Development in Three Generations. Cambridge, Mass, Schenkman Publishing, 1970, Chap 2
30. Litwak E: Occupational mobility and extended family cohesion. In Reiss IL (ed): Readings on the Family System. New York, Holt, Rinehart and Winston, 1972, pp 413–431
31. Billingsley A: Black Families in White America. Englewood Cliffs, NJ, Prentice-Hall, 1968, p 21
32. Sussman, MB: Family systems in the 1970s: Analysis, policies and programs. In Skolnick A, Skolnick JH (eds): Intimacy, Family and Society. Boston, Little, Brown, 1974, p 590
33. Sussman MB, et al: Changing families in a changing society. Forum 14 in Report to the President: White House Conference on Children. Washington DC, Government Printing Office, 1971
34. Woodward KL, et al: Saving the family. Newsweek, May 15, 1978, p 67
35. U.S. Bureau of the Census. Household and family characteristics, March 1974. Current Population Reports, Series P-20, No 276. Washington DC, Government Printing Office, pp 2, 4, 13
36. Woodward KL, et al, *op. cit.*
37. LeMasters EE: Parents without partners. In Skolnick A, Skolnick JH (eds): Intimacy, Family and Society. Boston, Little, Brown, 1974, p 523
38. *Ibid.,* pp 523–524
39. *Ibid.,* p 524
40. *Ibid.*
41. LeMasters EE: Parents with partners. In Skolnick A, Skolnick JH (eds): Family in Transition. Boston, Little, Brown, 1971, pp 403–408
42. Keller S: Does the family have a future? In Coser RL: The Family, 2nd ed. New York, St. Martin's, 1974, p 583
43. LeMasters EE, 1971, *op. cit.,* p 410
44. Herzog E, Sudia CE: Children in fatherless families. In Caldwell BM, Ricutti HN (eds): Review of Child Development Research, Vol. 3. Chicago, University of Chicago Press, 1973

45. Cogswell BE: Variant family forms and life styles: Rejection of the traditional nuclear family. The Family Coordinator 24:391–394, 1975

46. *Ibid.,* p 394
47. *Ibid.,* pp 400–404
48. Keller, *op. cit.,* pp 591–592

STUDY QUESTIONS

Choose all correct answers to the following questions.
1. Which of these characteristics belong in a broad definition of "family"?
   a. Composed of one or more persons.
   b. Geographic dispersion.
   c. Emotional involvement.

2. Which is correct?
   a. The family of parenthood/procreation is the family into which you were born.
   b. The family of orientation/origin is the family of marriage.
   c. The extended family includes the immediate community, including but not limited to the family plus relatives.
   d. None of the above.

3. The family functions to meet the *needs of society* by:
   a. Mediating between society's expectations and the needs of the individual.
   b. Providing recruits for society's needs.
   c. Reproduction and socialization.

4. The family functions to meet the *needs of its members* by:
   a. Providing recruits for society.
   b. Serving as a "buffer" between society and the individual.
   c. Facilitating the personality development of the individual.

5. Which of these is (are) example(s) of how the ill family member can adversely affect the family?
   a. Advent of handicapped child disrupts marital relationship.
   b. Emotional disturbance of husband disrupts the economic and emotional stability of the family.
   c. Family is brought together in common effort to help the ill member get well.

6. Which of these is (are) the main reason(s) for the community health nurse to work with the family?
   a. The entire family is affected by the health problem of a family member.
   b. Promotion of health functioning of the whole family will positively affect each family member.
   c. The family is the primary target of the community health nurse; individual family members are of secondary importance.

How does the family affect the health of its family members in each of the following six stages of health/illness?
7. Prevention of illness.

8. Symptom experience stage.

9. Care-seeking stage.

10. Medical contact stage.

11. Dependent-patient role.

12. Rehabilitation stage.

13. Some ways in which the family has been able to influence/change society's values, attitudes, or sanctions are:
    a. Birth control.
    b. Premarital sex.
    c. Election laws.
    d. Establishment of communal families.

Fill in the correct answers to the following questions.
14. Variant family forms refer to:

15. Give three examples of traditional variant family forms.

16. Give three examples of nontraditional (experimental) family forms.

17. Describe briefly three stressors which commonly impact on single-parent families.

Choose the correct answer(s) to the following question.
18. What are the usual ties between nuclear and extended family (circle all accurate descriptions)?
    a. A modified extended family exists within a network of generational interaction.
    b. Parents and siblings of spouses form the most important network of extended kinship relations.
    c. The extended family network provides significant support and continuing assistance to the nuclear families within the network.

STUDY ANSWERS

1. c

2. d

3. a, b, and c

4. b and c

5. a and b

6. a and b

7. *Prevention of illness.* Reinforces health provisions and preventive measures.

8. *Symptom experience stage.* Family defines meaning of symptoms.

9. *Care-seeking stage.* Family persuades individual to seek care.

10. *Medical contact stage.* Family is the primary health referral agent (to whom, when).

11. *Dependent-patient role.* Family defines appropriate activity (roles) of patient during this stage.

12. *Rehabilitation stage.* Family either supports rehabilitation efforts or hinders them by perhaps being neglectful, oversolicitous, fostering dependent behavior, etc.

13. a and b

14. Variant family form refers to all deviations from the traditional nuclear family.

15. Examples of traditional variant family forms are: nuclear dyad (childless couple), single-parent family, single adult living alone, and three-generation family.

16. Examples of nontraditional variant family forms are: commune family, unmarried parent and child family, unmarried couple and child family, cohabiting couple, and homosexual unions.

17. Role conflicts; role shifts; poverty; social stigma (see chapter for further description).

18. All (a–c)

GOALS OF FAMILY-CENTERED NURSING

Ideally, in all clinical areas of nursing practice we should be family-centered. In some settings, however, family involvement is more difficult to achieve than in others. In the episodic settings, especially in intensive care units and emergency rooms, where immediate life-saving measures are needed, a patient focus is often mandatory. The degree of family-centeredness also is dependent on the philosophy of the system within which the nurse works. Work environments (what leadership rewards and negatively reinforces) are major determinants of behavior.

Community Health Nursing: Definition and Scope of Practice

The 1975 statement of the American Nurses Association (ANA) Division of Community Health Nursing Practice relative to defining community health nursing and its scope of practice[1] provides a helpful introduction to family nursing goals. The ANA's definition of community health nursing and its scope of practice are as follows:

> Community health nursing is the integration of nursing practice and public health practice applied to the promotion and preservation of the health of the population. The nature of this practice is general and comprehensive, includes all ages and diagnostic groups, and is non-episodic and continuous. Community health nursing is directed to individuals IN FAMILIES [author's emphasis] and groups, and intrinsically relates to and contributes to the health of the total population. Therefore, the dominant responsibility of the community health nurse is to the population as a whole. The primary focus of community health nursing is on the prevention of illness and the promotion and the maintenance of health. Therefore, community health nursing practice includes the provision of needed therapeutic services, counseling, education, direction, and advocacy activities. The community health nurse who is in constant contact with people in groups who seek and need health care, has unique opportunities to identify discrete health problems, as well as potential health problems, and to evaluate current health status. The community health nurse is involved in the planning and coordination of community health programs and services. The community health nurse, therefore, has responsibility in general and comprehensive areas of health practice for: 1) determining health needs of the individual, the family and the community; 2) assessing health status; 3) implementing health planning; 4) evaluating health practice; and 5) providing primary health care.

The concepts of community health nursing developed by the ANA have three basic components: (1) the focus of community health nursing is on the prevention of illness and health promotion and maintenance; (2) the health of the larger community or population is the ultimate target of services; (3) the

Family-Centered Nursing: Goals and Roles

LEARNING OBJECTIVES

1. Describe several important components within the ANA's definition of community health nursing and its scope of practice.
2. Differentiate between how the priority of goals is set by the family-centered nurse in an institutional setting versus how goals are set and prioritized by the family-centered community health nurse.
3. Explain why health promotion and maintenance is the primary thrust of family nursing.
4. Briefly describe the three levels of prevention.
5. Identify the three recent health promotion movements, referred to as the "New Medicine."
6. Discuss the primary factors leading to increased interest in health promotion today.
7. Define high-level wellness (Dunn's definition) by explaining its major facets.
8. Explicate the five key dimensions of wellness, as described by Ardell.
9. Explain the purpose and contents of the health hazard appraisal tool used in preventive medicine.
10. Describe the nurse's role in primary, secondary, and tertiary prevention.
11. Discuss briefly each of the following family nursing roles:
    a. health educator
    b. coordinator
    c. deliverer and supervisor of physical care
    d. client advocate
    e. collaborator/team member
    f. consultant
    g. counselor
    h. case finder/epidemiologist
    i. environmental modifier.

"process" utilized in community health nursing practice is heavily emphasized (the ANA's Standards for Community Health Practice are solely composed of "process" criteria).

The above statement focuses on services to population as a whole (or the community). And many authors have stated that it is through families that community health nurses improve or preserve the health of communities. This is certainly true. Yet family nursing, if focused on community health, has a different mission and thus different priorities than does family nursing practiced in other settings. In clinical nursing or medicine, for example, the individual client or family is the unit of care. In contrast, the central unit of service in community health practice is a population group that is a defined community.[2] The implications of this difference are that in rendering personal health services to a family with mother and young children, the "noncommunity health-oriented" nurse would be concerned with the family's unique problems first and second with the community health problems common to young families (the first commitment being a client and family). In a community health setting, the nurse would be cognizant of the pressing maternal–child health problems in the community which were relevant to the client family (such as immunizations and family planning), and prioritize these needs. Obviously the dichotomy of services is not that clear-cut, as community health nurses do provide individualized nursing services, as well as programs and services which are developed to attack the major community health problems.

LEVELS OF PREVENTION

Leavell and Clark developed a framework, referred to as levels of prevention, by which one can look at the family-centered nursing role.[3] These levels of prevention refer to the entire spectrum of health–illness and speak of the health goals existent in each of the levels. The three levels of prevention are briefly defined below:

1. *Primary prevention* involves health promotion and specific preventive measures to keep people free of disease/injury.
2. *Secondary prevention* consists of early detection, diagnosis, and treatment.
3. *Tertiary prevention* covers the stage of convalescence and rehabilitation, designed to minimize the client's disability and maximize his or her level of functioning.

Primary prevention will be covered under health promotion. The nurse's role in secondary and tertiary promotion will be explored later in this chapter.

THE MAJOR THRUST OF FAMILY NURSING: HEALTH PROMOTION

As the ANA statement and other literature, notably, Tinkham and Voorhies,[4] make clear, the primary goal of family nursing is health promotion and maintenance. Primary prevention is included under health promotion as one of its important components, but the term health promotion is used rather than primary prevention, since this term is a much more positive, dynamic one, whereas prevention is seen as defensive and largely reactive. The preventive posture is designed to protect the individual from illness or ill health, whereas health promotion, in contrast, achieves the same end (health or wellness) in a dynamic, positive manner.

Health promotion covers both general health promotion and maintenance strategies and specific preventive measures such as immunization. Primary prevention, the prevention of an acute or chronic health problem, poses the greatest problem in our society, but also the greatest challenge. Perhaps our most important goal should be to assist people (individuals and families) to learn *how* to be healthy in a natural, enjoyable way, rather than focusing on how not to get sick, or worse yet, only on assistance *when* sick.

Thus the promotion of health, or primary prevention, may be viewed as a most exciting and important role. This role has, however, largely been overlooked in practice, although much rhetoric about the significance of health teaching and prevention is heard. The adherence of health professionals to the medical model—in which health and illness are looked on as discrete, separate entities and in which the client is seen as a set of physiological systems—has led us and society (the consumers) to view health care solely in terms of curative medical care. Individuals, when ill, "turn themselves over" to health providers. There has been little encouragement or reward from society or health professionals for assuming self-responsibility for staying well or striving to improve one's total functioning.[5] Moreover, most health professionals act as poor role models for their clients, e.g., they smoke and are overweight, sedentary, and under apparent stress, and thus are not in a position to speak effectively about improvements in life style.

Nurses and other health professionals have been taught to respond to illness and crisis but not how to teach/counsel "symptom-free" individuals and families to enhance their level of wellness. Interestingly enough, the present health promotion movement referred to as "the New Medicine" or alternative health care (including holistic health care, self-care, and wellness training) was for the most part not initiated and led by health professionals but by lay persons and groups.

Recently these health promotion movements have become "respectable" in most health professional circles; even the more esoteric modalities for stress reduction and pain control are being looked on as "possibly helpful" by the medical establishment. There is much more openness and acceptance of alternative modalities, including yoga, meditation, biofeedback, acupressure, acupuncture, guided imagery, visualization, and body therapies.

Wellness training, holistic health care, and self-care share in the fundamental belief in taking responsibility for one's own health. The basic assumption underlying self-care is that people have self-directing and self-healing powers that can be consciously mobilized and applied. Inherent also is the belief that individuals and families should have control over their own actions. In addition, it is felt that the responsibility for one's health lies not with the physician but with the individual.[6]

Factors Leading to Renewed Interest in Health Promotion

Several of the important factors that have led to the renewed interest in health promotion are discussed below.

Need for a Change in Focus. Our present health care system is crisis oriented, with treatment being given in many cases too little, too late. In the case of chronic illness, our prevailing cause of morbidity and mortality, one is not treating and eradicating disease, but only minimizing its impact, repairing the damage as much as possible, and treating its complications. Some now recognize that we are spending most of our money treating the end result of self-destructive life styles rather than focusing in on the causative factor of ill health, i.e., life style and environmental hazards.[7]

Rising Costs. There is a growing concern among lay persons, legislators, and some health professionals that the present system of health care is both *costly* and relatively *ineffective*, with no cost containment or conservation of health resources in sight. We spend enormous amounts of money for hospital and medical care with little improvement to show for it. Longevity has not significantly improved in recent years, even though we keep pumping more and more money into a leaky system. Compliance studies show that there is a widespread lack of medical compliance by patients, which naturally raises costs even more. Ardell reminds us that Americans spend vast amounts of money on the treatment of diseases that could be prevented for free.[8]

Demystification of Primary Health Care. There have been unprecedented public disclosures of the inadequacies and inequities of professional service. Iatrogenesis is becoming a familiar term among the lay person. For instance, the women's movement has focused national attention on the poor quality of care received by women in a male-dominated system. The downward transfer of functions (from physicians to nurse practitioners and physician assistants, and from registered nurses to vocational nurses, community workers, and nurse's aides) has helped with the demystification process.

Consumerism and Popular Demands for Increased Self-control. Consumers today expect to be informed of the findings of medical services and to be given more self-control over their lives. This usually translates into being given sufficient information to be reasonably informed so that they can make their own choices and evaluate services. The need for greater self-control is related to present societal values and antitechnology and antiauthority sentiments.

Changes in Life Style and Increased Educational Levels. A considerable number of educated, middle-class persons and families are placing a greater value on health, personal fulfillment, and the quality of their lives, and putting less importance on materialism, competitiveness, and achievement. Although the general level of health knowledge in our society is relatively low, these persons, through reading of a multitude of health-oriented articles and books and exposure to mass media, conferences, and so forth, have become quite informed about general health promotional strategies and environmental hazards and risks. This shift in values and the improvement of education level has led to improved life styles for many.[9]

Lack of Accessible and Available Professional Health Services. A major impetus to self-care may arise from situations where professional health services are not readily available or accessible.[10]

Growing Recognition of the Interrelationship Between Stress and Illness. It is estimated that 80 percent of all illnesses are stress induced, with stress at least aggravating all illnesses. Multiple studies have shown the negative role stress plays on one's emotional and physical health status.[11] Because of this, treatment of the disease alone is not adequate. The whole person—body, mind, and soul—must be considered, with an integration of body and mind being of prime importance for recovery and wellness. Stress reduction has become one of the five major dimensions of wellness training,[12] and perhaps the most important facet of holistic health care.

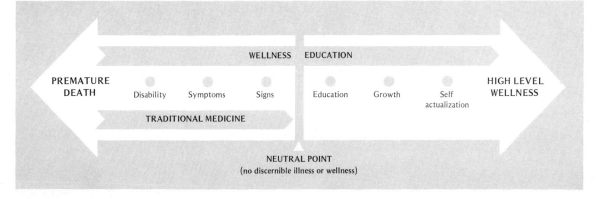

FIGURE 2.1
The health–illness continuum and its relationship to health care. (*From: Travis J: Wellness Inventory. Wellness Resource Center, 42 Miller Avenue, Mill Valley, California 94941.*)

What Does Health Promotion/Primary Prevention Involve?

The goal of health promotion or primary prevention is high-level wellness. In 1961 Halbert Dunn, the father of the wellness orientation, defined high-level wellness as: "An integrated method of functioning which is oriented towards maximizing the potential of which the individual is capable within the environment where he is functioning."[13] The key words are: (1) "integrated," meaning to function as a whole, be united, not disjointed, or in a situation where various facets of an individual are in conflict with other aspects of that person. Ardell speaks of an "integrated" life style, where each of the key dimensions of high-level wellness (self-responsibility, nutritional awareness, physical fitness, stress management, and environmental sensitivity) are balanced and consonant with each other, producing a synergistic effect. (2) "Maximizing potential" connotes a dynamic state where a person is continually striving to grow and improve his level of wellness. Abraham Maslow's hierarchy of needs has a similar connotation; here man is seen as striving to meet higher needs as the lower, more basic needs are met. And (3) "within his environment" suggests that we have to look at individuals within their psychosocial and physical environments when assessing their level of wellness. The primary group (family) is a critical part of this environment. In spite of poor and deprived environments, some individuals (in some literature they are referred to as the "invulnerables") may achieve high-level wellness. Dunn calls this status "emergent wellness." According to him, families and communities can be similarly assessed using the same definition of high-level wellness.

Ardell has written a most interesting and enlightening book for lay persons and health professionals alike, *High Level Wellness—An Alternative to Doctors, Drugs, and Disease.*[14] In this book he describes five key dimensions and a variety of alternative approaches, strategies, and techniques as part of a life style philosophy he calls high-level wellness. Travis, a "wellness doctor," gives this explanation of the meaning of high-level wellness:

> The ideas of measuring wellness and helping people attain high levels of wellness are relatively new. Most of us think in terms of illness and assume that the absence of illness indicates wellness. This is not true. There are many degrees of wellness as there are many degrees of illness. The diagram (Fig. 2.1) is a model used by well medicine.[15]

Travis explains his diagram as follows:

> Moving from the center to the left shows a progressively worsening state of health. Moving to the right of center shows increasing levels of health and well-being. Traditional medicine is oriented towards curing evidence of disease, but usually stops at the midpoint. Well begins at any point on the scale with the goal of helping a person to move as far to the right as possible.

Health has an enriched and extended meaning for Travis:

> Wellness is not a static state. It results when a person begins to see himself as a growing, changing person. High level wellness means giving good care to your physical self, using your mind constructively, expressing your emotions effectively, being creatively involved with those around you, being concerned about your physical and psychological environment and becoming aware of other levels of consciousness.[16]

Wellness Life Style

Ardell's five key dimensions delve into the vital aspects making up a wellness life style and are described below.

Self-responsibility

This is the basis on which the other four dimensions rest. Without a sense of active accountability for one's own health, the necessary motivation will be lacking to engage in a health-producing life style. Families also need a strong sense of accountability to avoid high-risk personal behaviors, for example, overeating, smoking, alcohol consumption, lack of rest or sleep, inactivity, and excessive stress.

Families have to be convinced that their health lies primarily in their hands and that a wellness life style fueled by a strong sense of self and family responsibility can be more gratifying than living a life filled with high-risk behaviors.[17]

A major factor accounting for insufficient self-responsibility is the lack of effective health education. In fact, the health professions discourage their clients from engaging in independent actions on their own behalf. Ardell writes that part of self-responsibility and self-care is knowing how to use the health system effectively, coupled with creating a life style which keeps us well and out of the medical system as much as possible. Vickory and Fries in their *Take Care of Yourself*[18] express these same sentiments and do not recommend annual histories and physicals as preventive measures, except for some specific exceptions such as skin testing for tuberculosis, pap smears for women over 25, blood pressure checks for adults, tonometry readings for those over 40 for detection of glaucoma, and sigmoidoscopy after age 50. Thus the wellness-oriented physicians do not believe that the annual comprehensive physical examination is very helpful.

Nutritional Awareness

The United States Senate Select Committee, chaired by Senator George McGovern, recently concluded years of fact-finding studies and testimony relative to our dietary habits and nutritional status. Here are the conclusions of this survey report:

> We have reached the point where nutrition, or the lack or the excess or the quality of it, may be the nation's number one public health problem. The threat is not beri beri, pellagra, or scurvy. Rather we face the more subtle, but more deadly, reality of millions of Americans loading their stomachs with food which is likely to make them obese, to give them high blood pressure, to induce heart disease, diabetes, and cancer—in short, to kill them over the long term.[19]

Five of the ten leading causes of death are related to faulty diets (heart disease, stroke, diabetes, arteriosclerosis, and cirrhosis of the liver).[20] The Senate Committee formulated nutritional goals. They advocate changing the proportion of fats, carbohydrates, and proteins as follows:

	Present Diet	Dietary Goals
FAT	42%	30%
	16% as saturated fats	10% as saturated fats (6% decrease)
	26% unsaturated	20% unsaturated (6% decrease)
PROTEIN	12%	12% (no change)
CARBOHY-DRATES (CHOs)	46%	58%
	22% complex CHOs (starches, vegetables)	43% complex CHOs (21% increase)
	24% sugars	15% sugars (9% decrease)

It is within the context of family that faulty dietary habits are learned, involving familial behavioral patterns which are central to daily life. Though difficult, it is within this context that such patterns may be changed.

Stress Management

According to Brown, 80 percent of our present illnesses are stress induced, and all of our health problems can be aggravated by stress.[21] Hans Selye, the father of the stress theory, points out that it is the effects of prolonged stress (or "distress") which are particularly deleterious on the body, causing such problems as migraine headaches, peptic ulcers, heart attacks, hypertension, mental illness, and suicide.[22] Selye recently coined the word "eustress," referring to the positive aspects of stress. Because of today's prevalent stressors, stress has to be managed so that eustress (an appropriate amount of stress for enjoying life and being stimulated and productive) exists.

One component of stress management involves the use of some skill or techniques that can be used to gain mental relaxation in times of duress. A multiplicity of such strategies and techniques for stress reduction and relaxation is discussed in the literature.* Families need to be sensitive to the amount of stress within the home environment and how as a group to provide an environment and opportunity for stress reduction.

Physical Fitness

The benefits of regular exercise are so substantial and wide-ranging that increased numbers of adults have taken up a variety of sports—jogging, swimming, biking, tennis, hiking, dancing, golf, and walking. Inactivity is linked with hypertension, obesity, chronic fatigue, back pain, premature aging, poor musculature,

---

*McQuade W, Aikman A: Stress. New York, Bantam, 1975. This book describes the primary strategies used for stress reduction and management.

inadequate flexibility, tension, a lower general health status, and shortened longevity. Unless an individual is reasonably fit, high-level wellness cannot exist.[23]

The positive effects of regular exercise and a state of being physically in shape are mood elevation (reinforcing a healthy self-concept, greater self-confidence), better eating habits, fewer risk behaviors, and an overall ability to relate effectively to other people. Physiological benefits include the lowering of the heart rate, blood pressure, percentage of body fat, stress level, and lipids and cholesterol in the blood.[24]

Through the values they live by and the behavior they reinforce, families set the stage for individual members to be either physically active or sedentary and apathetic toward physical activity. Much healthy physical activity can be done while participating in family recreation activities, an excellent way to also promote healthy family relationships.

Environmental Sensitivity

Environmental sensitivity encompasses the physical, social, and environmental influences—that is, how the environment either enhances or limits health and well-being. The air we breathe, the community in which we reside, and the neighborhood characteristics are all examples of the physical and social environments affecting us. The smaller spatial circle surrounding us is the personal environment. This includes the personal space which one "owns" and works or lives in (bedroom, office, etc.), as well as a person's primary group and network of friendships. In order to achieve the level of environmental sensitivity needed to enhance health, one must first be cognizant of the effects of the environment on health and well-being.[25] Just as individuals need to be aware of their environment and its effects on them, so do families need to look at their home, neighborhood, school, community, and sets of relationships and seriously consider how these settings and groups affect them as a unit and as individual members.

A large-scale health survey conducted in the middle 1960s of 7,000 adults in California who were later followed for 5½ years demonstrates the values of a healthy life style. Belloc and Breslow demonstrated that (1) an individual's overall health status was improved, and (2) an 11.5 year greater life expectancy could be achieved for men age 45 whose life style incorporated six or seven of the "old health habits" traditionally stressed versus men of the same age who followed only three or less "habits." These life-lengthening habits were: (1) no smoking, (2) no alcohol or only in moderation, (3) seven or eight hours of sleep nightly, (4) regular meals with no snacking in between, (5) daily breakfast, (6) normal weight, and (7) moderate, regular exercise. For women the same positive cor-

relation between habits and longevity appeared, although only seven years were gained by incorporating six or seven "habits" into their lives versus three or less.[26]

When working with a family during the child-rearing years, the above suggestions on life-style improvements are certainly needed. However, what clinical implications are there for promoting the health of the children and family as a whole? First of all, many of the life-style principles apply equally well to the family and individual, and by the adult family members stressing the values and habits inherent in this way of living, the children, through identification and imitative learning, should also learn a more healthy life style. In fact, role modeling by significant others (parents, important peers, teachers, etc.) has been found to be the best learning device. As the old adage says, "actions speak louder than words." Parents also need to understand normal growth and developmental patterns, including the important developmental tasks their children are struggling to achieve, so that they, in turn, can encourage and foster healthy growth patterns.

Primary Preventive Approach

The more specific preventive measures subsumed under primary prevention involve maintaining and improving the level of family resistance. Such measures connote a degree of protection against disease versus immunity and denote absolute protection. In epidemiology this would be referred to as "increasing the resistance of the host." Level of immunization can refer broadly to increasing resistance to social, emotional, and biological forces which precipitate disease. A wellness-oriented life style, as described previously, should accomplish this "resistance." Specific preventive measures need also be considered. This encompasses preventive measures related to specific diseases such as immunization.

In preventive medicine the most common way in which primary prevention and health promotion are practiced is by determining long-term risks to which a client is exposed and prescribing measures which will hopefully reduce the risk factors. In many cases a health-hazard appraisal method or tool is used.* Here the total personal risks to a patient are estimated by identifying the average risk for the cause of death in the patient's own age, sex, and racial group. From this, one can develop a prognosis for the well patient. Using this appraisal, therefore, the health practitioner would make an estimation of those causes most likely to

---

*The health-hazard appraisal tool is used for both primary prevention—to counsel clients regarding risk exposure—and secondary prevention, since it also consists of screening for present problems—weight, hypertension, and so forth.

TABLE 2.1
Health Hazard Appraisal Tool

Name:　　　　John Doe
Age:　　　　43
Race and Sex: White male
Occupation: Small businessman

Rank— Disease/Injury	Prognostic Criteria	Patient Findings	Treatment (Rx)
1. Arteriosclerotic heart disease	Blood pressure	120/70	
	Cholesterol level	300	Reduce saturated fats and calories
	Diabetes	No	
	Exercise	Sedentary—none	Initiate regular exercise program
	Family history	None	
	Smoking	3 packs a day for 20 years	Referred to stop-smoking clinic
	Weight	200 lb. (5 ft, 10 in)	Weight reduction diet. Reduce to 165 lb.
2. Auto accidents	Alcohol	Occasional	
	Drugs	None	
	Mileage	30,000/year	
	Seat belts	100%	
3. Suicide	Depression	None observed	
	Family history	Negative	
4. Cirrhosis of liver	Alcohol use	Occasional	

Source: Adapted from Robbins LC, Hall JH: How to Practice Medicine. Methodist Hospital of Indianapolis, Indiana, 1970.

bring about death and disability and prescribe those procedures most likely to reduce the risk of death and disability. Table 2.1 gives an example of the use of the health-hazard appraisal method.

SECONDARY PREVENTION

Case finding is the key to secondary prevention so that early diagnosis and prompt treatment can be instituted. If the nature of the disease precludes cure, then the goal is to control the progression of the disease and prevent disability.

The nurse's role here would be screening through visual and auditory testing of children, for example, and the completing of health histories and physical examinations of all family members; additionally she would initiate and follow through on referrals for diagnosis and treatment "tailor made" to suit the patient, his health problem, and family's needs. Health teaching along with careful referral and follow-up are concomitant functions at this time.

The Issue of the Yearly Physical

What has been the efficacy of the annual or periodic health examination completed by an asymptomatic patient? This is a hotly disputed subject and one in which there is no firm evidence showing that the annual physical examination is warranted either in terms of cost effectiveness or in terms of detecting significant numbers of diseases in their early stages. Although many family practitioners and internists practicing preventive medicine still advocate the annual physical for detection of problems, many other physicians and health planners question its value.[27]

Cost effectiveness of the multitude of screening procedures done in some physical examinations and multiphasic examinations (history, all the components of a physical, laboratory, and other diagnostic tests) has been seriously questioned by Kaiser-Permanente after studying their multiphasic examination program. It has been found that only a relatively few diseases or risk factors can reasonably be found in a preclinical state such that the disease's natural outcome could be altered or palliated, and so benefit the patient or society.[28] There has been a proliferation of unvalidated procedures prescribed in physical examinations, and it may be a disservice to clients to engage in "evangelical" advocacy regarding annual health examinations until firmer positive evidence has been obtained regarding their value. However, selective screening of ostensibly well clients, using a limited number of tests and at a frequency of screening which has proven beneficial, is felt to be of practical significance.

TERTIARY PREVENTION

Rehabilitation is the primary focus of tertiary prevention. Convalescence and maintenance care for chronically ill persons are also included. Rehabilitation involves restoring individuals disabled by disease or injury to a level of functioning optimal for them—or to their greatest usefulness—physically, socially, emotionally, and vocationally. In learning to live with a permanent disability, the client and his family need tremendous support and extensive teaching of self-care. The nurse plays central roles in tertiary prevention. In addition to direct care-giving, the nurse's most significant roles are that of team member, coordinator, patient/family advocate, teacher, and counsellor.

ROLES OF FAMILY-CENTERED NURSE

A description of specific roles which are of special importance to family-oriented community nursing practice follow.

Health Educator

The family-centered community nurse must be able to undertake effective teaching of families, both formally and informally. In order to teach, we must have current information or know where to get it. To teach successfully, it follows that we should know some essential things about the learner and the teaching–learning process. The aim of learning is to support healthy behavior or to change behavior, albeit alterations of behavior are not always immediate or observable. More specifically, the purposes of health education are: (1) teaching of health promotion and disease prevention and (2) assisting families to develop skills to cope with their present health problems or needs.

When formally teaching (in contrast to the spontaneous teaching which goes on in our client–nurse interactions), the establishment of objectives and the ability to measure how well the objectives are met are essential to the teaching–learning process. The simple imparting of information cannot be considered teaching, particularly if there is no evidence that the client has learned or met the objective of the teaching. It is crucial that the health educator and client share the same objective; otherwise internalized learning by the client will not occur.

Anticipatory guidance is an important facet of health teaching. Discussing probable events, feelings, and situations with the family provides for clarification of ideas, reduction of anxiety, and future role change adaptability. Anticipation of and preparation for the coming event will make it less traumatic and allow it to be better handled. An example of the success of antici-patory guidance is the huge success which Lamaze classes enjoy. When labor begins, both parents are fully prepared and usually sail through the process with excitement and positive feelings, and they are better able to handle their future roles as parents.

Health teaching today needs to be geared toward assisting the patient and family to engage in self-care and self-responsibility. No longer should we as health professionals foster dependency and immaturity. People need to feel they have the capacity for self-care and the right to sufficient information so that they can make their own decisions. If this philosophy is established, then the traditional superordinate–subordinate positions no longer are appropriate. We need to play the role of facilitator and resource person to clients who will decide which options are best for them.

Coordinator

The ANA[29] characterizes community health nursing practice as "general, comprehensive and continuous." Continuous nursing services can be implemented only if continuity of care is planned for and coordinated. Coordination is one of the major roles of the nurse working with families. The community health nurse is often *the key person* in the provision of comprehensive, continuous health care. In addition to the particular functions the nurse is carrying out in working with a family, she or he supports other team members, supports and interprets their objectives and service, and coordinates nursing services with the various other services the family is receiving.

Without coordination the client may receive a duplication of some services from different agencies or, even more distressing, a gap in other essential areas of need. An illustration of this problem follows. A rehabilitation clinic patient once remarked to various members of the health team that she was having difficulty getting out of the bathtub and had no shower facilities to switch to. Each time she mentioned this to the team members they noted her response, but "no one made any suggestions of what to do." A social worker, sanitarian, homemaker-home health aide, and visiting nurse may all be visiting a family concurrently. In this situation it is the nurse's responsibility to make sure that collaboration is taking place and coordinated efforts are being achieved.

Promoting continuity of care for long-term, chronically ill patients and their families is a particularly great need. Anderson found that much wasted effort and patient regression occurred with interruptions in services to patients with long-term illness.[30] The community health nurse must make continuing efforts to improve referral systems between the various health and welfare agencies in the community, and be willing to share knowledge about clients' needs and progress with others to whom she or he is referring or from whom she or he has received the referral. Referral is a two-way street, and communication must flow in both directions for the system to be functional.

In summary, the community health nurse functions as a bridge between family and various services by acquainting the family with available community resources, effecting continuity of care, and coordinating services patients are receiving.

Deliverer and Supervisor of Physical Care

The nurse working with clients in home/clinic and inpatient facility has direct responsibility for providing physical care or supervising and directing others who provide care, with the exception of where agency policies preclude the carrying out of this function. Agencies which limit nurses in giving direct physical care are usually official health agencies in large metropolitan areas where visiting nurses' associations and other home health agencies have often assumed this role.

Many long-term and disabled patients require a high level of physical care in order to continue living at home. Especially important is the prevention of the deterioration resulting from immobility. For the bedfast patient the nurse must work at maintaining muscle strength and joint mobility and preventing deformities, metabolic disturbances, decubital ulcers, urinary tract infections, and respiratory complications. The community health nurse often teaches and supervises the patient, homemaker-home health aide, and/or family member to provide the necessary care. The improvisation of gadgets, equipment, and strategies for rehabilitation is also an important facet of this role.

Archer and Fleshman point out that nursing students often feel that they are not doing anything for their patients unless they physically "do something" such as change a dressing, take a blood pressure, or give an injection. Although we know that teaching, counseling, making referrals, etc., are often the most important service the nurse is providing, it is true that families also often tune in to the tangible services given. According to Archer and Fleshman, a visible direct service may often be the act that lends credibility to the other services rendered.[31] Fagin confirms that meeting physical needs and performing visible acts are extremely important when working with poor families. Without the capacity to give on-the-spot attention to physical needs and concerns, a helper is at a disadvantage in meeting psychosocial needs. Ability in this area brings the nurse to a level of intimacy with the realities of family life.[32]

Nevertheless, Archer and Fleshman caution us in often failing to make credible our indirect nursing services, thus reinforcing the fallacy that nursing is not nursing unless something is done directly to and for the client.[33]

Client Advocate

According to the dictionary, an advocate is one who speaks for and on behalf of some other person or group. It is also someone who vindicates or espouses a cause by argument, a defender or intercessor, such as the position a defense attorney would assume. Kosik's definition of advocacy goes further, involving deeper commitment.[34] Client (patients and families) advocacy is basic to comprehensive care and concern for the whole person and family. She explains:

> For me, patient advocacy is seeing that the patient knows what to expect and what is his right to have, and then displaying the willingness and courage to see that our system does not prevent his getting it. The goals of patient advocacy are, first, making a person more independent because he knows the what, why, and how of the system and, second, changing the system to make it more sensitive and relevant by revealing injustices and inadequacies, thereby making complacent continuation of the status quo impossible. The nurse may have to make waves. She may have to see that workers and agencies do their jobs and expose the indifference and inhumanity of care givers.[35]

Although a goal of client advocacy is client independence, the advocate may have to accept and perhaps even foster dependency temporarily, for many persons, especially the poor, have never had their dependency needs met. And thus we need to start there and assist the person or family to grow.

Community health nurses are in a strong position to act as advocates. They are out there in the community working with families who are often poor and feeling powerless and hopeless. Not only is there a greater need for the community health nurse to assume this role because of client needs, but unless this position is assumed, often one cannot go on to render the other essential services the family needs.

Supervisors and administrators have a critical role here, too: first, in supporting the nurse acting in this capacity and, second, by keeping tallies of the problems clients are experiencing in various agencies. Then as specific patterns become well documented, the administrator is able to communicate to the leadership of that community agency her or his concerns. By working together in this way the identified problems can often be ameliorated.

Thus the community health nurse can be a client advocate in at least two ways: (1) by assisting the client to obtain what he or she is entitled to from the system and (2) by trying to make the system more responsive to client needs in general. Client/family advocacy can range from calling the welfare department before referring a family in an effort to pave the way for them, to testifying in court on behalf of a client, or calling a meeting with representatives from several agencies to coordinate and improve services to the community.

Collaborator/Team Member

Nursing is only one health service vital to comprehensive health care. As members of a health team, nurses collaborate and plan comprehensive family-centered care with other health team members. The composition of the health team (or health and welfare team) may vary depending on an agency's available resources and the family's needs. In a home health agency the team is commonly composed of community health nurse, licensed vocational nurse, homemaker-home health aide, social worker, and physical therapist. The occupational therapist and nutritionist are also often members—or act as consultants to the team. The family physician acts partially as a team member, since he or she is not present and is often difficult to reach. Many independent health goals need to be formulated by the home health team based on the medical information and directives the physician has provided. The family and patient can frequently be included on the team also. (Ideally, the patient and family should be central members of the team.)

In primary health care, the team often involves the physician, nursing practitioner, clinic nurse, social worker, nurse's aide/vocational nurse; in the official health agency, on the other hand, the team may be broader or smaller in size depending on the family's particular health, welfare, and educational needs. The community health nurse may be a member of a community team working with a young, child-rearing family in which the school nurse and teacher, probation officer, caseworker, and psychologist are a part.

Collaboration implies a professional, collegial relationship—in which there is mutual respect and egalitarianism. An authoritarian type of relationship, where the leadership and direction flow from the physician to nurse to nurse's aide to patient, cannot be considered a team or collaborative relationship. It might be best named "the pecking order." Here communication is neither open, direct, nor two way, and team members' contributions and effective functioning are seriously stifled.

Kindig points out that the structure of each health care system and the mix of people working on a health care team depends on the needs of the patient population and on the available resources. Where a health team continually works together there is a great need for health care members to work out the process by which decisions are made, communications channeled, procedures adopted, and role identification of each of the team members defined. If a health team runs smoothly, this frees more energy for client care, since less energy will be needed for team maintenance and coping with member's interpersonal problems.[36]

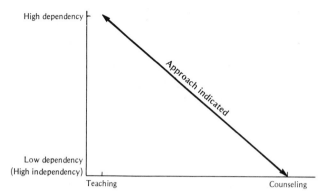

FIGURE 2.2
Variation of the interpersonal approach indicated by the family's degree of dependence—independence.

Consultant

Family-oriented nurses often serve as consultants to the client. Consultative relationships occur with physicians, school teachers, legislators, probation officers, or anyone else who carries on a helping relationship with the client. Although many community nurses maintain a generalist approach in their work, others develop special expertise in such areas as family planning, nurse practitionering, tuberculosis, venereal disease, drug abuse, chronic illness, crisis intervention, behavior modification, cultural diversity, nutritional counseling, or growth and development.

Counselor

Closely allied to teaching is the counseling role. Teaching and counseling have been described as ends of a continuum, with teaching the appropriate mode for working with a more dependent family (one which needs structure and specific directions) and counseling at the other end of the continuum and indicated when the nurse is working with a mature and independent family (therefore needing little structure and minimal "direction"). The role in this case would be assisting the family to utilize its own problem-solving skills and strengths. Figure 2.2 illustrates this role.

In this model, teaching would be defined in a traditional sense, rather than the more enlightened definition presented under health educator role. Here teaching would be described as "instructor-directed" (goals and methods set *by* the teacher) with information and skills taught *to* the client. In the counseling role the nurse would act as resource person and facilitator, leaving family members to make their decisions independently. Encouraging the family and its members to explore feelings and alternatives for coping would be prime goals. The supportive/caring role is crucial for many families adjusting to significant loss or crisis.

Case Finder/Epidemiologist

As part of the community health nurse's responsibilities in disease control, early identification of disease by case finding is a central role. When initially visiting or working with a family, the nurse should use the family and patient histories as tools for eliciting symptoms of unrecognized health problems or risks to which the individuals or the family as a whole is being exposed. One may also pick up situations where a person has been improperly treated, which is another form of case finding.

The initial visit to the home is usually elicited by an identified problem—"the entree into the home" problem. But countless more opportunities exist for case finding in families, extended families, and neighborhood families. The community health nurse is an active epidemiologist, especially in communicable disease control, when she or he is functioning in an official public health agency.

Environmental Modifier

When working in home health agencies, where a large proportion of clients are older persons and disabled, another significant role becomes necessary—that of a home "improvisor." Disabled patients often need modifications in their home environment to enable them to remain there. Families are often not knowledgeable or may not be present to help (unless the nurse or patient specifically enlists the aid of extended-family members). Some of the activities nurses assist families with are room and furniture arrangements, arrangement of kitchen equipment and food, borrowing or purchasing of special aids (beds, chairs, supports, handgrips), and building of ramps and removal of door sills—all various adaptations needed to minimize physical exertion, increase accessibility and mobility, and maximize safety.

REFERENCES

1. American Nurses Association, Division on Community Health Nursing Practice: Concepts of Community Health Nursing Practice, 2nd rev. Kansas City, Mo, A.N.A. Publication Code CH-6, 1975
2. Kark S: Epidemiology and Community Medicine. New York, Appleton, 1974, p 319
3. Leavell H, Clark EG, Gurney B, et al: Preventive Medicine for the Doctor in His Community: An Epidemiologic Approach, 3rd ed. New York, McGraw-Hill, 1965, pp 19–28
4. Tinkham C, Voorhies E: Community Health Nursing: Evolution and Process, 2nd ed. New York, Appleton, 1977, p 167
5. Bruhn J, Cordova FD: A developmental approach to learning wellness behavior. Part II. Adolescence to maturity. Health Values: Achieving High Level Wellness 2(1):20, 1978
6. Leonard G: The Holistic Health Revolution. Los Angeles, New West, May 10, 1976, p 43
7. Ardell D, Newman A: Health promotion—Strategies for planning. Health Values: Achieving High Level Wellness 1(3):100, 1977
8. Ardell D: High Level Wellness—An Alternative to Doctors, Drugs and Disease. Emmaus, Pa, Rodale, 1977, p 4
9. Levin LS, Katz A, Holst E: Self-Care—Lay Initiatives in Health. New York, Prodist Press, 1976, pp 20–22
10. Ibid., p 23
11. Pelletier K: Mind as Healer, Mind as Slayer. New York, Dell, 1977
12. Ardell, op. cit., p 93
13. Dunn HL: High-Level Wellness. Arlington, Va, RW Beatty, 1961
14. Ardell, op. cit.
15. Travis J: Wellness Workbook. Wellness Resource Center, Mill Valley, California, 1976
16. Ibid.
17. Ardell, op. cit., pp 95–180
18. Vickory D, Fries J: Take Care of Yourself—A Consumer's Guide to Medical Care. Reading, Mass, Addison-Wesley, 1976
19. U.S. Senate Select Committee on Nutrition and Human Needs: Nutrition and Health—An Evaluation of Nutritional Surveillance in the U.S. Washington, D.C., Government Printing Office, 1975, p 5
20. Ardell, op. cit., p 56
21. Brown B: New Mind, New Body: Biofeedback, New Directions for the Mind. New York, Bantam, 1974
22. Selye H: Stress Without Distress. New York, Lippincott, 1974, pp 14, 18, 111
23. Ardell op. cit., p 146
24. Ibid., pp 145–159
25. Ibid., pp 162–177
26. Belloc NB: The relationship of health practices and mortality. Prev Med 2:67, 1973
27. Spitzer W, Brown B: Unanswered questions about the periodic health examination. Ann Intern Med 83:257, 1975
28. Ibid., p 258
29. American Nurses Association, op. cit.
30. Anderson EM: A continuity of care plan for longterm patients. Am J Public Health 54:308, 1964
31. Archer S, Fleshman R: Community Health Nursing. North Scituate, Mass, Duxbury Press, 1975, pp 10–11
32. Fagin C: Concluding discussion. In Fagin C (ed): Family-Centered Nursing in Community Psychiatry. Philadelphia, Davis, 1970, p 163
33. Archer and Fleshman, op. cit., pp 10–11
34. Kosik SH: Patient advocacy or fighting the system. Am J Nurs 72:694, 1972
35. Ibid., p 694
36. Kindig D: Interdisciplinary education for primary health care team delivery. J Med Educat 50:102, 1975

STUDY QUESTIONS

Choose the characteristic that is most correct

1. According to the ANA Division of Community Health Nursing Practice, community health nursing has the following qualities:

   a. Episodic   or   b. Distributive

   c. Integration of nursing   or   d. Combination of nursing
   and public health   and public health

   e. Specialist focus   or   f. Generalist focus

   g. Directed toward   or   h. Directed toward individ-
   families   uals, families, and
                                          communities

   i. Main goal—health   or   j. Main goal—resolution
   promotion and disease   of community health
   prevention   problems

   k. Provides acute health   or   l. Provides primary health
   care   care

2. What is the different mission of the family-centered community health nurse versus the family-centered nurse working in an institutional setting?

3. Which of the following statements are true about the levels of prevention? The levels:
   a. specifically identify the nurse's role in prevention of disease,
   b. cover the entire spectrum of health and disease,
   c. identify goals for each of the three levels of prevention,
   d. are generally synonymous with preventive, curative, and rehabilitative phases of health care.

Match the correct level of prevention from the right-hand column with the description in the left-hand column.

4. Case finding.   a. Primary prevention.

5. Health promotion.   b. Secondary prevention.

6. Specific preventive measures.   c. Tertiary prevention.

7. Early detection and treatment.

8. Convalescence.

9. Minimizing the complications of the disease.

10. Rehabilitation.

11. Health maintenance.

12. Risk avoidance and reduction.

13. List the three movements within "New Medicine."

14. Identify five factors that have led to increased interest and involvement in health promotion.

15. What are three important components of Dunn's definition of high-level wellness?

16. Discuss briefly each of the five key dimensions making up a wellness life style.

17. The health-hazard appraisal tool contains and asks for what kinds of information?

18. The nurse is working with a family referred by a physician. Sammy, the eight-month-old son, was recently diagnosed as having leukemia. When the nurse arrives at the home, she discovers that the mother has little knowledge of leukemia, a limited income, and no transportation to medical services. The mother is overprotective and terribly solicitous in her care of her infant son. Identify the nurse's roles (give three).

19. Nurse B is visiting the Jeffers family to discuss Mrs. Jeffers' prenatal status. Mary, the 10-year-old daughter, is sick in bed. The nurse goes into the bedroom saying, "Oh, Mary, you look so uncomfortable. Let me help you." She straightens the bottom sheet, fluffs the pillows, and repositions Mary. "Your Mom tells me she thinks you have a fever. I'm going to take your temperature." After taking temperature, checking skin for rashes, and questioning both for other pertinent information, she says, "I think you ought to call your doctor and discuss Mary's condition."
Identify the nurse's roles (give three).

20. Nurse C is present when Mr. J is examined by the physician, Dr. Mays. The doctor has finished the examination and is talking with Mr. J. Dr. Mays says, "Tom, you need surgery." "But I can't go into the hospital now, I've just started a new job," says Tom. "Now Tom, it's essential that you have surgery." "But I can't now." The nurse, seeing Tom has a problem, decides to speak in his behalf. She says, "Dr. Mays, Mr. J. says he has a new job. I can see how surgery now poses a problem for him." "That's true," says Dr. Mays. "Can you arrange for surgery by the end of the month, Tom?" "Well, that would give me more time to arrange things. Let me talk it over with my wife."
Identify the nurse's role (give one).

21. The community health nurse has stopped by Mrs. Smith's home because her daughter, Susan, age 4, has missed her important appointment in the Pediatrics Clinic to follow up on a severe streptococcal tonsillitis and pharyngitis problem. The mother said she had not been able to attend because her two other children, ages 1 and 5, felt "hot" and were not feeling well.
Identify three nursing roles.

22. The visiting nurse has made her first home visit to an elderly couple. The husband, Mr. Paul, age 80, has severe emphysema and has just been discharged from a local general hospital. The wife is also 80 and has assumed the caretaker role. In completing a nursing assessment, one of the observa-

tions the visiting nurse made is that Mr. Paul is seeing three doctors (a chest physician, an internist for his "heart condition," and a general practitioner who is a lifelong friend and seen for immediate problems or "anything else"). His bathroom is filled with prescriptions—new, old, same drugs with different doses, and several drugs which have similar actions—prescribed by the different physicians. The patient, being quite concerned regarding his health, is complying by taking all of these. The wife is confused and finds caring for her bedridden husband alone a real burden. She complains of a continual backache and fatigue.

Identify five important nursing roles.

STUDY ANSWERS

1. b, c, f, h, i, and l

2. The ordering of priorities is different. The community health nurse would be committed to providing services to families to help resolve major *community health* problems, in addition to services designed to meet unique health needs of family, whereas the family-centered nurse in hospital setting would prioritize the family's particular health needs.

3. b and d   8. c

4. b   9. b

5. a   10. c

6. a   11. a

7. b   12. a

13. 1. Wellness training.
    2. Self-care.
    3. Holistic health care.

14. 1. Recognition of need to change priorities in health care—from crisis-oriented acute care (often the end result of self-destructive life patterns and environmental hazards) to causative factors of major chronic illnesses (life-style and environmental improvements).
    2. Growing costs of present health care system with little cost effectiveness.
    3. Demystification and discontentment with primary health care.
    4. Life-style changes and increased educational levels (a better informed middle class).
    5. Problems with accessibility and availability of primary care health services.

15. 1. "Integrated functioning."
    2. Continually striving to grow and "maximizing potential" (dynamic state).
    3. "Within person's environment." Showing importance of our interaction with the environment.

16. 1. Self-responsibility, self-accountability, and self-care.
    2. Nutritional awareness—nutritional patterns which promote health and personal enjoyment.
    3. Stress management—learning how to handle stress (keeping it at healthy level).
    4. Physical fitness—maintaining a regular exercise program so that physiological and psychological benefits are attained.
    5. Environmental sensitivity—to be aware of environmental surroundings and their effects, modifying the physical, social, and personal environments, again, so that positive benefits to health and happiness are accrued.

    (See chapter text for a more thorough discussion of these dimensions.)

17. The health-hazard appraisal tool lists basic identifying data on individual (name, age, race, sex, and occupation) and the rank and nature of the major health problems (causing death) for persons of that age and sex. Prognostic criteria for each of these major health problems are also identified adjacent to problem. The tool then asks for information of patient relative to each of these criteria and has space next to patient data for treatment (Rx) advised to reduce risks.

18. 1. Teacher/health educator
    2. Referral agent
    3. Counselor–supportive role

19. 1. Deliverer of services
    2. Case finder
    3. Coordinator/referrer

20. 1. Client advocate

21. 1. Case finder
    2. Health educator
    3. Coordinator-referral agent

22. 1. Health educator
    2. Counselor–supportive role
    3. Coordinator
    4. Environmental modifier
    5. Team member

Comprehensive family nursing is a complex process, making it necessary to have a logical, systematic approach for working with families and individual family members. According to Yura and Walsh, "The nursing process is the core and essence of nursing. It is central to all nursing actions, applicable in any setting, within any frame of reference, any concept, theory, or philosophy."[1] Process is described as a deliberate and conscious act of moving from one point to another (through a series of steps) toward goal fulfillment. It is basically a problem-solving process which is utilized whether the nurse is working with individuals, families, groups, or communities.

FAMILY NURSING PROCESS

There is no major difference between the nursing process used in working with families and that used in working with individual clients. The sole difference is that the recipient of nursing services for the family-centered nurse is both the individual and the family, thus enlarging the scope of practice. This means that the family-health nurse will be utilizing the nursing process on two levels—that of individual family member and that of the family. Assessment, diagnosis, planning, implementation, and evaluation will, therefore, all be more extensive and complex because of this additional charge.

Some nursing authors have spoken of the family as the unit of service, without specifically mentioning its members. But it is important to assess and focus on both levels. A full understanding of the family cannot be developed if we learn only from each member what he or she is like. Conversely an understanding of each member can be gained only when we view that individual within his or her primary group (family) context. Therefore, nursing care must be directed at both the family as a whole *and* the individual clients within the family.

This two-level approach to planning family-nursing care—assisting the family and its members to achieve high-level wellness—is illustrated in Figure 3.1. In reality, the steps in the diagram are interdependent and not strictly sequentially or linearly organized. In practice, one or more steps may overlap and take place simultaneously with movement back and forth among the various steps.

ASSESSMENT

The process of nursing assessment is highlighted by continuous information gathering and professional judgments which attach meaning to the information being gathered. In other words, data is collected in a systematic fashion, classified, and analyzed as to its

3

The Family-Centered Nursing Process

LEARNING OBJECTIVES

1. Explain the difference of using the nursing process in family nursing in contrast to using the nursing process in working with individuals.
2. Describe each of the five basic steps within the nursing process relative to its purpose and meaning.
3. Discuss the preparation needed to adequately visit a family.
4. Describe briefly the basic findings of the interactional study conducted by Conant.
5. Define the PES syndrome and enumerate the advantages for using this method in family health nursing.
6. Describe several variables the family health nurse would consider when determining priorities for nursing care.
7. Identify within what phases of the nursing process the identification of resources is included.
8. Apply the premise that "families have the right and responsibility to make their own health decisions" at each step of the nursing process.
9. Compare Freeman's three types of nursing interventions with specific roles delineated in Chapter 2.
10. Define the term "contracting" when it is used as a method of intervention by the family health nurse.
11. Summarize the philosophy underlying the use of contracting in a community health nursing setting.
12. Identify four characteristics an effective contract should have.
13. List two family problems which confront community health nurses and interpret the meaning of these problematic behaviors.

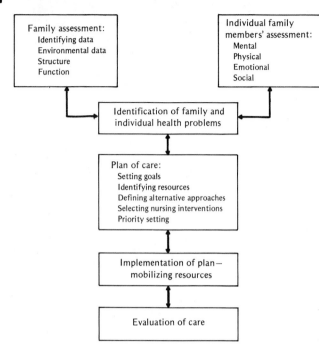

FIGURE 3.1
Steps in the family-centered nursing process.

meaning.* Often much cursory data is collected on each of the major areas, and when the assessor then finds significant/probable/potential problems, she or he will probe them more deeply. The amount of information is also dependent on the client, who may need to convey more in one area than another. Data collection is the *sine qua non* of problem identification. Although assessment is the first step of the nursing process, data continues to be gathered throughout the provision of services, showing the dynamic and flexible quality of this process.

Family data collection comes from many sources: client interviews relative to past and present events, objective findings (e.g., observations of home and its facilities), subjective appraisals (e.g., responses of individuals and family members), and information from referrals, various agencies working with family, and other health team members.

The establishment of a trusting relationship in which there is mutual respect and open, honest communication has also been included in the assessment or the preassessment process. It certainly sets the stage for and is the cornerstone of effective nursing care.

---

*Most recent authors of nursing process texts[2-4] have included the reaching of conclusions or the formulation of nursing diagnosis under assessment. I have separated nursing diagnosis (which I call identification of family and individual health problems) only because of the greater complexity posed by having both family and individual health problems, thus the academic need for a discrete step for purposes of discussion.

When visiting the family in the home, careful preparation must precede the actual visit. Since the community health nurse is out there on her or his own without immediate access to resources (except by phone), the preparatory aspect of the home visit is critical to success. Since home visits are quite costly in terms of both time and money, the most efficient and cost-effective method is to be as prepared as time constraints and other reality factors permit. This implies the reading of available records, discussing the family with health team members who know the family well, and anticipating the types of needs that the family might have (i.e., both common developmental and unique situational needs). In this way the nurse can gather whatever teaching supplies, information, assessment, and intervention tools (e.g., tongue blades, developmental screening kit, dressings, etc.) are needed before leaving the agency. Flexibility, of course, is essential, since unanticipated or priority needs often become apparent, and part of the preparation may not be needed—or at least not on the particular visit. When the family has a telephone, calling to introduce oneself and stating the reason for the visit and making arrangements is preferable.[5] Much wasted time and effort have been expended by needless visits to families not at home or when the nurse has not been adequately prepared.

One of the important roles of the family health nurse is that of a participant observer in the family. While the nurse is actively working with families, she or he must also have the ability to "stand back" and objectively observe the conditions and situations existing in the home.

The nurse's sensitivity will add to her observation. Sensitivity has to do with the ability to role take and empathize with others. Dyer points out that families operate on two levels of activity: one level is the activity of work (what the family is overtly doing, who is doing what, and how they are doing it), and the other is the feeling level (how the family members feel about what they are doing). It is crucial to understand both levels.[6]

The nature of client–nurse interactions also needs some exploration. Conant relates the findings of a research study she conducted in which 48 nursing visits to 24 families were observed and interactions rated.[7] Client–nurse interactions were categorized during each visit. Analysis of these visits showed that some nurses asked many questions and provided few answers, while in another large group of visits the opposite was observed—relatively few questions and much giving of information and suggestions. The patients tended to evaluate the visits on the basis of the help they thought they received. Thus, parts of the visit in which the nurse asked fewer questions and supplied more answers were reported to be highly satisfying to clients. Nurses who had a high rate of questioning also tended to be less active in giving, particularly in the positive social–emotional area.

The author suggests that greater client satisfaction is due to the nurse's willingness to give (and not just "take," which the asking of a lot of questions implies to the patient). She also expresses the view, which I support, that providing incidental assistance to the client, which although not central to nursing goals is important to the client, will help cement the relationship. When the family-centered nurse renders the help the client desires, both the relationship and nursing services may be facilitated.[8]

After having collected the data needed pertaining to both the family and its family members, the next step is analyzing the data. The family health nurse needs to summarize and collate data, then group similar data together and arrange it in orderly form so that accurate conclusions and problems can be identified. It is also at this time that gaps in data become obvious, indicating where further probing and detailing of information are needed.

IDENTIFICATION OF FAMILY AND INDIVIDUAL HEALTH PROBLEMS

The assessment culminates in a nursing diagnosis.* The family health nurse and the family are together responsible for identifying individual and family health problems. Nursing diagnosis is considered the end product or outcome of nursing assessment. It can be an expression of family and client health status, with an identification of strengths and assets, as well as of deficits and weaknesses. A nursing diagnosis may indicate either that no health problems exist that suggest health team, including nursing, intervention or that certain present or potential health problems exist which interfere with the family's level of wellness.[9] The nursing diagnosis may describe the family's problem(s), the family's needs, or both. At the family level, the nursing diagnosis can be derived from any of several approaches: the structural–functional framework, as presented in this text, e.g., role problems, value conflicts, communication problems; the systems framework, e.g., closed boundaries, lack of intact parental subsystem; the interactional framework, e.g., role transition problem, decision-making conflicts; or the developmental framework, e.g., communication gap between father and son, caretaker problems with an elderly parent in the home, and so forth.

I have used Gordon's components in defining the

nursing diagnosis,[10] which consists of the health problem (or health need); the etiological factor(s) (including contributory factors), which I term variables; and the symptoms of the problem (and signs). The nursing care plan at the end of the chapter illustrates how this aspect is schematically handled in a nursing care plan tool. Gordon refers to these components as making up the PES syndrome—the problem, etiology, and symptoms. When behaviors (symptoms) and variables (etiological factors) are included in the diagnosis, richer and broader avenues for both goal setting and intervention strategies are provided. Goals and interventions can then be aimed directly at the problem, modifying symptoms or manipulating variables (etiological or contributory factors).

One of the problems in determining health needs or problems of families is that all the information gathered is interrelated, and there are almost insurmountable difficulties involved in sorting out the cause-and-effect relationships. Also, there is an overlapping of problems such as role and power conflicts, and certain problems are not of the same type or level of generality or specificity as others. Pulling out the cardinal health problems and showing other related problem areas (economic, housing, community, education) as variables has often assisted in the listing of discrete problems (they are discrete for purposes of planning, but in real life never are).

The problems identified in family nursing often focus on the family's ability to cope with a health or environmental problem. In many situations there will be no present illness or disability at all. In these cases the most frequent diagnoses are preventive or health promoting, such as reduction of risks (nutritional modification—salt, caloric, sugar, and fat reduction; lowering stress levels) and life-style improvements (regular exercise program, more rest and relaxation, better communication).

A diagnosis may also involve potential health problems originating in existing or anticipated conditions. Freeman calls these "foreseeable crisis or stress points."[11] Because of these anticipated periods of unusual demand on the family and its members, anticipatory guidance or health teaching, health counseling, and the initiation of referrals to community resources are often indicated. Examples of foreseeable stressors are pregnancy, movement into a new community, retirement, adolescence, wife beginning full-time employment, and the progressive deterioration of an aging parent.

What are family health problems? These are problems which involve either the total family or two or more of its members (a subsystem of the family). An example of a common family health problem is: "Poor communication between mother and daughter

---

*This chapter will not cover the meaning of nursing diagnosis or the basic discussion needed to differentiate this from a medical diagnosis. Chapter references 2–4 all cover this subject well.

characterized by mutual hostility; causative factors: value, control, and limit-setting conflicts and mother's low self-esteem" (this is full nursing diagnosis). Other common family health problems (not fully described) are parenting or child-rearing problems, role conflicts or role change problems, affectional problems, poor family health practices, lack of preventive health care, and inadequate nutritional, sleeping, and cleanliness patterns. In the discussions of each assessment area that follow (Chapters 8–17) the reader will be able to gain insight into the types of family health problems which may result from a deficiency in fulfilling a family function and/or in meeting familial structural needs (family interactional needs).

Some identified family or individual problems are primarily within the domain of other related disciplines such as medicine, social service, recreation, or education. In this case the family health problems still need to be identified and discussed with family, which serves to verify that the need or problem is mutually perceived. Often the nursing role here is to refer the family to appropriate resources and to provide the necessary teaching/support related to the problem and referral. Other problems are the concern of several health professionals, with each health professional having a different way of assessing and a different approach to working with the family. In these instances, collaboration with the other health team members is imperative to avoid unnecessary client confusion and lack of efficient, effective services.

One word of caution is necessary concerning the problems identified by a referring agency. The presenting problem, or reason for referral to the agency, is rarely the only problem. In fact, it may be the least serious problem the family faces. Archer and Fleshman recommend that community health nurses use a sorting or triage process when working with families, since there is always too much to do and a scarcity of resources.[12] The triage process they recommend is based on a hierarchy of needs, as described below.

Of low priority and hierarchy relative to providing services are those needs that are impossible to do anything about, because of either client or agency constraints. Thus it is fruitless for individual nurses to "spin their wheels." Other needs or problems will resolve themselves or can be handled by the family's support system or someone less costly and more available, e.g., the homemaker–home health aide. Again, valuable health professional services should not be committed to these problems. Some needs require more resources than the agency or community can commit, and if a nurse attempts to meet these needs, other families will probably suffer from neglect. Thus realistic priorities, given limited resources, must be established. There are also needs and problems that

are beyond the control of the client or the control and/or level of expertise of the nurse. These limitations must be recognized. If the problem is not within our area of expertise, it needs to be referred. The needs for which family health nurses can effect change or on which she or he can make a discernible, positive health impact in an efficient manner are the problems we should be assisting families to alleviate or ameliorate.

As Archer and Fleshman point out, community nurses have long been considered "generalists," engaging in all sorts of problem areas. But this characterization has resulted in frustration, case overload, and cost ineffectiveness.[13]

Diagnosis involves the process of putting information together with the family to formulate the problem and to explore a possible course of action. It is not enough for the nurse working with a family to observe that the family is under stress and not following their plan for bringing in family or friends to help with, for instance, necessary child-care responsibilities. Together with the family, the nurse needs to generate a diagnosis as to what is happening and why the family is not able to follow through with their intended action. If the nurse has collected adequate information and verified it with the family, the diagnosis will be reasonably correct. His or her diagnosis should then lead to goals and intervention aimed at assisting the family to cope more effectively.[14]

Once family and individual health problems have been identified, they should be listed in order of priority, according to their magnitude and importance to the client. There is often a disjuncture between how the professional views client needs and what a client wants. Only by ranking needs and priorities from the client's perspective can plans for intervention have any chance of success. The widespread use of problem-oriented records provides a ready vehicle for listing problems. These identified problems will then form the basis for nursing goals and intervention.

PLANNING

Goal Setting

After the family nurse and family members have identified and validated health problems, the question then is posed: "In light of the information I have and the problems the family and I have identified, what goals and actions could we take that would be effective?"

Planning means determining what needs to be accomplished to assist the family and its members. This involves the mutual setting of goals, identifying possible resources, delineating alternative approaches to meet goals, selecting specific nursing interventions, mobilizing resources, and operationalizing the plan (setting of priorities and phasing plan in). The nursing care plan serves as a blueprint for action.

Goal setting has been increasingly recognized as a highly important component in planning. The development of clear-cut, specific, and acceptable goals is crucial. If the nursing goals are not clear, it does not make much difference what activities are carried out because the end point is not known. To the extent that the stated objectives are defined and accepted as valid by all concerned, the desired action is likely to follow. In addition to the acceptability, clarity, and specificity of goals, they also need to be stated in behavioral terms so that they can be measured (evaluated).

There are several levels of goals. The first level includes the specific, immediate, and measurable short-term goals; in the middle of the continuum are immediate goals; and at the other end of the continuum are the long-term, more general, ultimate goals that indicate the broad purposes the nurse and family hope to achieve. Short-term goals are necessary to motivate and give confidence to family and individuals that progress is being made, as well as to guide the family toward the larger, more comprehensive goal.

Freeman distinguishes between the setting of goals and then securing compliance of others and true mutual goal setting, where the resources and commitment of nurse and family are actually merged to produce a mutually acceptable and viable objective.[15] Even though families are often hard put to verbalize goals explicitly, the family nurse needs to motivate them to develop health goals that are explicit, tangible, time related, measurable, and realistic.

Tinkham and Voorhies help families determine their own health goals by providing them with all the relevant information about the family and its members. This allows them to make sound decisions about what goals and services they wish to plan.[16] Thus the main forces of the identified goals is the family and what they are able and willing to do, not the nurse and what she or he hopes to achieve.[17]

In goal setting it is desirable to work with the family in differentiating those problems which need to be resolved by nursing intervention, those problems which should be handled by themselves, and those which need to be referred to other members of the health team or handled on a collective basis. A case in point would be an elderly couple who might need (1) assistance in obtaining Medicaid, (2) diet counseling, and (3) basic nursing care for the nonambulatory husband. The nurse may decide to handle diet counseling herself, refer the couple to a social worker for Medicaid assistance, and suggest a home health aide to provide the routine nursing care needed for the husband. As a member of the health team serving families, the family-centered community nurse must also be contin-

ually alert to situations where team conferences (formal or informal) might be beneficial to the clients. Sharing of the nurse's plan of care with other team members helps to foster a better understanding of client, in addition to enhancing collaborative efforts.

Generating Alternative Approaches and Identifying Resources

After setting goals, the health professional and family need to generate alternative ways for reaching the stated goals. As these are delineated, possible resources for handling needs are identified. Such resources include inner family strengths, the family's support system, and physical and community sources of assistance.

Otto has made a comprehensive list of family strengths, resources, and potentials which are useful in assisting nurse and family in resolving family health problems. These inner and external strengths and resources include physical, emotional, and spiritual strengths; healthy child-rearing practices and discipline; meaningful and clear communication in the family; support, security, and encouragement among family members; growth-producing relationships and experiences; active community relationships; parental growth; assumption of self-responsibility and accepting assistance when needed; flexibility of family functions and roles; mutual respect for the individuality of family members; the family's use of crisis for growth; and family unity, loyalty, and cooperation. Otto reports that he has successfully used these family strengths in counseling of families. He explains that family strengths are first identified and then progressively shared with family members so as to increase their awareness of their resources and to take inventory of further potentials or strengths they have. Members are encouraged to discover latent strengths and unfulfilled potentials as part of their problem-solving efforts.[18]

Specific nursing actions or approaches are selected from the available alternatives and resources. These are approaches which both family and nurse feel are appropriate and, hopefully, have a high probability of success. Strategies might involve family members, other health team members, or extended family and friends, as well as the nurse.[19]

In thinking through the planning of nursing approaches, the nurse needs to ask the following questions:

Will my proposed approaches result in increased dependence or increased independence on the part of the family?
Is this action within the information and skill level of the family members or their own resources?

Will this action diminish or strengthen the coping abilities of the family?[20]

Does the family and/or its members have sufficient commitment and motivation to adhere to the plan?

Are there adequate resources available to carry out the plan?

One of the basic premises of family-centered nursing states that families have the right and responsibility to make their own health decisions. In carrying out this premise, there will be certain actions that families choose for which they must understand the possible consequences and with which we may personally disagree. So important is the issue of client information and understanding of possible consequences of action (so that he or she can make a reasonable decision), that we now have informed consent laws in most states. Archer and Fleshman cite the example of a client who was exposed to rubella during the first trimester of pregnancy, with tests showing no immunity to the rubella virus. The nurse's responsibility in such an instance would be to discuss with the parents the risk of having an infant who is deformed and to inform them of possible alternatives (abort, continue pregnancy, seek further consultation, etc.). The parents need time and an opportunity to discuss their feelings and thoughts, as well as assistance with problem solving. However, we cannot make decisions for them. We may draw on professional judgment and knowledge to recommend a particular course of action after hearing their concerns, but we should in no way reject or withdraw our support if the client makes a decision counter to our advice.[21]

Some of the approaches we plan with families are less than ideal, but are hopefully realistic and an improvement to the client's (family's) situation. Seeking obtainable ways to reach goals is both realistic and pragmatic.

Priority Setting

The operationalization of the nursing care plan follows the selection of approaches designed to reach each of the stated goals. Priority setting of interventions and a phasing in and coordinating of the plan leads to its implementation.

Ordering nursing interventions by priority will provide an efficient, effective, and safe means for reaching goals and differentiating between short-term goals needing present attention and long-term goals.

The nurse uses professional judgment, coupled with consideration of the client's views on priorities. Some nurses assign planned intervention low-, medium-, and high-priority ratings, with high-priority actions being those which must be carried out

immediately or very soon. Reality factors such as agency policies, time and money constraints, and availability of personnel and other resources also influence priorities. In addition to client safety or life-threatening situations, two important factors to consider in assigning priorities are (1) the client's sense of urgency (this is important in building of rapport) and (2) actions that will, or might have, therapeutic effects on future actions. Some actions are prerequisite to others.

IMPLEMENTATION

The implementation phase begins with the completion of the nursing care plan. Implementation may be carried on by a number of team members: the client (individual or family), the nurse(s), other health team members, and extended family or significant others. In mobilizing resources which emanate from the nursing care plan, more extensive utilization of the client's social support system is often indicated, since the nuclear family is often isolated from family support or such support is nonexistent.

Freeman classifies nursing intervention as being supplemental (doing things that the family cannot do for itself); facilitative (removing economic, transportation, or social barriers to care); and developmental (goals aimed at improving the capacity of the recipient to act on his or her own behalf, e.g., self-care, self-responsibility). Nursing actions most often involve all three types of intervention, although an emphasis on developmental or self-care actions should be encouraged as the ultimate aim of nursing intervention.[22]

During the execution of nursing intervention, new data will be continually coming in. As this information (client's responses, changes in situation, etc.) bombards the nurse, she or he needs to be sufficiently flexible and adaptable to make modifications to the plan extemporaneously. Careful observation must continue while carrying out nursing strategies so that unanticipated outcomes can be detected and dealt with.

Dyer discusses the need for family-centered nurses to take risks in their practice.[23] Doing so involves taking actions that have unpredictable and uncertain consequences. As the nurse faces problems and generates plans, a certain amount of personal risk is often called for if they are to be implemented. It often demands a certain degree of risk to confront people, to express important feelings, to engage in programs that are unpopular. The nurse, in working with families, faces such situations constantly: if she tells the family the truth, she may be rejected, or bringing families together may cause further conflict or anger to be directed at her. Nevertheless, there are significant gains to be made by taking risks. There is the possibility that positive decisions will be made, that the family will respond to the new information, and that family relationships will be strengthened. Each person must decide whether the positive side of the risk outweighs the negative possibilities.[24]

An effective means by which a family-centered nurse can realistically assist individuals and families to engage in self-care for their own well-being is the use of contracts. In community-health nursing a contract is a working agreement made between client and health worker. It is continuously renegotiable and covers the following areas: goals, length of contract, client responsibilities (commitments), and health team members' responsibilities. If it is a formally written contract, it includes signatures of those involved; there may also be a fee determination, depending on the agency.[25]

The philosophy underlying the use of contracts is that of client involvement and the encouragement of self-care and self-responsibility. The contract draws the client in as a partner (the chief partner) in his or her health care. The effective use of this process is dependent on family involvement in its development and the implementation of specific activities as agreed on.

Barriers to Implementation

In reporting his work with families in the community, Dyer mentions two related problems with which family nurses are confronted—family apathy and indecision. The first of these problematic behaviors must not only be recognized as a major problem, but more importantly, must be interpreted as to its possible meaning.[26]

Behavioral manifestations of apathy are apparent. When the nurse finds health problems which she or he feels vitally affect the family and discusses these problems and recommendations, the family responds with a "so what" attitude and gives no signs of action or concern. Does the family really not care? Not usually. It is often the case that there are differences in values, especially if the family is of a different socio-economic or ethnic background. Whereas the nurse feels health should be a top priority, the more basic physiological and safety needs for economic security, livable housing, and adequate food may have a greater urgency for such families. Health practices (dietary patterns, cleanliness, preventive health care) are not part of the general life experiences of the poor. What the nurse may perceive as apathy is really just a continuation of the family's life experience. What the nurse is faced with is the educational task of trying to get families to change behaviors, attitudes, and values so that they will be more receptive to health needs. The educational task is even more difficult if the family's social network or social system (relatives, friends, and neighbors) does not support the activities advised by the nurse. Some research shows that if members of a group adopting new practices support each other, the possibility of changing their behavior is greater. Based on this understanding, many therapeutic self-help groups have been formed to assist group members adopt new behavioral patterns (e.g., Alcoholics Anonymous, Parents Anonymous, Weight Watchers, Colostomy Club, Reach for Recovery, psychotherapy groups, and so forth).

In addition to value differences, apathy may also be the outcome of a sense of hopelessness—the belief that "whatever the family does, it won't matter anyway" or feeling that "what will be, will be." Fatalism is a central theme among the poor and powerless. Certain problems may be just too overwhelming for individuals to know where to begin. Breaking a task up into small, sequential steps may help a family proceed successfully toward a goal which at first seems insurmountable. Not trying to accomplish is a common way of coping to "save face," since it avoids the embarrassment of being found to be inadequate or rejected.

The third explanation for apathetic behavior on the part of a family is that family members may have a sense of futility about the effectiveness or availability of services: "So I have tuberculosis? There is nothing that can be done if they do find it!" Without a perception that effective and accessible treatment exists, clients are not going to seek health services.[27] The family-centered nurse will need to probe a situation where apathy exists to attempt to determine what is going on. Is faulty information the problem, or finances, or management of their resources, or excessive fear (and thus avoidance)?

Dyer describes indecision as the second behavioral area nurses in the community find problematic.[28] This behavioral problem is related to apathy. The family does not appear completely apathetic, but they cannot seem to make a decision. What are the causes of this type of behavior? Dyer identifies several. First, indecision often results from the inability to see the advantage of one action compared to another. Whatever is done, the advantages or disadvantages seem to be equal. In this case the nurse needs to help the family problem solve, so that the pros and cons, in addition to feelings, are explored thoroughly. It is hoped that this process results in one approach gaining superiority in the family's mind so they can take action. Some clients desperately want direct advice on what to do. Very careful consideration should be given to their requests. Temporary dependence is sometimes the best avenue, but generally this approach only solves a particular problem, and the family will not have learned how to

TABLE 3.1
Student Tool Used to Assess, Plan, and Implement Nursing Care

I. Assessment
   A. Assessment of Individual Family Members
   B. Assessment of Family*
      1. Identifying Data   3. Structural Analysis
      2. Environmental Data   4. Functional Analysis

II. Nursing Care Plan (Family)

Nursing Diagnosis Including Major Variables	Signs and Symptoms of Problem (Behavioral Manifestations)	Goals	Intervention	Evaluation
Family overprotection of son, Bobby, due to: Parental 1. guilt about unwanted pregnancy 2. anxiety about child's health condition: asthma	Mother dresses Bobby even though at age 4, he is able to do this himself. Mother wouldn't let Bobby play outside for fear of his hurting himself. Child is clinging to mother when strangers present. Parents view Bobby as a special, "fragile" child.	Mother will let Bobby dress himself, with help only in realistically difficult tasks. Mother will let Bobby play with brother and friends outside in the afternoon.	*Modifying Behavior* Helped explore her feelings and behavior toward child. Discussed with the parents their child's developmental needs. Discussed with sibling activities they might enjoy playing together. *Manipulation of Variables* Advised mother to discuss with her doctor child's health condition and prognosis.	Mother is letting Bobby dress himself when there is time. Bobby enjoys doing so. Under mother's supervision, Bobby is playing in the outside garden of house. Father is beginning to play ball at the park with both of the boys.

* To be discussed in later chapters.

cope with the next problem independently. Being a supportive resource person is the preferable role.

Indecision may also be the result of unexpressed fears and concerns. Marked anxiety and fear immobilize problem-solving abilities.

De facto decision making (letting things just happen) may also be a part of the family's life style. This type of decision making has been found to be predominant in disorganized families and many poor families.

EVALUATION

The fifth component of the nursing process is evaluation. The evaluation approach used in working with families is based on evidence of the effectiveness of services provided and is determined by how the client responded to the planned interventions. Thus evaluation is not based on nursing performance, but on family responses, although it is assumed that client responses reflect the quality of nursing intervention received. Although a client-centered approach to evaluation is most relevant, it is also frustrating because of the difficulties in establishing objective criteria for desired outcomes and because of factors other than nursing activities that intervene to effect family/client outcomes. Because of such factors, one never gets a clear-cut, "pure" look at the quality of nursing intervention.

The nursing care plan contains the framework for evaluation. If clear, specific behavioral goals have been delineated, these can then serve as the criteria for evaluating the degree of effectiveness achieved. In some instances there may be a need to develop even more specific criteria for evaluation of goals. For example, the goal, "The family will seek medical services for their sick baby," may need more specific criteria to judge whether the goal has been attained. Criteria for evaluation might include the fact that the family has been seen by a pediatrician and has received treatment for illness. In many cases, however, the goal can be written in more specific terms to avoid further criteria development, such as, "The child will obtain diagnostic and treatment services from pediatrician within one to three days."

Evaluation is an on-going process that occurs each time a nurse updates the nursing care plan. Before care plans are expanded or modified, certain nursing actions will need to be looked at to see if they are really helpful to the client. Unless family responses to nursing intervention are evaluated, ineffective nursing action may persist.

The following questions should be contemplated when evaluating:

Were family expectations set in realistic and accurate goals?

Do the family and other health team members agree with evaluation?

What additional data need to be collected?

Were the nursing diagnosis, goals, and approaches realistic and accurate?

If the family's behavior indicates that the problem has not been satisfactorily resolved, what are the reasons?

Were there any unforeseen outcomes which need to be considered?

Cost-Effectiveness Questions

If the goals were attained, could they have been reached without nursing intervention?

Were the results commensurate with the expenditure of time, money, and other resources?

There are various methods of evaluation used in nursing; the most important factor is that the method needs to be tailored to the goals being evaluated.

MODIFICATION

Modification is incorporated into and also follows the evaluation plan. Modification results in revision and refinement activities, returning to assessment and reassessing—feeding in the new information obtained from previous encounters, and then continuing to revise each phase in the cycle as needed.

Modification is often difficult to do, as it can be frustrating and ego deflating to admit our plan and implementation were ineffective. So often in working with families in the community we see only very slow results or perhaps no movement of a family at all—at least not when we are working with them. At this point we need to make sure that if we continue our search for a more accurate diagnosis or a more effective plan, our efforts have some chance of success and the resources to be expended will be commensurate with the gain achieved.

Table 3.1 summarizes the information presented in this chapter.

REFERENCES

1. Yura H, Walsh M: The Nursing Process. New York, Appleton, 1978, p 1
2. *Ibid.*, p 28
3. Lewis L: Planning Patient Care, 2nd ed. Dubuque, Iowa, William C Brown, 1970
4. Bower FL: The Process of Planning Nursing Care, 2nd ed. St. Louis, Mosby, 1977
5. Leahy K, Cobb M, Jones M: Community Health Nursing, 3rd ed. New York, McGraw-Hill, 1977, pp 176–178
6. Dyer W: Working with groups. In Reinhardt A, Quinn M: Family-Centered Community Nursing. St. Louis, Mosby, 1973, pp 146–147
7. Conant L: The give and take in home visits. In Stewart D, Vincent P: Public Health Nursing. Dubuque, Iowa, William C Brown, 1968, pp 51–64
8. *Ibid.*, p 53
9. Bower, *op. cit.*, p 13
10. Gordon M: Nursing diagnoses and the diagnostic process. Am J Nurs 76:1298, 1976
11. Freeman RB: Community Health Nursing Practice. Philadelphia, Saunders, 1970, p 58
12. Archer S, Fleshman R: Community Health Nursing. North Scituate, Mass, Duxbury Press, 1975, pp 47–49
13. *Ibid.*, p 50
14. Dyer, *op. cit.*
15. Freeman, *op. cit.*, p 63
16. Tinkham C, Voorhies E: Community Health Nursing: Evolution and Process, 2nd ed. New York, Appleton, 1977, p 161
17. *Ibid.*, p 167
18. Otto H: A framework for assessing family strengths. In Reinhardt A, Quinn M (eds): Family-Centered Community Nursing. St. Louis, Mosby, 1973, pp 87–93
19. Bower, *op. cit.*, pp 81–102
20. Dyer, *op. cit.*
21. Archer, Fleshman, *op. cit.*, p 50
22. Freeman, *op. cit.*, pp 58–60
23. Dyer, *op. cit.*
24. *Ibid.*, p 148
25. Sloan M, Schommer B: The process of contracting in community nursing. In Spradley B (ed): Contemporary Community Nursing. Boston, Little, Brown, 1975, pp 221–222
26. Dyer, *op. cit.*, p 150
27. Becker MH: The health belief model and personal health behavior. Health Educ Monogr 2:326–327, 1972
28. Dyer, *op. cit.*, p 151

Choose the correct answer(s) to the following question.

1. The primary difference between the nursing process when working with families versus working solely with individual clients is (select the best answer):
   a. The community setting must be assessed.
   b. The level of assessment, diagnosis, planning, implementation, and evaluation is broadened to include both the family and its members.
   c. The level of assessment, diagnosis, planning, implementation, and evaluation is the family system.
   d. Prevention and health promotion are the aim versus cure and rehabilitation when working with individuals.

2. Match the correct process characteristics in the left-hand column with the nursing phase/component on the right.

Process Characteristics	Phase/Components of Nursing Process
a. Continuous data collection.	1. Assessment
b. Approaches based on identi-fied goals.	2. Diagnosis
c. Client outcome appraisal.	3. Goal setting
d. Anticipated behaviorally-stated client responses.	4. Plan of care
e. Setting of priorities.	5. Implementation
f. Nursing action, therapy, or approaches.	6. Evaluation
g. Execution of the nursing care plan.	7. Modification process
h. Existing or potential family and individual health problem.	
i. Mobilizing community resources.	
j. Identification of resources.	
k. Refinement and revision efforts.	
l. Defining alternative approaches.	

Choose the correct answers to the following questions.

3. The nursing assessment is (choose the best answer):
   a. Done on initial gathering of data.
   b. Done by all persons involved in providing client care.
   c. A sensitive and continuing process conducted by all involved health providers.

4. One objective of the nursing assessment process is priorities for intervention.
   a. True.
   b. False.
   c. Uncertain.

Match the nurse's statements with the appropriate step in intervention.
   a.   Establishing a relationship.
   b.   Obtaining information.
   c.   Identification/clarification of focal problem.
   d.   Assessment of strengths and resources.
   e.   Formulation of a therapeutic plan and mobilization of client's and others' resources.

5.   "How have things been with your family?"

6.   "I'm concerned about your problem and would like to know more."

7.   "Can you tell me more about the fight with your wife?"

8.   "Tell me how I can help you."

9.   "Do you feel you can talk easily with your sister about your worries?"

10.   List the three activities the family health nurse should carry out in preparation for a home visit.

Choose the correct answer(s) to the following question.
11.   In her study of interactional patterns of community health nurses with families at home, Conant found that:
   a.   Families were more satisfied when they were permitted to speak more.
   b.   Families perceived the value of a visit in terms of what they thought they received in benefits.
   c.   Families felt they benefited more from visits where the nurse asked many questions and answered few questions.
   d.   Families felt they benefited more from visits where nurse asked relatively fewer questions but gave more suggestions and answers.

Fill in the spaces in the following question.
12.   The PES syndrome stands for _____
_____ and is part of the identification of
_____ and _____ health problems. One advantage to
using this method of diagnosing is _____
_____

Choose the correct answer(s) to the following question.
13.   In planning nursing intervention, priorities need to be established. These variables are significant when establishing priorities:
   a.   Family/individual interests and perceptions.
   b.   Degree of urgency or acuteness of problem.
   c.   Availability of resources.
   d.   Agency policies.
   e.   Actions which are prerequisite to other actions.

Fill in the space in the following question.
14.   Family involvement in the nursing process should occur during _____
_____
_____ phase(s)
of the nursing process.

15. What nursing roles, as discussed in Chapter 2, can be subsumed under each of Freeman's types of nursing intervention? For Supplemental, give two roles; for Facilitative, six; and for Development, two.

Are the following statements True *or* False?

16. a. Contracts can be unwritten or written.
    b. Contracts are legal agreements between two sets of individuals.
    c. Contracts encourage self-responsibility and self-care.
    d. Using contracts greatly aids in the evaluation process.
    e. A contract must contain time limitations.
    f. A contract is made by the nurse and signed by the patient.
    g. A contract spells out goals to be achieved and the respective responsibilities of the involved members.

After reading the vignettes, answer the following study questions.

17. Mr. and Mrs. Wade's daughter, age five, has been observed several times by kindergarten teachers in grand mal seizures. The school nurse, while visiting family, discusses the convulsions and need for medical follow-up at a special clinic in a nearby community. She notes that the parents change subject, brushing off observed seizures as temper tamtrums. They state that the family does not have time to take her to a doctor.
    a. What type of problem does the school nurse have in working with this family?
    b. What may be the basis for this problem?

18. Mrs. J., a single parent with limited income, is having difficulty raising only son, age ten. She describes him as rebellious, disobedient, and irresponsible. Because of this parenting difficulty, she feels that she is a failure in the mothering role. The community health nurse, who is visiting because Mrs. J. is pregnant, listens to her concerns regarding son. For several years, teachers and church minister have encouraged her to take the child for counseling, but she could never decide whether this would be helpful or more damaging.
    a. This type of behavior problem is called _____.
    b. What may be the basis for the problem?

STUDY QUESTION ANSWERS

1. b.

2. a. 1   g. 5
   b. 5   h. 2
   c. 6   i. 5
   d. 3   j. 4
   e. 2 and/or 4 k. 7
   f. 5   l. 4 or 5

3. c

4. b

5. a and b

8. e

6. a and b

9. d

7. b or c

10. Any three:
    a. Review written records.
    b. Discuss family with other health team members who know family well.
    c. Gather whatever information, teaching supplies, and assessment and intervention equipment needed or anticipated.
    d. Call family on phone to set up visit if possible.

11. b and d

12. The PES syndrome stands for *problem, etiological factors, and symptoms of problem* and is part of the identification of *individual* and *family* health problems. One advantage to using this method of diagnosing is *that the symptoms and etiological factors lead to more comprehensive setting of goals and approaches.*

13. All choices (a–e) are correct.

14. All phases, since the family and its members are the crucial, central focus of our services and must be involved in all phases in order for each phase to be accomplished.

15. *Supplemental*
    a. Direct physical care and its supervision.
    b. Case finder/epidemiologist.
    Facilitative
    a. Coordinator.
    b. Collaborator with team members.
    c. Referral agent.
    d. Environmental modifier.
    e. Client advocate.
    f. Consultant.
    Developmental
    a. Counseling.
    b. Health education.

16. a. True
    b. False
    c. True
    d. True
    e. True
    f. False
    g. True

17. a. Apathy.
    b. Any of the following:
       Difference in value system
       Difference in perception of problem due to ignorance or fear
       Sense of futility about available resources

18. a. Indecision.
    b. Family fears/unexpressed concerns.

APPROACHES TO FAMILY ANALYSIS

Nye and Berardo in their book, *Emerging Conceptual Frameworks in Family Analysis*, delineate the following approaches utilized to study the family: anthropological, structural, functional, situational, psychoanalytic, economic, institutional, interactional, social-psychological, developmental, Western Christian, and legal.[1] As one can readily see, this list of conceptual frameworks is impressive. For our purposes there are only five well-established frameworks which need to be described because of their relevance to family-centered practice.

Systems Approach

The family is viewed as an open social system with boundaries, self-regulatory mechanisms, interacting and superordinate systems, and subcomponents. Chapter 6 is devoted to an in-depth discussion of this framework.

Structural-Functional Approach

This approach is an elaboration of the structural and functional dimensions of systems theory. Again the family is viewed as a social system, with the analysis of its functional and structural dimensions receiving primary attention. This approach has been selected as this text's organizing and theoretical framework and, as such, will be discussed in Chapter 7. In addition, Part II (Chaps. 9–17) elaborates on and describes the operation of the structural–functional framework, modified here to bring under this rubric the various content areas needed for family nursing.

Interactional Approach

In the interactional approach the general focus is on the ways in which family members relate to one another. Thus the family is viewed as a set of interacting personalities, and internal family dynamics are dealt with in detail in this approach.

The interactional conceptual framework for studying families is a social–psychological approach. It is concerned with the relation between the individual and the family group.[2] Schraneveldt explains that

> within the family, each member occupies position(s) where a number of roles are assigned. The individual perceives norms or role expectations held individually or collectively by other family members for his attributes and behaviors.... It is this tendency to shape the phenomenal world into roles which is the key to role-taking as a core process in interaction. An individual defines his role expectations in a given situation in terms of a reference group and by his own self-conception. Individual family members role-play. The family and its individual members are studied through the analysis of overt inter-

4

Approaches to Family Analysis

LEARNING OBJECTIVES

1. Identify five basic approaches utilized in the behavioral sciences for analyzing families.
2. Discuss the interactional approach to family analysis.
3. Trace major alterations which occurred in family functions during the change from an agrarian, nonindustrialized society to that of the present day.

actions. Each family is not only supported, but limited by family life pattern which has evolved in its interaction in society. Through this limitation or support, each family in interactional process achieves its own tempos or rhythms of family living. A unique, differentiating characteristic of the interactional approach is that it is based on the action of the family resulting from communication processes. It views family behavior as an adjustive process: cues are given, individual members respond to these stimuli.[3]

In other words, the interactional approach strives to interpret family phenomena in terms of internal dynamics. These processes or dynamics consist of role playing, status relations, communication patterns, decision making, coping patterns, and socialization, with the assessment of roles and communication processes forming the core of the framework. Both personality and socialization are also viewed as central concerns of the interactional framework.[4] However, this approach does not examine the family within its external environment nor how the external social system interfaces with the family.

When studying the family from an interactional frame of reference, wherein families are seen as a unity of interacting personalities, a shift takes place from viewing the family broadly—as a social institution—to viewing the family more narrowly—as an internal association. With this approach the family practitioner centers his or her attention on how the family functions as they interact between and among each other. The approach is useful not only in providing a practical way of assessing the family, but also in isolating and specifying potential sources of difficulty as family members relate to one another and their community.

The same processes focused on within the interactional framework are considered as a part of family structure in the structural-functional framework of this text, since these family dynamics are crucial in understanding a family's behavior. By itself, the interactional approach is limited by the fact that the family does not operate in a vacuum, but rather is active within an environment, and that environment must be included for assessment if comprehensive family nursing care is to be provided. Therefore, this approach was not selected as the text's organizing framework, although its vital content has been retained in the chapters dealing with family structure and functions.

Developmental Approach

The developmental approach focuses on an analysis of the family as a small group progressing and changing through a life cycle—from its inception through old age and dissolution. Chapter 5 describes this approach in detail.

Institutional Approach

The fifth framework for analyzing the family is the *institutional* or *historical* approach. Using this approach the family is assessed as an institution and how it relates to other institutions in society, including religious, educational, governmental, and economic systems.

The primary focus is on the functions that the family carries out for society and how these dovetail with the functions which other institutions provide for the family. The family is also studied as its functions change over time. Certain functions have naturally changed over time in response primarily to societal changes. If one examines the American family as it existed before industrialization—when an agrarian life style and culture predominated—and compares the present-day family and its functions, profound changes become apparent.

Urban industrialized society has intruded forcefully on the family, and its institutions have assumed many functions that were once the family's domain. The old now live apart in old-age homes, housing projects for senior citizens, or their own apartment or house isolated from the family. Economic support is now provided to the old, unemployed, disabled, and dependent through Social Security or welfare programs. The young are no longer trained at home, but are educated by schools, mass media, peers, and various other associations and groups. Activities that traditionally took place within the home or involved the entire family now take place elsewhere and engage family segments. For instance, economic activity, which traditionally the family engaged in at home as a whole, has until recently been the father's responsibility—and one that took him out of the home and away from family life. Table 4.1 compares the American family before and after industrialization.

The institutional or historical framework also includes comparisons between different settings, especially of urban versus rural environments, and their effects on the family. Some of the significant forces facing families of rural and urban environments are outlined below. Each of the items listed should be understood as representing one end of a continuum describing the differences between rural and urban life. Obviously, no single community fully conforms in all respects to the somewhat exaggerated characteristics given here. For instance, city life is certainly more "urban" in New York than in Los Angeles.[5]

Rural Setting	*Urban Setting*
1. Geographic and social isolation	1. Geographic and social proximity
2. Homogeneity of community residents	2. Heterogeneity of community residents

TABLE 4.1:
Changes in Family Functions: Pre- and Postindustrialization Periods

Family Function	Family Functions Before Industrialization	Present-Day Family Function
1. Economic	Family served as sole economic unit. It was a self-contained, self-sufficient unit: home and business were combined; all family members helped. Family both produced and consumed its product. Family was supported by strong kinship associations (the extended family).	The family's economic function is much more limited. Food and clothes are bought outside of home. Children are no longer economic assets. Single individuals survive quite well. Head of household works outside of home, bringing home money to buy outside products and services.
2. Status Conferring	Family conferred privilege, honor, and status on persons. Family affiliation crucial in locating and placing someone in society.	Function still present but much decreased in importance. Persons are seen primarily as individuals, not as family members.
3. Education	Education ("schooling") done primarily in home. Father taught son vocation. Mother taught daughter homemaking and child-rearing skills.	Education is carried on outside of home to great extent; very formalized and institutionalized which has a pervasive influence on children, in both school and extracurricular activities, e.g., sports, music, school clubs, etc. Occupational skills are learned outside of home.
4. Socialization of Children	Child rearing occurred in the home and was the responsibility of mothers, grandmothers, aunts, and older female children.	Socialization function remains, although shared with outside institutions, e.g., nursery schools, baby sitters, child-care centers, teachers, counselors.
5. Care of Ill/Older Family Members	Protection and supervision of family members, especially of dependent, disabled, or aged individuals was by the family. The aged, dependent, and infirme were cared for at home.	This function has decreased greatly, depending on ethnic background and degree of acculturation to white Anglo-Saxon Protestant (WASP) culture. With older or disabled persons, society takes responsibility when family cannot or will not care for these dependent members.
6. Religious	Religious activities and beliefs were taught in home.	This is largely accomplished in outside agencies or is lacking.
7. Recreational	Since family was without commercial recreation, family-centered activities predominated.	Commercialization of recreation is ubiquitous. Family-centered activities are greatly curtailed.
8. Reproduction (procreation)	Marriage and family were necessity for survival.	Having child creates family, but marriage or having a family is not necessary. Reproduction is still a *vital* family function.
9. Affective	Primary group relationships were not as strong; extended family was more important.	This function not only remains, but has an increased importance. The usual American family has weakened extended family ties, whereas emotional relationships between the mates and parent–children are very intense. The result is a great emotional strain on relationships. Historically there existed an economic basis for marriage which now is usually an affective basis.

Rural Setting (cont.)

3. Agricultural employment
4. Sparsely populated
5. A subsistence economy
6. Personal

Urban Setting (cont.)

3. Industrial employment
4. Densely populated
5. A consumer economy
6. Impersonal

It can easily be seen that more disruptive forces are part of city living, although it is also apparent that life styles in the two settings are quite different and that a change in residence from urban to rural setting or vice versa could also be very disruptive.

The institutional approach adequately explains broad patterns of family life occurring over a long time scale. It is not concerned with individual family members or with single family units or their individual differences.[6] Except for providing a broad, macroscopic understanding of the family, this approach cannot satisfy the need of clinical family nursing for a guiding framework, since it does not allow for or interpret individual, family, or sociocultural differences.

In summary, five conceptual frameworks used to explain family dynamics have been discussed. Two frameworks, the interactional and the historical frameworks, were briefly elaborated upon in this chapter. Chapters 5 to 7 will deal in depth with the remaining three frameworks. The systems approach and the structual-functional framework are particularly important in that the systems approach provides the broader perspective for the text's organizing framework: structural-functionalism.

REFERENCES

1. Nye I, Bernardo F: Conceptual Frameworks for the Study of the Family. New York, Macmillan, 1966
2. Stryker S: The interactional and situational approaches. In Christensen HT (ed): Handbook of Marriage and the Family. Chicago, Rand McNally, 1964
3. Schraneveldt JD: The interactionist framework in the study of the family. In Reinhardt A, Quinn M (eds): Family-Centered Community Nursing. St. Louis, Mosby, 1973
4. Eshelman JR: The Family: An Introduction. Boston, Allyn & Bacon, 1974, pp 53–68
5. *Ibid.*
6. Rodgers RH: Family Interaction and Transaction: The Developmental Approach. Englewood Cliffs, NJ, Prentice-Hall, 1973, pp 9–11

STUDY QUESTIONS

1. Match approaches used in studying family on the left with *best* descriptions in column on the right.

Approaches

a. Systems approach.
b. Interactional approach.
c. Developmental approach.
d. Institutional approach.
e. Structural–functional approach.

Descriptions

1. Studies family relating to present situation, i.e., behavior vis-à-vis "triggering" event.
2. Studies family progressing through life cycle.
3. Family viewed as an open social system.
4. Deals with internal family dynamics.
5. Studies family functions in society as they change over time.
6. Describes family as having predictable natural history common to families and associated with changing ages and member composition.
7. Family viewed as social system with emphasis on purposes family achieves and its internal organization.

Fill in the correct answer to the following question.

2. The interactional approach analyzes the family in respect to: _____ .

3. Give three important areas the interactionist would assess using the above framework.

4. Match each function on the left with the appropriate description on the right of how the function has changed (as society changed from an agrarian to industrialized state):

Function	*Description*
a. Affective.	1. Continues to be crucial.
b. Socializing.	2. Decreased in importance or limited.
c. Economic.	
d. Religious.	3. Increased in importance.
e. Care, disabled family members.	4. Function important; function shared with other institutions in society.
f. Educational.	
g. Status conferring.	
h. Reproduction.	

STUDY ANSWERS

1. a. 3
   b. 4
   c. 2 and 6
   d. 5
   e. 7

2. Its internal dynamics or the interaction between the family members.

3. a. Role structure.
   b. Power structure (decision-making processes).
   c. Communication patterns.
   Stress reaction, status relations, and socialization problems are also correct.

4. a. 3   e. 2
   b. 4   f. 2
   c. 2   g. 2
   d. 2   h. 1

THE DEVELOPMENTAL APPROACH

One of the more recent frameworks generated for studying families is that of family development. This approach attempts to account for change over time in the family system and thus of interactions among family members. The developmental approach is based on the observation that families are long-lived groups with a natural history, or life cycle, that must be assessed if the dynamics of the group are to be fully and accurately interpreted.[1] Although each family goes through each stage of development in its own unique way, all families can be considered as examples of an overall normative pattern[2] and to follow a universal sequence of development.[3] The family takes one kind of structure when children are infants or of preschool age; a second when the parents enter into the prime of life and the children reach adolescence, and finally another when the children mature, marry, and go their own ways. Rodgers describes these changes further:

> The structure of the group changes during its history. . . . As members interact with one another over a variety of matters happening in the group, a whole set of learned and shared experiences develop which become precedents for further interactions. Although many of these experiences are unique, a great many are related to the normal and inevitable issues that arise in living together. Recently married couples must work out a set of relationships which are mutually satisfactory concerning many matters. Once established, however, the relationships do not remain constant, but change subtly or perhaps dramatically because of later events, which may occur in the family or outside of it. . . . Many happenings are anticipated and prepared for, whereas many are unexpected—though not peculiar to that family alone. Thus, though each family's history is unique, it is also common. Furthermore, it has a certain quality of inevitability though not necessarily of predictability as to exact time or circumstance. The developmental approach does not seek to explain family dynamics in terms of its unique elements, but in terms of the common quality of its experience over its history. There exist many more events that are common than are unique.[4]

Although developmental theory is based on the common, general features of family life and can be criticized for its assumption of homogeneity, its middle-class bias, and its lack of adequate attention to family diversity, the use of this framework for assessment is exceedingly helpful, since it provides us with ways of anticipating what to expect. If one knows (1) about a family's composition and its members and their relatedness; (2) the family's ethnic, religious, and social class status; and (3) the family's particular life cycle, it is possible to predict somewhat reliably the overall pattern of the family's activities, what significant elements to look for, and what forces one may expect to find.[5] Thus by assessing the family's developmental stage and its performance of the tasks

5

The Developmental Approach

LEARNING OBJECTIVES

1. Discuss three basic observations and/or concepts which form the basis for the developmental approach.
2. Discuss the usefulness of the developmental approach in assessing and working with families.
3. Define the meaning of family developmental tasks and family life styles.
4. Identify and describe each of the developmental stages within the life cycle of the family.
5. Identify three health promotion needs or health concerns of the family commonly experienced within each of the family's stages of development.
6. Describe developmental tasks of parents and how they relate to the family's stages of development.
7. Discuss adolescence and its impact on family.

appropriate to that stage, one is provided with guidelines for analyzing family growth and health promotion needs. The family health nurse is able to better provide the support needed for smooth progression from one stage to another.

The Family Life Cycle

There are predictable stages within the life cycle of every family. Just as individuals go through successive stages of growth and development, so do families as a unit go through successive stages of development. The most widely used formulation of the developmental stages of family life is the eight-stage family life cycle devised by Duvall and Hill in 1948 and recently updated by Duvall. In this paradigm, Duvall uses the age and school placement of the oldest child as a guidepost for the life cycle intervals (Fig. 5.1). Of course, when there are several children in the family, some overlapping of different stages will occur.[6]

Obviously, not everyone "fits" into the normative family life cycle stages. Variations in family life cycle include those persons who never marry, couples who never have children, and homosexual unions. For these persons the life cycle stages are attenuated or modified. For instance, the couple without children would go through stage I (marriage), stage VII (middle-age family), and stage VIII (the contracting family).

Family Developmental Tasks

Just as individuals have developmental tasks* which they must achieve in order to feel satisfied during a stage of development and to be able to proceed successfully to the following stage, each stage of family development has its specific developmental tasks. Family developmental tasks refer to growth responsibilities that must be achieved by a family during each stage of its development so as to meet (1) its biological requirements, (2) its cultural imperatives, and (3) its own aspirations and values.[7]

How do the developmental tasks of the family differ from those of the individual family member? While in reality many of them dovetail, family developmental tasks are generated when the family strives as a unit to meet the demands and needs of family members who in turn are striving to meet their individual developmental requisites. Family tasks are also created by community pressures for the family and its members to conform to the expectations of the family's reference group and the wider society.

---

* Examples are the developmental tasks which are inherent within the following frames of reference: (1) Erikson's stages of emotional development, (2) Piaget's stages of cognitive development, (3) Kohlberg's stages of moral development, and (4) Freud's stages of psychosexual development.

Stage I	Beginning Families (referred to also as the stage of marriage).
Stage II	Early Childbearing Families (the oldest child is an infant through 30 months).
Stage III	Families with preschool children (oldest child is 2½–5 years of age).
Stage IV	Families with school children (oldest child is 6–13 years of age).
Stage V	Families with teenagers (oldest child is 13–20 years of age).
Stage VI	Launching Center Families (covering the first child who has left through the last child leaving home).
Stage VII	Families of Middle Years (empty nest through retirement).
Stage VIII	Family in Retirement and Old Age (retirement to death of both spouses).

FIGURE 5.1
The eight-stage family life cycle. (*Adapted from Table 7-3, p. 144, in Marriage and Family Development, 5th edition by Evelyn Millis Duvall.* © *1957, 1962, 1967, 1971, 1977,* by J. B. Lippincott Company. Reprinted by permission of Harper & Row Publishers, Inc.)

In addition, family developmental tasks also include the tasks specific to each stage inherent in accomplishing the five basic functions of the family, consisting of (1) affective function (personality maintenance function), (2) socialization and social placement function, (3) provision and allocation of physical necessities and care, (4) reproductive function, (5) economic function, and (6) family coping patterns or strategies (see Chap. 7 for a complete discussion of these functions).

The real challenge in family life is to be able to meet each of the member's needs, as well as the general family functions. The meshing of individual developmental needs and family tasks is not always possible. For instance, the toddler's tasks involving the exploration of the environment are often in opposition to the mother's tasks of maintaining an orderly home.

STAGE I: BEGINNING FAMILIES

The marriage of a couple marks the beginning of a new family—the family of marriage or procreation—and the movement from their former family of origin to this new intimate relationship.

Family Developmental Tasks

Establishing a mutually satisfying marriage, relating harmoniously to the kin network, and family planning constitute the three critical tasks of this period.

Establishing a Mutually Satisfying Marriage

When two people become united in marriage, their initial concerns are preparing for a new type of life together. The resources of the two people are combined, their roles altered, and new functions assumed. Learning to live together while providing for each other's basic personality needs becomes a crucial developmental task. The couple has to develop a mutual accommodation in many small routines. For example, they must develop routines for eating, sleeping, getting up in the morning, cleaning house, sharing the bathroom, recreational pursuits, and going places they both enjoy. In this process of mutual accommodation, a set of patterned transactions are formed and then maintained by the couple, with each spouse triggering and monitoring the behavior of the other.

The success of the evolving relationship depends on the mutual accommodation just discussed and on a complementarity, or the fitting together of the needs and interests of the mates. Just as important, individual differences need to be acknowledged and may, in fact, enrich the marital relationship. Achieving a satisfying relationship is dependent on the development of satisfactory ways to handle "differentness" and conflicts. A healthy way of resolving problems is related to the mates' ability to empathize, be mutually supportive, be able to communicate openly and honestly,[8] and approach a conflict with feelings of mutual respect.[9]

Many couples experience problems in sexual adjustment, often because of ignorance and misinformation leading to unrealistic expectations and disappointment. Moreover, many couples bring their own unresolved needs and desires into the relationship and these can adversely affect the sexual relationship.

Relating Harmoniously to Kin Network

A basic role shift occurs in the first marriage of a couple, as they move from their parental homes to their new setting. Concomitantly, they become members of three families—those of their respective families of origin in addition to the one they have begun to create. The couple faces the tasks of separating themselves from each family of origin and working out different relationships with parents, siblings, and in-laws, since their primary loyalty must shift to their marital relationship. This entails that the couple form a new relationship with each set of parents that allows not only for mutual support and enjoyment, but also an autonomy that protects the newly formed family from outside intrusion that might undermine the building of a satisfying marriage.

Family Planning

Whether to have children and the timing of pregnancies becomes a significant area of concern. Littlefield[10]

underscores the importance of considering the whole family pregnant when one is working in maternity care. The type of health care the family as a unit receives during the prenatal period greatly influences the family's ability to cope effectively with the tremendous changes after the baby's birth. This text will not deal with the specific supportive, teaching, and counseling roles of the family-centered nurse who works with the pregnant family, since excellent chapters are available in this area in maternity texts.[11]

Health Concerns

The primary areas of concern are sexual and marital role adjustment, family planning education and counseling, prenatal education and counseling, and communication. It becomes increasingly apparent that counseling should be provided premaritally. Lack of information often results in sexual and emotional problems, fear, guilt feelings, unplanned pregnancies, and venereal disease either before or after marriage. These unfortunate events do not allow the couple to plan their lives and begin their relationship with a stable foundation.

Traditional marriage concepts are being challenged by love relationships, common-law marriages, and homosexual unions. People entering into these nonmarriage unions need as much if not more help from health workers who may be called on to assist such couples. It is perhaps at this point that family health workers are caught between two "families," the family of orientation and the forming union. In such a situation, they need not make value judgments, but must help each of the two groups to understand themselves and each other.[12]

Family Planning

Because family planning is such a cardinal responsibility for the nurse working with families, a more in-depth discussion of this area follows. The absence of informed, effective family planning affects family health in many ways: maternal–infant morbidity and mortality; child neglect; ill health of parents; child development problems, including intelligence, and learning ability; and marital discord. Informed and intentional family formation involves making decisions regarding the circumstances and timing of marriage, first pregnancy, birth spacing, and family size. People have the right to make personal decisions about when and/or whether to have children, even aside from any family health considerations. A planned, uncrowded family has the number of children wanted by parents, each born at a time desired, and causing no harm to the mother or the rest of the family.

In 1972 half of the first births in the United States

were to women under 22 years of age, and 1 in every 10 girls in this country will give birth before reaching 18, at present rates. Pregnancy is, not surprisingly, the chief cause of girls leaving school, as well as a frequent cause of premature marriage. Within marriage, early pregnancy (before 2 years) detracts from marital adjustment. All of these are important mental health factors for children and parents.[13]

The physical health of mother and child is a major issue, documented in obstetrical and perinatal studies. Birth intervals of between 2 and 4 years and a maternal age in the 20s are the most favorable factors for reducing maternal and infant mortality and morbidity. A recent review concludes that optimal family size, spacing, and timing of births might reduce the infant mortality of the United States by as much as 30 percent.[14]

The issue of world overpopulation must be a consideration in any discussion of family planning. On the national level, it is estimated that even when couples barely replace themselves (2.1 births per woman), our population will have grown from 211,909,000 in 1974 to 262,494,000 by the year 2000. The President of the National Academy of Sciences has warned, "The greatest threat to the human race is man's procreation. Hunger, pollution, crime, and overlarge, dirty cities—even the seething unrest that leads to international conflict and war—all derive from the unbridled growth of human populations."[15] However, overpopulation and its attendant crowding and overburdening of resources can also be seen at the level with which this text is concerned—the individual family.

The rate of planned pregnancies is growing, as is the number of women or couples who are using contraceptives. Forty-five states, as well as the District of Columbia, have enacted legislation allowing teenage girls under the age of 18 to obtain contraceptives without parental consent.

According to Manisoff, a well-known leader in family planning, the disparity between the poor and more advantaged groups in their use of effective contraception is related to accessibility of services. "Wherever free or low-cost family planning services have been offered at convenient locations under considerations of respect, dignity, and free choice, unusually high patient acceptance has been found."[16] She estimates that although family planning services are expanding, there are still about two million poor or near-poor who do not have medically supervised family planning services available to them. As indicated above, sexually active teenagers constitute the group of women for whom family planning services are most needed.[17] In addition to medical clinics and permissive legislation for teenagers to receive care, more effective and understanding sex and family planning health education

programs need to be devised and implemented in schools, churches, and health agencies.

Such services should be focused not on the general premise that family planning is an end in itself, but on the health benefits of family planning to the individual and to the growth and development of the family. Counseling for family health must also include health needs of existing children and potential ill effects on them of family "overpopulation."

Forcing birth control on families, however, is not ethical, since doing so destroys the sense of initiative, integrity, and competence. Teenage girls who want babies need to be counseled on physical and emotional readiness for parenthood and realistic protection from pregnancy along with good health supervision. Little has been done to balance the societal pressures toward sex and marriage with realistic contraception education.[18]

STAGE II: EARLY CHILDBEARING

Stage II begins with the birth of the first child and continues through the infant's 30th month. Usually the parents are thrilled about their first-born, but also quite apprehensive. This apprehensiveness about the baby usually decreases by about the third day—the day the mother often goes home—as the mother and baby begin to get to know each other. This unadulterated elation ends, however, when the mother arrives home with baby. She and father are suddenly confronted with the all-engrossing roles that have been thrust upon them. It is especially difficult in the beginning because of the feelings of inadequacy of new parents, the lack of help from family and friends or the conflicting advice of helpful friends and family and health professionals, and the frequent waking up of the baby at night—which usually continues for about 3 to 4 weeks. Also, the mother is fatigued psychologically and physiologically and often feels she has returned to the burdens of all the other household duties in addition to caring for the baby. It is especially difficult if the new mother has been ill or has had a long, difficult labor and delivery or a cesarean section.

The arrival of a new baby into the home creates changes for every member of the family and for every set of relationships. A stranger has been admitted into a close-knit group, and suddenly the balance of the family shifts—each member takes on new roles and begins new relationships. In addition to a baby being born, a mother, father, and grandparents are born. The wife must now relate to the husband as both a spouse and a father and vice versa. And in families with previous children, the impact of the new baby is as significant on the siblings as on the married couple. Telling a child to adjust to a new brother or sister may be equivalent to a husband telling his wife that he is bringing home a mistress whom she is to love and accept as an equal![19] It is truly a time of developmental crisis for all involved.

Although parenthood may represent an extremely important goal for a couple, most find it a very difficult life change. The adjustment to marriage is not nearly as hard as the adjustment to parenthood. Although a very meaningful and gratifying experience to most parents, the advent of the baby calls for a sudden change to an incessantly demanding role. Two important factors complicating the difficulty of assuming the parental role are that most persons today are not prepared to be parents and that many deleterious, unrealistic myths romanticizing rearing of children are current in our society.[20] Parenthood is the only major role for which little preparation is given, and the main family toll which the lack of preparation and romanticizing of parenthood takes is the diminution in the quality of the marital and the parent–infant relationships.

The Crisis of Parenthood

Thus, the coming of the first-born is a crisis and a critical family experience, as studies of families during this stage of the life cycle consistently illustrate.[21-24]

To discover how the introduction of new children affected families, LeMasters studied family adjustment to the birth of the first child by interviewing 46 urban middle-class parents (ages 25 to 35) and determining crisis severity. He found that 17 percent of couples experienced no or only moderate problems, but that the remaining 83 percent experienced extensive and/or severe problems.

The common problems found were as follows:

1. Husbands felt neglected (mentioned most frequently by husbands).
2. There was an increased number of mate quarrels and arguments.
3. Interruptions in schedules (e.g., "so tired all the time") were continual.
4. Social and sexual life were disrupted and diminished.[25]

In summarizing this and subsequent studies, it was found that families interviewed had an idealized, erroneous notion of parenting prior to the birth of the first child and that marital satisfaction dropped sharply with the coming of the first baby.

Clark conducted a study of families after the birth of a new baby which underscored both the difficulty in adjusting to parenting and the critical need for continuity of nursing services after delivery into the home and via clinic services.[26] Professional nursing given at home and in primary care settings is eminently suited to provide the emotional support and guidance needed by new mothers and families during this critical period. Thus, continuation of professional nursing care at home is indicated.

Developmental Tasks of the Childbearing Family

After the coming of the first-born, the family has several important developmental tasks. These are primarily related to setting up the young family as a stable unit, reconciling conflicting developmental tasks of the various members, and jointly facilitating the developmental needs of mother, father, and baby in ways that strengthen each other and the family as a whole. Husband, wife, and baby must all learn new roles, while the family unit expands in functions and responsibilities. This involves the simultaneous meshing of the developmental tasks of each family member and the family as a whole.[27]

The birth of a child makes radical changes in family organization. The functions of the couple must differentiate to meet the new demands of the infant for care and nurturance. These 24-hour responsibilities of feeding, bathing, nurturing, laundering, house cleaning, shopping, and cooking must be accomplished. And while the fulfilling of these responsibilities varies tremendously with the sociocultural position of the couple, a common pattern is for the parents to assume more traditional roles or division of responsibilities.

The most important role to assess when working with the childbearing family is the parental role—including both parents, not just the mother, as was once the case. To fulfill this role, a good parent–infant relationship is vital. Much has been written in the past describing the dire effects of maternal deprivation on infants and children.[28, 29] More recent studies of Klaus,[30] Kendall,[31] Rubin,[32] and others further verify the impact of early attachment and a beginning warm, positive parent–child relationship on the future parental relationship with the child. Areas needing assessment include the parents' attitude about themselves, their attitudes about the baby, and the characteristics of parental communication and stimulation of the infant.[33]

Role changes and adaptation to new parental responsibilities often are more rapidly learned by the mother. The child is a reality to the expectant mother much earlier than for the husband, who usually begins to feel like a father at the birth, but sometimes even later than that.[34] The way in which most fathers have traditionally been left out of the perinatal process has certainly delayed men from taking on this important role change and hindered their emotional involvement. Thus the husband often remains initially uncommitted while the woman is rapidly adjusting to a new family structure.

The mother and father grow and develop their parental roles in response to the continually changing demands and developmental tasks of the growing youngster, the family as a whole, and themselves. According to Friedman, parents go through five successive stages of development.[35] The first two stages fall into this phase of family life. First, during the child's infancy, parents learn cues their baby expresses in making his or her needs known. With each successive child, parents will go through this same stage as they adjust to each infant's unique cues.

The second stage of parental development, learning to accept child's growth and development, occurs in the toddler years. Just prior to and during this stage, parents, particularly parents with their first child, need guidance and support. They need to understand tasks the child is attempting to master and his or her needs during this time for safety, limits, and toilet training. They need to understand the concept of developmental readiness, or "the teachable moment." At the same time, parents need guidance in understanding the tasks they themselves are mastering during this stage.

New communication patterns evolve with the coming of a child, with mates relating to each other both as mates and parents. Spouse transactional patterns have been found to change drastically. Feldman observed that parents of infants talked less with each other and had less fun, less stimulating conversation, and a diminished quality of marital interaction. Some parents can become overwhelmed with the added responsibilities.[36]

The reestablishment of creative communication patterns—including personal, marital, and parental feelings and concerns—is critical. Mates must continue to meet each other's personal adult psychological and sexual needs as well as sharing and interacting with each other about parental responsibilities.

The sexual relationship of the mates generally declines during pregnancy and through the six-week postpartum period. Sexual difficulties during the later period are also common, arising from such factors as the mother's absorption in her new role, fatigue, and feelings of loss of sexual attractiveness, as well as the husband's feeling of being "left or pushed out" by the new baby.

Family communications now include a third member, making for a triad. Parents must learn to perceive and discern the communication cries of the infant. For instance, the baby's cries need to be differentiated into expressions of discomfort, hunger, overstimulation, sickness, or fatigue. And the baby begins responding to cuddles, fondling, and talking, which then is received and reinforced by the parents.

Family planning counseling usually occurs at the six-week postpartum examination. Parents should then be encouraged to openly discuss family spacing and planning and to realize that frequent, closely spaced pregnancies can be harmful to the mother, as well as to siblings and the family unit.

This life cycle stage requires an adjustment of relationships within the extended family and with friends, as when other family members try to support, guide, and assist with the new functions. Although grandparents, for instance, can be of great help to the new family, the potential for conflict exists because of differences in values and expectations existing between the generations.

Despite then the importance of having a social network or social support system in achieving satisfaction with and positive feelings about family life, the young family needs to know when they need help and from whom to accept it and when to depend on their own inner resources and strengths.[37]

Thus a strong, viable marital relationship is essential to the stability and morale of the family. A satisfying husband–wife relationship will give the mates the strength and energy to "give" to the infant and to each other. Conflicting pressures and demands such as between the mother's loyalty to infant and to husband are problematic and can be agonizing. This type of conflict can become the central source of unhappiness during this life cycle stage.

Health Concerns

A major portion of a community health nurse's practice is devoted to families in the expansion stage. The main concerns of these families are family-centered maternity education, well-baby care, early recognition and appropriate handling of physical health problems, immunizations, child development counseling, family planning, and family interaction.

Other health concerns during this period of a family's life are inaccessibility and inadequacy of child-care facilities for working mothers, parent–child relationships, or parenting problems.

STAGE III: FAMILIES WITH PRESCHOOL CHILDREN

The third stage of the family life cycle commences when the first-born child is about 2½ and terminates when he or she is 5 years of age. The family can now possibly consist of three to five persons, with the paired positions of husband-father, wife-mother, son-brother, and daughter-sister. The family is becoming more complex and differentiated.[38]

Family life during this stage is busy and demanding for parents. The mother may be working part or full time, and so both parents will have greater demands on their time. Nevertheless, realizing that parents are the "architects of the family," designing and directing family development,[39] it is critical for them to strengthen their partnership—in short, to keep the marriage alive and well.

Preschool children have much to learn at this stage, especially in the area of independence. They must achieve sufficient autonomy and self-sufficiency to be able to handle themselves without their parents in a variety of places. Experience in nursery school, kindergarten, Project Head Start, a day-care center, or similar programs is a good way to foster this kind of development. This is especially important to remember when assisting parents with preschool children from inner-city, low-income families, where a considerable rise in both IQ and social skills has been reported to occur after children have completed a two-year nursery school experience.[40]

There exist a large number of single-parent families within this particular life cycle stage. By 1974 the number of preschoolers without fathers in the home had risen to 13.2 percent; in black families this figure was 35.2 percent.[41] The role strain on the single parent is very great, and low-cost, quality day-care centers for working parents are difficult, if not impossible, to locate.

Family Developmental Tasks

Because the family is now growing in both numbers and complexity, the need of preschoolers and other young children to explore the world around them, and parental needs for their own privacy, housing, and adequate space often become major problems for the family. Equipment and facilities also need to be child-proofed, for it is at this stage that accidents become the most common causes of both mortality and disability. Assessing the home for safety hazards is of prime importance for the community health nurse, and health education must then be included so that the parents and children are cognizant of the risks involved and of ways of preventing accidents.

Due to both lack of specific resistance to the many bacterial and viral diseases and increased exposure, preschoolers are frequently sick with one minor infectious illness after another. Frequent visits to the doctor, caring for sick kids, and running home from work to pick up an ill child from the nursery school are common weekly crises. Additionally, these infections usually spread through the family. Thus children's contacts with infectious and communicable diseases and their general susceptibility to disease are prime health concerns. Accidents, falls, burns, and lacerations are also quite common occurrences. These are even more frequently seen where there are large families, families where an adult caretaker is not present, and in low-income families. Environmental safety and adequate child supervision are the keys to reducing accidents.

The husband-father assumes more involvement in the household responsibilities during this stage of family development than during any other, the largest percentage of this being spent in child-care activities. The father's role at this time is especially important in achieving the proper sexual identification of the children. It is particularly critical for boys in the first five years of life to associate closely with a strong, limit-setting, warm father or father substitute so that their masculine role identity can be established.[42]

A more mature role is also assumed by preschooler, who gradually takes on more responsibility for his or her own care, plus helping mother or father with household jobs. It is not the productivity of the child which is important here, but the learning which occurs.

Contrary to expectations, research has shown that the advent of the second child into the family has an even more deleterious effect on the marital relationship than does the first birth. Feldman reports that parental roles make the marital roles difficult, as exhibited by the following observations: couples perceive negative personality changes in each other; they are less satisfied with the home; there is more task-oriented interactions; fewer personal conversations and more child-centered conversations take place; more warmth is exhibited toward the children and less toward each other; and there is a lower level of sexual satisfaction.[43]

This well-recognized study parallels reports and observations of family counselors—that the marital relationship is often troubled at this phase of the cycle. In fact, many divorces occur within these years due to weak or unsatisfactory marital ties. Privacy and time together are prime necessities. Marriage counseling and marriage encounter groups have become important resources among the middle class. For the family without economic resources, however, limited assistance is available for strengthening a salvageable marriage; the marriage or family most often has to be in a state of real crisis and dysfunction before members of this group are considered eligible for counseling services.

A major task of the family is socializing the children. Preschoolers are developing critical self-attitudes (self-concepts) and rapidly learning to express themselves, as seen in their rapid grasp of language.

Another issue during this period deals with how to integrate a new family member (second or third child) while still meeting the needs of older child(ren). The displacement of a child by a newborn is psychologically a very traumatic event. Preparation of children for the arrival of a new baby helps ameliorate the situation, especially if the parents are sensitive to the older child's feelings and behavior. For example, sibling rivalry is often expressed by hitting or negatively relating to new baby, regressive behaviors, and attention-getting activity. The best way to handle sibling rivalry is for the parents to spend a certain amount of time each day exclusively relating to the older child to give him or her the assurance that he or she is still loved and wanted.

About the time their children become preschoolers, parents enter their third parenting stage, one of learning to separate from the children as they toddle off to nursery school, a day-care center, or to kindergarten. This stage continues during the preschool and early school years. Separation is often difficult for parents and children, and parents need support and an explanation of how the preschoolers' mastery of developmental tasks contributes to their increasing autonomy. Setting limits should be discussed, for as children learn to handle their own bodies more effectively and potentially dangerous situations increase, the needs for limits will be altered. Children must be given limits for their protection, but within these limits they should find the freedom to explore and satisfy their insatiable curiosity. Separation may also occur as parents go to work or due to trips, vacations, or hospitalizations. Family preparation for separation is important in helping the children adjust to change.

Assisting parents to obtain family planning services after the arrival of a new baby or to continue with contraception if there has been no intervening pregnancy is also indicated. It is, for instance, not unusual for a woman to have stopped using contraceptives because of a missed period with the belief that she was pregnant, only to find out later that her eventual pregnancy resulted from sexual intercourse without contraceptive protection.

Both parents need to have some outside interests and contacts to rejuvenate themselves to carry on the multitude of home tasks and responsibilities. The lower-class parent often does not have the opportunity to do this, and these families have the least satisfactory associations with the wider community in the health, recreational, educational, vocational, and social areas due to their alienated position and the paucity of resources available to them.

Health Concerns

Numerous health concerns have been identified throughout our discussion of the preschool family. As indicated earlier, the major physical health problems concern the frequent communicable diseases of the children and the common falls, burns, poisonings, and other accidents which occur during the preschool age. The prime psychosocial family health concern is the marital relationship. Studies verify the diminished satisfaction many couples experience during these years and the need for working to strengthen and reinvigorate this vital unit. Other important health concerns involve sibling rivalry, family planning, growth and developmental needs, parenting problems, environmental safety, and communication. Of course, general health promotion strategies continue to be germane during this stage.

STAGE IV: FAMILIES WITH SCHOOL-AGE CHILDREN

This stage commences when the firstborn is 6 years old and begins elementary school and ends at 13, the beginning of adolescence. Families usually reach their maximum number of members, and so of relationships, at the end of this stage.[44] Again these are busy years. Now children have their own activities and interests, in addition to the mandatory activities of living and the parents' own activities. Each person is working on his or her own developmental tasks, just as the family attempts to fulfill its tasks. According to Erikson, parents are struggling with twin demands of finding fulfillment in rearing the next generation (generativity) and being self-absorbed in their own growth, while school-age children are working at developing a sense of industry—the capacity for work enjoyment—and trying to eliminate or ward off a sense of inferiority.[45]

The parental task at this time is that of learning to deal with the child's separation or, more simply, letting the child go. More and more, peer relationships and outside activities play larger roles in the life of the school-age child. These years are filled with family activities, but there are also forces gradually pushing the child to separate from the family in preparation for adolescence. Parents who have other interests outside of their children will find it much easier to make the gradual separation. In instances where the mothering role is the central and only significant role in a woman's life, however, this separation process may be a very painful one and strongly resisted.

Parents feel intense pressure from the outside community via the school system and other extrafamilial associations to have their children conform to the community's standards for children of school age. This tends to influence the middle-class family to stress more traditional values of achievement and productivity, and to cause some working-class families and many poor families to feel alienated from and at conflict with school and/or community values.

Children's handicaps may come to light during this period of a child's life. School nurses and teachers will detect many visual and hearing defects, in addition to learning and behavior problems. Working with the family in the role of health educator and counselor, in addition to initiating an appropriate referral for follow-up screening, assumes much of a school nurse's energies. She or he also acts as a resource person to the school teacher, enabling the teacher to handle the common and more individualized health needs of her or his pupils more effectively.

There are a number of other handicapping conditions occasionally detected during the school years, including epilepsy, cerebral palsy, mental retardation, speech problems, and orthopedic conditions. The family health nurse's primary function here—in addition to referral, teaching, and counseling parents regarding these conditions—would be to assist the family in coping so that any adverse impact of the handicap on the family will be minimized.

Family Developmental Tasks

One of the critical tasks of parents in socializing their children at this time involves promoting school achievement. Another significant family task is maintaining a satisfying marital relationship. Again it has been reported that marital satisfaction is diminished during this stage. Two large studies reinforced these observations.[46, 47] Promoting open communication and supporting the spouse relationship is vital in working with the school-age family.

STAGE V: THE FAMILY WITH TEENAGERS

When the first-born turns 13 years of age, the fifth stage of the family's life cycle commences. It usually lasts about 6 or 7 years, although it can be shorter if the child leaves the family early or longer if the child remains home later than 19 or 20 years of age. Other children in the home are usually of school age. "The overall family goal at the teenage stage is that of loosening family ties to allow greater responsibility and freedom, preparatory to releasing young adults in-the-making."[48]

This stage of the family's life is probably the most difficult, or certainly the most discussed and written about. The American family is affected by the tremendous developmental tasks of both the adolescent and parents and the inevitable conflicts and turmoil these create. The developmental tasks of adolescence demand a movement from dependence on and control by the parents and other adults, through a period of in-

tense peer group activity and influence, to the assumption of adult roles.[49]

The major challenges in working with a family with teenagers revolve around the developmental conflicts and crises. Adams delineates three aspects of the adolescent process upon which much attention has been focused, namely, emancipation, youth culture, and the generation gap.[50]

Emancipation

As Douvan and Adelson explain, "The period begins with the child almost entirely dependent on the family . . . still tied to his parents emotionally, still clinging to their ideas and ideals."[51] At the end of the period the teenager is usually transformed into a person freer to make decisions, committed to his or her own beliefs and values, and looking outside of the family for love and support. Thus there are three types of independence and autonomy achieved by adolescence at the end of this developmental period: emotional autonomy, behavioral autonomy, and value autonomy. Individuals vary greatly in both the speed at which they move through this process and the extent to which they become emancipated. Emancipation can be developed within the bounds of the parental values or outside the bounds of the parental value system, involving the rejection of parental beliefs and expectations.[52]

Youth Culture

During the preteen years, children become aware of the differences between themselves and their parents. Moreover, they are not only aware of the differences, but now have defined their own set of standards distinct from the parents. Many studies have documented the extent to which key socializing agents shift from home to peers.[53, 54] During the teen years, the school and peer group are the powerful and pervading forces in the socialization of the adolescent. Furthermore, youth culture or the peer group assists its members to achieve adult status.

The Generation Gap

In spite of the basic similarity in values between youth and their parents, many authors have noted the inevitable conflicts which arise between parents and adolescents. Davis, in a classic article, describes parent–youth conflicts as being an outcome of societal conditions. If society were a stable rural society, with autonomy from parental control marked by gradual and institutionalized steps and with little delay of marriage and adulthood following puberty, parent–youth conflicts would be small. But in present-day American urban culture, with its weak or unclear parental role models, strong socialization forces outside the family, rapid societal changes, postponed adulthood, and a choice of adult roles, conflict is inevitable and extensive.[55] Society and its values change so dramatically from one generation to the next that parents and children do not have the ability to empathize with each other.*

Other authors see the generation gap as the direct outcome of a power struggle revolving around the question of how much control adults can rightfully exercise over adolescents.[56] The implied ideal relationship between parents and their teenage children is one of consensus and harmony. Adolescents, however, often feel no need to hide or disguise their rebellious thoughts and actions out of deference to parents. As they defy parents, this contributes directly to growing frustration and feelings of inadequacy in the parents. This rebellion is often seen as a threat to an established order essential to the well-being of adults. However, it must be remembered and emphasized in counseling parents that it is through the process of rebelling that the adolescent asserts his or her own self-identity. While negatively viewed by parents, rebellion, within limits, is actually "functional" and beneficial for the adolescent.

Parental Roles, Responsibilities, and Problems

Needless to say, parents find it a most difficult task to raise teenagers today. Nonetheless, parents need to stand firm against unreasonable testing of the limits that have been set in the family as they go through the process of gradually "letting go." Duvall also identifies the critical developmental task of this period to be the balancing of freedom with responsibility as teenagers mature and emancipate themselves.[57] Friedman similarly defines the parental task of this stage as learning to accept rejection without deserting the child.[58]

When the parents accept themselves as they are, with all their weaknesses and strengths, and when they accept their several roles at this stage of development without undue conflict or sensitivity, they set the pattern for a similar sort of self-acceptance in their children.[59]

Schultz and others have expressed the view that the increasing complexity of American life has made the role of parents unclear. Parents may feel in competition with a variety of social forces and institutions—from school authorities and counselors to birth control

and premarital sex options. Other factors add to their considerably diminished influence. Because of specialization of occupations and professions, parents are no longer able to help children with their vocational plans. The residential mobility and lack of continuing trustworthy adult relationships for both adolescents and parents, in addition to the inability of many parents to discuss sexual concerns openly and nonjudgmentally with their children, has also contributed to parent–youth problems.[60]

Family Developmental Tasks

As with the last three stages, the marital relationship is a focus of concern. Many couples have become so preoccupied with their parental responsibilities that their marriage no longer plays a central role in their lives. The husband usually spends much time away from home working and furthering his career, while the wife feels bogged down and engrossed in her domestic responsibilities. Many wives now also work, which leaves little time or energy for the marital relationship.

The positive side of this stage is that since the children are more responsible for themselves, the couple can more easily leave home to engage in their careers or establish postparental interests. Thus they can begin to build a foundation for the future stages of the family life cycle.

The most pressing family need now is open communication between parents and children. Because of the generation gap, open communication is often an ideal, rather than a reality. There is often mutual rejection by parents and adolescents of each other's values and life styles. Parents in multiproblem families have been found to frequently reject and then to disengage from their older children.

Family ethical and moral standards need to be maintained by parents. While the young are searching for their own beliefs and values, it is of paramount importance for parents to defend and adhere firmly to their own sound principles and standards. Adolescents are very sensitive to incongruities between what is "preached and practiced." Conformity to family values and standards is now questioned by the teenager, so that understanding and sound reasons must be given for parental decisions. Parents and children can learn from each other in the fast-changing and pluralistic society of today. Value transformations of youth are also transforming families. The adoption of a freer and more casual life style symbolizes a value transformation affecting every phase of life.[61]

Health Concerns

At this stage the physical health of the family members is usually good, but health promotion remains an im-

---

* Volumes of literature have been written about rapidity of cultural-social change. Alvin Toffler's *Future Shock* (Random House, New York, 1970) is a culmination of thinking in this area. Toffler indicates that the rapid rate of social change threatens personalities and social relationships and that the concomitant stress may result in the breakdown of one's biological system.

portant concern. Risk factors should be identified and discussed with families, as well as a healthy life style. From age 35 on, the risk of coronary heart disease rises appreciably in males, and at this point both adult members are beginning to feel more vulnerable to ill health as part of their developmental changes and are usually more receptive to health promotion strategies. With teenagers, accidents, particularly automobile accidents, are a great hazard, and broken bones and athletic injuries are also common.

Drug and sex education and counseling are relevant areas of concern. In discussing these topics with families, the nurse may get caught squarely in the middle of a parent–youth dispute or problem. Such questions arise as whether a health worker should report drug usage, venereal disease, or sexual relations of minor children to parents, or how parents and teenagers can be helped to communicate more effectively. For more productive discussions, separate interviews with the teenagers and parents prior to bringing them together are often indicated.

The other area of health need is again in the area of support and assistance in strengthening the marital relationship. Direct supportive counseling or referral to community resources for recreational, educational, counseling, and other services may be needed.

STAGE VI: LAUNCHING CENTER FAMILIES

The beginning of this phase of family life is characterized by the first child leaving the parental home and ends with "the empty nest," when the last child has left home. The stage could be quite short or fairly long, depending on how many children are in the family or if any unmarried children remain at home after termination of high school or college. The usual length of this stage is six or seven years.

This phase is marked by the culmination of years of preparation of and by the children for an independent adult life. Parents, as they let their children go, are relinquishing 20 years or so of the parenting role and returning to their original marital dyad. Family developmental tasks are critical while the family is shifting from a household with children to a husband–wife pair. The major family goal is the reorganization of the family into a continuing unity while releasing matured young people into lives of their own.[62] During this stage the marital pair take on grandparent roles—another change in both roles and their self-image.

Early middle age, which is about the average age of parents during the launching of their oldest child, has been characterized as a "caught" period of life: caught between the demands of youth and the expectations of the elderly and caught between the world of work and the competing demands and involvement of the family, with the often seeming impossiblity of meeting the demands of both realms. Studies indicate, however, that while the middle-aged may feel squeezed between the poles of youth and aging, at least for middle- and upper-class individuals, they can often appreciate their own importance and achievements: "They often know that they are the nation's decision-makers; they set the tone for life in this society. Society depends on middle-aged people's leadership and productivity."[63]

Family Developmental Tasks

As the family assists the oldest in his or her launching, the parents are also involved with their younger children, helping them to become independent. And when the "released" son or daughter marries, the family task involves expanding the family circle to include new members by marriage and becoming accepting of the couple's own life style and values.

With the emptying of the nest, parents have more time to devote to other activities and relationships. Hopefully, they have not grown so far apart from each other that they cannot reinstitute or reestablish the wife and husband roles to the place of primary importance these roles once held. LeShan also views this stage as a challenge to the marital relationship: "When the children leave, marriage faces a moment of truth; is there strength enough to sustain it without the excuse of parenthood?"[64]

This period is usually much more difficult for the woman than for the man. In most families the central and enduring role—enduring in the sense that the role has existed 20 some years—for the woman has been the role of mother. Although less prevalent today, the woman's identity and feelings of competency have been based on being a good mother, and despite the years of gradual separation of children preceding this stage, the launching often comes psychologically quite suddenly. With the children gone or going, the mother now finds herself with a clean house (not much work here anymore) and no place to go or purpose for her existence. Typically, middle-class husbands are at the peak of their careers and are spending long hours away from home, putting in a concentrated period of years to attempt to succeed occupationally, financially, or professionally, to fulfill their aspirations before it is too late. Many women have been so absorbed in their children that they have not prepared for this phase of their life and do not have other equally fulfilling commitments in which to invest their energies and talents. The middle-age crisis is more severe for women not only because of the children leaving home and the unavailability of their husbands, but also due to feelings of loss of femininity with the beginning of menopause (usually between 45 and 55) and loss of beauty when discernible signs of aging appear. If a woman has commitments outside of home (work, an avocation, etc.), she usually has fewer problems than if she has remained home in the traditional role of housewife and full-time mother.

Men in middlescence also face potential developmental crisis: the drive to get "ahead" in their careers with the realization that they have not succeeded or have not reached their aspirations; signs of diminished masculinity such as lower energy levels and lessened potency and sexual excitation; figure, hair, and skin aging signs; and financial worries. The frequency of extramarital affairs, divorces, mental illness, alcoholism, and suicide all rise among adults of these age groups, underscoring the middle-age developmental crises which occur.

Friedman reiterates the significance of the marital relationship by characterizing the parental developmental stage at this point in the family life cycle as the building of a new life together.[65]

Another important developmental task of the middle-years family is that of assisting aging and ill parents of the husband and wife. Even though the actual care of aging and/or dependent parents is not an expected function of the American family with the exception of certain ethnic groups, the husband and wife are expected to assist and support elderly family members as much as they feel is feasible. Such activity takes all forms: from frequent telephoning and supportive calls to assisting financially, providing transportation, and visiting and caring for their parent(s) in the home. In America the family is seen as primarily responsible for the succeeding generation, the offspring, and only secondarily for the previous generation, the parents.[66]

Three-generation families, although not the usual pattern, are not uncommon, particularly in "traditional" Asian, Hispanic, Greek, Italian, and Jewish families. Most often in the United States the multigenerational family seems to develop primarily when the nuclear family is disrupted by death or divorce, but financial expediency or child-care needs may also encourage such living arrangements. In fact, older parents typically desire to live independently so as not to impinge on their children's lives and, more importantly, to retain their own feelings of competence, independence, and privacy.[67] Parents may also have to wrestle with the decision to place their parents in a nursing home or retirement or board-and-care facility during these years.

In summary it can be seen that as children disperse, parents must again learn independence. In readjusting, the marriage must be viable if parents' needs are to continue to be fulfilled. Parents have to readjust their relationship—to relate to each other as marital partners rather than primarily as parents. For this stage to be complete, children must be independent while maintaining ties and bonds with parents.

Health Concerns

The primary health concerns involve communication problems between young adults and their parents; role-transitional problems for wife and husband; caretaker concerns (for aging parents); and the emergence of chronic health conditions or predisposing factors such as high cholesterol levels, obesity, or high blood pressure. Family planning remains important. Menopausal problems among women are common. The effects associated with prolonged drinking, smoking, and dietary practices become more obvious. Finally, the need for health promotion strategies and a "wellness life style" become more pressing for the adult members of the launching center family.

STAGE VII: FAMILIES OF MIDDLE YEARS

The seventh stage of the family life cycle—the stage of the middle years—begins when the last child departs from the home and ends with retirement or death of one of the spouses. This stage usually starts when parents are about 45 to 55 years of age and ends with the retirement of a spouse, usually 16 to 18 years later. Typically, the marital couple in their middle years constitutes a nuclear family, although still interacting with their aging parent(s) or other members of their own family of origin, as well as with the new families of marriage of their own children and their offspring. The postparental couple is not usually isolated today; more middle-age couples are living out their full life span and spending a greater portion of it in a postparental phase, with extended kin relationships between four generations not being unusual.[68]

To many such families, these years are seen as the prime of life. Other couples disagree, stating that because of problems of aging, the loss of children, and a sense of themselves as failures in parenting and work efforts, these years are generally difficult and onerous ones. Deutscher conducted extensive interviews with 45 postparental spouses to determine the extent of satisfaction in this period of life.[69] Only three of the couples felt the period to be clearly negative; 22 of the spouses felt the period was better than previous life cycle stages; and an additional 22 evaluated this period as equal to preceding phases or were not certain of their feelings. The positive comments relative to the middle years revolved around the freedoms this time period permitted—freedom from heavy financial responsibilities, freedom of mobility, freedom to think of self first. Even more important seemed to be the new, enhanced marital relationships and self-concepts resulting from having the other freedoms.[70]

Family Developmental Tasks

By the time the last child leaves home, many women have rechanneled their energies and lives in preparation for the empty nest. For some women, a middle-age crisis (discussed in the stage VI family) is experienced during the early period of this life cycle. Now the woman works at encouraging her grown children to be independent by redefining her relationship with them (not intruding on their personal and family life). She needs to maintain a sense of well-being physiologically and psychologically by living a healthful life—weight control, balanced diet, regular exercise program, and adequate rest—and to attain and enjoy a career or other creative accomplishments. Occupationally, men may find the same frustrations and disappointments present as discussed in the launching center family. On the one hand, they may be at the peak of their career and not have to work as hard as previously or, on the other hand, may find their job monotonous after 20 to 30 years at the same type of work. Many middle-class workers suffer from the "plateau phenomenon"—where salaries and promotions are no longer available—leaving them to feel in a rut. Career discontent is supposed to reach alarming proportions under these conditions, with many persons making mid-life job changes due to the feelings of discontentment, boredom, and stagnation. Because work has traditionally been man's central role in life, this common experience greatly influences his stress level and general health status.

The cultivation of leisure-time activities and interests are significant, since more time is now available and preparation for retirement must take place in a more planned fashion.

An important developmental task for this stage is the provision of a healthy environment. It is in this period that taking on a healthier life style becomes more prevalent for couples, despite that the individuals concerned have probably been engaging in many self-destructive habits for 45 to 65 years and that the toll of these indiscretions have begun to be visible. Although not inadvisable to start now, since "better now than never" is always true, it is largely too late to reverse many of the physiological changes which have already taken place, changes such as arthritic changes due to inactivity; high blood pressure due to lack of exercise, prolonged stress, or poor dietary habits; and vital capacity diminution due to smoking. What usually motivates middle-age persons to improve their life style? The primary motivation, unfortunately, appears to be a feeling of susceptibility or vulnerability to illness and

disease generated when a friend or family member of the same age group has a heart attack, stroke, or cancer. In addition to fear, a belief that regular checkups and healthful living habits are effective ways of reducing susceptibility to various diseases are also powerful motivating forces. Heart disease, cancer, and stroke account for two-thirds of all causes of mortality between the ages of 45 and 64 years of age, with accidents the fourth cause of death.[71]

A second developmental task relates to sustaining satisfying and meaningful relationships with aging parents and children. By accepting and welcoming grandchildren into the family and promoting satisfying intergenerational relationships, this developmental task can be highly rewarding.[72] It allows the middle-age couple to continue feeling like a family and brings the joys of grandparenthood without the 24-hour responsibilities. The more problematic role is that of relating to and assisting the aging parents and sometimes other extended family members.

The third developmental task to be discussed here is that of strengthening the marital relationship. Now the couple is really alone after many years of being surrounded with other family members and relationships. Although appearing as a welcome relief, for many mates it is a difficult experience, and their relationship needs much strengthening to be able to meet the test of time and satisfaction.

Recent studies have shown that postparental couples, after recultivating their relationship, have often found greater marital satisfaction and higher marital adjustment than during previous stages.[73] Mutually enjoying leisure activities and companionship was most frequently mentioned as the prime factor leading to marital happiness. Sexual satisfaction was also positively correlated with both good communication and marital satisfaction,[74] even though middle-age husbands may experience a decline in sexual adequacy in the middle years. Intimate husband–wife communication is essential for maintaining understanding and interest in each other throughout these years.

For couples who experience problems, the reduced pressure of life in postparental years may lead not to marital bliss, but to marital "blahs." According to Kerckhoff, marriage counselors have long observed that when trouble arises in the marriage during the middle years, it is often related to boredom of the union, not to its traumatic qualities. A common characteristic of this period relative to marriage is "smug complacency" and "comfortable rot."[75]

Health Concerns

The health concerns mentioned throughout the description of the life cycle stage include the following:

1. Health promotion needs: adequate rest, leisure activities, and sleep; good nutrition; regular exercise program; reduction of weight down to optimum weight; cessation of smoking; reduction or cessation in use of alcohol; and preventive-health screening examinations.
2. Marital relationship concerns.
3. Communication with and relating to children, in-laws, grandchildren, and aging parents.
4. Caretaker concerns: assisting in care of aging or disabled parents.

STAGE VIII: FAMILY IN RETIREMENT AND OLD AGE

The last stage of the life cycle of the family begins with the retirement of one or both spouses, continues through the loss of one spouse, and ends with the death of the other spouse.[76] The number of aging individuals—persons 65 and older—in our country increases slowly each year, and they now account for about 10 percent of the total population. As a result of improved longevity over the last two decades, declining birth rates, and expectations that birth rates will continue to drop, the aged will likely constitute an even larger proportion of the population in the future.

Perceptions of this stage of the life cycle differ significantly among aging families. Some persons are miserable, while others feel it is the best years of their lives. Much is dependent on the adequacy of financial resources, the ability to maintain a satisfactory home, and the individual's health status. Those who have lost their independence due to ill health generally have low morale; and poor physical health is often an antecedent to mental illness among the elderly.[77]

In spite of this stage's potential advantages, many aging families find this stage of the life cycle to be extremely difficult. Society's devaluation of the aged, a lack of socialization and preparation for aging, and the many losses common to aging make this period of life problematic.

Society's Devaluation of the Aged

Our society emphasizes the achievements of those in the young adult years, glorifying the period of youth. Therefore, adults, through grooming, dress, and styles, try to maintain their youthful appearance as long as possible. Aging has always meant losing hair, friends, aspirations, and strength. For both the community at large and individual families, dealing with the aged has had a negative connotation, one loaded with feelings of being burdened down with imposing problems. Additionally, society has not allowed the aged to remain productive. Hence, society's negative appraisal of older persons has negatively affected their self-image. Of course today many associations and organizations and much literature advocate and illustrate the strengths, resources, and other positive aspects of aging, which has begun to diminish the negativism and stereotypic thinking about the aged and to help us recognize the assets of the older person and the great diversity of life styles among members of this age group.

Lack of Socialization and Preparation for Aging

With the loss of both the parental and the occupational roles, a substantial reorientation on the part of individuals and couples becomes necessary. What such changes entail, however, is not entirely clear, since the roles and norms for the older person are ambiguous. Women who have been completely engrossed in their mothering role and husbands who have been completely engrossed in their work role predictably have the greatest degree of difficulty adjusting. All in all, not enough is understood about the actual movement into old age.

Losses Common to Aging Persons/Families

As aging progresses and retirement becomes a reality, there are a variety of stressors or losses experienced by the majority of older persons and couples which confound the role transition. These include the following:

Economic—Adjusting to a substantially reduced income; later perhaps adjusting to economic dependency (depending on family or government for subsidy).

Housing—Often moving to smaller quarters and later perhaps forced to move to an institutional setting.

Social—Loss (death) of siblings, friends, and spouse.

Work—Mandatory retirement and loss of the work role.

Retirement

Retirement poses a problem of resocialization to new roles and a new life style. To fill the vacuum, many men increasingly engage in domestic activities and assume a more expressive role, a change demanding a role shift on the part of the wife as well. The retired husband's adjustment to the sharing of household tasks depends on his value system. If he sees this type of activity as "woman's work" and considers it demeaning to him, he will feel devalued in such activity. Troll found this more true of the working-class man, who values the traditional breadwinner role, but not as true for the middle-class man.[78] Retirement for women tends to be less difficult to adapt to as they still have their domestic roles to fall back on. Furthermore, women are more likely to retire by choice.

In any case, retirement necessitates role modification and is a time when, at least temporarily, declines in self-esteem, income, status, and health are frequently seen. The multiplicity of loss creates a situation among many aged where they are depleted of the coping energies needed to meet the challenges and adjustments with which they are faced.

Family Developmental Tasks

Maintaining satisfying living arrangements is a most important task of aging families. Housing after retirement often becomes problematic. In the years immediately following retirement, the couple usually remains in their home until either property taxes, neighborhood, size or condition of house, or health forces them to find more modest accommodations. Although a majority of older persons own their own homes, a high proportion of these are extremely old and often rundown, and many are located in high-crime areas where older persons are likely to be victims. Often, the elderly remain in these homes because no suitable options exist.[79] Nonetheless, older persons living in their own homes are generally better adjusted than those who live in their children's homes. Older people usually move in with one of their children because of a decline in health or economic status, and this has proven to be a less satisfying arrangement for the elderly.

The infirm often are forced to enter board-and-care, retirement, or nursing homes where there is a loss of personal privacy, freedom, and independence and an imposition of strict conformity to institutional living. The provision of full-time help in the home or, more feasibly, part-time health and homemaker services through a home health agency or homemaker agency is more humane and protective of the older person's need to remain in his or her own home and retain his or her independence as long as possible, as well as less costly than institutionalization. Albeit difficult, one of the mates and/or grown children of the couple (or the remaining parent) often have to decide what is the best path to take—home health services, retirement home, nursing home, or living with grown children.

Adjusting to a reduced income is a second task for the aging family. When men retire, there is an immediate drop in income, and usually as the years pass by, this income becomes less and less adequate because of the steady rise in cost of living and the depletion of savings. Six out of every ten older Americans are poor.[80]

Because of the frequency of long-term health problems, health expenses are a major financial concern.

Medicare has certainly alleviated part of this problem, but there are still unpredictable, and many times substantial, out-of-pocket expenses to be paid. For instance, Part B of Medicare covers only 80 percent of "reasonable" costs for medical services. And because of a fee-for-service type of payment system, some physicians will also have the patient return many more times for office visits than is absolutely necessary to provide safe and effective medical care. Medicaid is also available to those persons who are medically indigent and qualify for Supplementary Security Income (SSI). This health insurance program then supplements Medicare coverage.

As average life expectancy increases, more older people will spend more years with severely limiting medical problems. Even though women outlive men, and the gap in life expectancies between men and women is increasing, more married couples are surviving longer. Problems of caring for an elderly couple are often more difficult than providing for a widowed pensioner. Little consideration has been given to providing for the family unit in this phase of the life cycle, during which people have an increased likelihood of living in poverty as a result of the increased costs of health and social problems. The process of aging and declining health makes it necessary for the couple to help each other. Since women live longer than men, on the average, they are usually the ones to take care of their ailing or disabled husbands. In most cases the illnesses are chronic and progressively disabling, so that there is time to adjust to the eventuality of the situation. Husbands find the task of caring for a wife more difficult, since the caretaker, nurturant, and homemaker roles are still seen largely as female roles.

Nutritional deficiencies are extensive among the elderly and contribute to many problems associated with aging (fatigue, confusion, depression, and constipation to name a few). The incidence of falls and other accidents in the home are great, so that environmental safety measures are an important need.

Marital relationships continue to be paramount to the family's happiness. Marriages which were perceived of as satisfying in the later years usually had a long positive history, and vice versa. Research has also shown that marriage contributes greatly to both morale and continued activity of both older spouses.[81]

One of the myths of old age is that sex drives and sexual activities are no longer possible (or should not exist). Considerable research has shown just the reverse, however. Such studies have found that although there is a slowing down of sexual capacity, the pleasure in sexual activity continues and may even increase.[82] Ill health sometimes diminishes the sex drive, but usually the lack of sexual activity is due to socioemotional problems.

Adjusting to the loss of spouse is, in general, the

most traumatic developmental task. According to the statistics for 1976, four times as many women as men in the United States were found to be widowed (16 versus 4 percent, respectively).[83]

In comparison with younger groups, the aged are aware of dying as part of the normal process of living. One study reported that only 3 out of 80 dying elderly patients found it hard to discuss death.[84] The awareness of death does not, however, mean that the spouse left behind will find adjustment to loss easier. Loss of spouse takes its toll: the widowed die earlier than their married counterparts while the living are more likely to have a serious health problem (social isolation, being suicidal or mentally ill). In addition, the loss of a spouse demands a total reorganization of family functions. This is especially difficult to achieve satisfactorily, since the loss has depleted the emotional and economic resources needed to deal with the change.[85] For women this means a shift from mutual dependency and sharing activities of family living to being alone or associating with a group of unattached older women. For men the loss of spouse means the loss of a companion, as well as linkage to kin, family, and the social world in general. The aged widower does not have the same interest in or the ability to perform the homemaker-housekeeper roles and is often likely to need assistance in meal preparation, homemaking, and general care.

The extent of the difficult adjustment can be seen by the increase in suicides within the group of individuals over 65. Even though there is some increase in suicides among women over 65, the preponderance of suicides is found within the older male population. A review of suicide studies among this group showed that attempted and completed suicides often followed the loss of the mate.[86]

Studies of the widowed have consistently verified the difficult living conditions and life of the widowed. The widowed have lower morale and fewer social roles and ties than the married of the same age group. They have significantly less money to live on and are found to take poor care of themselves in terms of diet, exercise, alcohol, and tobacco consumption.[87] Bild and Havighurst, in a large study of the elderly in Chicago, reported that the loss of a spouse removed the strongest support of the elderly person, though children, when available, usually stepped in to fill the vacuum somewhat. Much more isolated still were the "never marrieds" and the childless widowed.[88]

With the maintenance of intergenerational family ties, much reciprocal aid and support is given. Family members are an important source of emergency assistance and social interaction. Older families are found generally to reciprocate in the giving of help to the extent to which they are capable.

As people age they must continue to make sense out

of their existence. Reminiscing about one's past life, called life review, is a common and vital activity, since it represents a search for the central meaning of life. It also eases the adjustment to difficult situations and provides insight into past events. The elderly are concerned with the quality of their life and being able to live with respect, meaning, and dignity.[89]

Health Concerns

Elderly persons make up 10 percent of the total population, but use 27 percent of the total cost of health care. Factors such as diminishing physical vigor and function, inadequate financial resources, social isolation, loneliness, and the many other losses that the older person experiences demonstrate some of the psychophysiologic vulnerabilities of human aging.[90] Therefore, multiple health concerns exist. Assisting the aging couple or individual with all phases of a chronic illness, from the acute phase through the rehabilitation phase, is needed. Both medically related functions (physical assessment, reporting untoward reactions) and nursing functions (assessing the client's response to illness and treatment and his or her coping abilities) are relevant here. Health promotion continues to be of critical importance, especially in areas of nutrition, activity, rest, eye, dental, and health examinations, and home safety measures.

Social isolation, depression, and other psychological problems are serious health concerns, particularly when in combination with physical ill health. Assessment and use of the family's or individual social support system should be an integral part of family health care.

Related problems of housing, a suitable income, adequate recreational and health care facilities adversely affect the elderly's health status. Government programs do not adequately provide secure retirement, as clearly demonstrated in problems concerned with the use of nursing homes, long-term board and care facilities, and mental hospitals as dumping grounds for the aged.

Family-centered health professionals can provide much indirect help by referring the older couple or individual to appropriate community resources to ameliorate their problems. Some of these community resources are

1) senior centers that offer recreation, continuing-education programs, some health and (occasionally) legal services. . . ; 2) information and referral services that give relevant information in response to a telephone call or visit; 3) homemakers' services, including cooking and cleaning and providing social relationships—services that enable some elderly people to remain in their own homes rather than be relocated in institutions. . . ; 4) geriatric day-care facilities, in which older persons receive super-

vision and a variety of services during the day—usually restricted to individuals who are not capable of using senior centers; 5) nutritional programs, some of which transport recipients to a central location to eat and some of which, like the Meals-on-Wheels program, transport food to people who are not ambulatory; 6) the Foster

Grandparent program, a federally subsidized program that pays low-income elderly people a small amount to care for, tutor, or play with institutionalized children; 7) the Retired Senior Volunteer Program, also federally subsidized, helping elderly persons to provide community services.[91]

REFERENCES

1. Duvall EM: Marriage and Family Development, 5th ed. Philadelphia, Lippincott, 1977, p 20

2. Rodgers RH: Family Interaction and Transaction. Englewood Cliffs, NJ, Prentice-Hall, 1973, p 12

3. Goode WJ: The sociology of the family: Horizons in family theory. In Merton RK, et al (eds): Sociology Today. New York, Basic, 1959

4. Rodgers, *op. cit.*, p 13

5. Duvall, *op. cit.*, p 131

6. *Ibid.*, p 145

7. *Ibid.*, p 177

8. Raush H, Goodrich W, Campbell JD: Adaptation to the first years of marriage. Psychiatry 26:368, 1963

9. Jackson D, Lederer W: Mirages of Marriage. New York, Norton, 1969

10. Littlefield VM: Emotional considerations for the pregnant family. In Clausen JP, et al (eds): Maternity Nursing Today, 2nd ed. New York, McGraw-Hill, 1977, pp 385–387

11. Books with excellent chapters on prenatal family: Clausen JP, et al: Maternity Nursing Today, 2nd ed. New York, McGraw-Hill, 1977; Jensen MD, Benson RC, Boback IM: Maternity Care: The Nurse and the Family. St. Louis, Mosby, 1977; Moore M: Realities in Childbearing. Philadelphia, Saunders, 1978

12. Williams JI, Leaman TL: Family structure and function. In Conn H, et al (eds): Family Practice. Philadelphia, Saunders, 1973, p 9

13. Cohn HD, Lieberman EJ: Family planning and health. Am J Public Health 3:226, 1974

14. *Ibid.*, pp 226–229

15. Duvall, *op. cit.*, p 202

16. Manisoff M: Psychosocial and cultural factors in family planning. In Clausen JP, et al: Maternity Nursing Today, 2nd ed. New York, McGraw-Hill, 1977, p 223

17. *Ibid.*, p 223

18. Cohn, Lieberman, *op. cit.*, pp 226–229

19. Williams, Leaman, *op. cit.*, p 9

20. Fulcomer DM: The family of today. In Clausen JP, et al (eds): Maternity Nursing Today, 2nd ed. New York, McGraw-Hill, 1977, p 55

21. LeMasters EE: Parenthood as crisis. Marriage and Family Living 19:352, 1957

22. Duvall, *op. cit.*, p 215

23. *Ibid.*

24. Clark AL: Adaptation problems and the expanding family. Nurs Forum 5:98, 1966

25. LeMasters, *op. cit.*, pp 352–355

26. Clark, *op. cit.*, pp 91–98

27. Duvall, *op. cit.*, pp 231–247

28. Bowlby J: Maternal Care and Mental Health. New York, Schocken, 1966

29. Ainsworth MD, et al: Deprivation of Maternal Care. New York, Schocken, 1966

30. Klaus MH, Kendall JH: Maternal-Infant Bonding. St. Louis, Mosby, 1976

31. Kendall JH: Maternal behavior one year after early and extended postpartum contact. Dev Med Neurol 16:172, 1974

32. Rubin R: Attainment of the maternal role. 1. Processes. Nurs Res 16:237, 1967; Attainment of maternal role. 2. Models and referrants. Nurs Res 16:342, 1967

33. Davis OS: Nursing approach to the postpartum family. In Moore ML: Realities in Childbearing. Philadelphia, Saunders, 1978, pp 653–654

34. Minuchin S: Families and Family Therapy. Cambridge, Mass, Harvard, 1974, p 19

35. Friedman DB: Parent development. California Med 86:25, 1957

36. Feldman H: The development of the husband-wife relationship. Unpublished study supported in part by the National Institute of Mental Health, 1961

37. Duvall, *op. cit.*, pp 245–246

38. *Ibid.*, p 249

39. Satir V: Conjoint Family Therapy. Palo Alto, Calif, Science and Behavior Books, 1967

40. Kraft I, Fushello J, Herzog E: Prelude to school: An evaluation of an inner-city preschool program. Washington, DC, Children's Bureau Research Reports, No. 3, 1968

41. Duvall, *op. cit.*, p 258

42. Walters J (ed): Special issue: Fatherhood. Family Coordinator 25:2, October 1976

43. Feldman H: Parent and marriage: Myths and realities. Paper read at the Merrill-Palmer Institute Conference on the Family, 21 November, 1969, Mimeographed, pp 18–19.

44. Duvall, *op. cit.*, p 273

45. Erikson EH: Childhood and Society. New York, Norton, 1950

46. Burr WR: Satisfaction with various aspects of marriage over the life cycle. J Marriage Family 32(1):29, 1970

47. Rollins BC, Feldman H: Marital satisfaction over the family life cycle. J Marriage Family 32(1):20, 1970

48. Duvall, *op. cit.*, p 293

49. Adams BN: The American Family. Chicago, Markham Publishing, 1971, p 161

50. *Ibid.*

51. Douvan E, Adelson J: The Adolescent Experience. New York, Wiley, 1966, p 125

52. Adams, *op. cit.*, p 162

53. Coleman JS: The Adolescent Society. Glencoe, Ill, Free Press, 1962

54. Gottlieb D, Ramsey C: The American Adolescent. Homewood, Ill, Dorsey Press, 1964 (see also Douvan, Adelson, *op. cit.*)

55. Davis K: The sociology of parent-youth conflict. Am Sociol Rev 5:523, 1940

56. Schwartz G, Merton D: The language of adolescents: An anthropological approach to the youth culture. Am J Sociol 72:459, 1967

57. Duvall, *op. cit.*, pp 179, 306
58. Friedman, *op. cit.*
59. Duvall, *op. cit.*, p 306
60. Schultz DA: The Changing Family. Englewood Cliffs, NJ, Prentice-Hall, 1972, pp 324–326
61. Yankelowich D: How students control their drug crisis. Psychology Today 9(5):39–42, October 1975, p 41
62. Duvall, *op. cit.*, p 322
63. Kerckhoff RK: Marriage and middle age. Family Coordinator 25(1):7, 1976
64. LeShan EJ: The Wonderful Crisis of Middle Age. New York, McKay, 1973
65. Friedman, *op. cit.*
66. Kalish RA: Late Adulthood: Perspectives on Human Development. Monterey, Calif, Brooks/Cole, 1975, pp 78–79
67. Troll L: The family of later life: a decade review. J Marriage Family 33:263, 1971
68. *Ibid.*
69. Deutscher I: The quality of post-parental life: definitions of the situation. J Marriage Family 26:52, 1964
70. *Ibid.*
71. National Center for Health Statistics: Mortality Reports, 1972–73
72. Duvall, *op. cit.*, p 376
73. Rollins, Feldman, *op. cit.*, p 24
    Hayes MP, Stinnett N: Life satisfaction of middle-aged husbands and wives. J Home Economics 63(9):669, 1971; Saunders LE: Social class and postparental perspective. PhD dissertation, University of Minnesota, 1969, p 131
74. Levin RJ, Levin A: Sexual pleasure: The surprising preferences of 100,000 women. Redbook, September 1975, pp 51–58
75. Kerckhoff, *op. cit.*, p 9
76. Duvall, *op. cit.*, p 385
77. Lowenthal MF: Some potentialities of a life-cycle approach to the study of retirement. In Carp FM (ed): Retirement. New York, Behavioral Publications, 1972
78. Troll, *op. cit.*, p 274
79. Kalish, *op. cit.*, p 97
80. Atchley RC: The Social Forces in Later Life, 2nd ed. Belmont, Calif/Wordsworth, 1977, p 125
81. Lee GR: Marriage and morale in later life. J Marriage Family, 40:131, 1978
82. Lobsenz NM: Sex after sixty-five. Public Affairs Pamphlet, No. 519. New York, Public Affairs Committee, 1975
83. Department of Health, Education and Welfare. Monthly Vital Statistics Report 23:13, May 30, 1975
84. Duvall, *op. cit.*, p 413
85. Duvall, *op. cit.*, pp 424–425
86. Rushing W: Individual behavior and suicides. In Gibbs JP (ed): Suicide. New York, Harper & Row, 1968, pp 96–121
87. Hutchison IW: The significance of marital status for morale and life satisfaction among low-income elderly. J Marriage Family 35(2):287, 1975
88. Bild BR, Havighurst R: Senior citizens in great cities: The case of Chicago. Gerontologist 16(1):63, 1976
89. Duvall, *op. cit.*, pp 405–406
90. Kelley JT et al: What the family physician should know about treating elderly patients. Geriatrics 32(9):97, 1977
91. Kalish, *op. cit.*, p 117

STUDY QUESTIONS

1. The developmental approach to family analysis contains three or more basic elements or tenets. What are these? (List at least three.)

Choose the correct answer(s) to the following questions.

2. Usually reliable predictions can be made regarding the common health concerns and forces which are at play within a family if the family-centered nurse knows:
   a. The developmental tasks of each member.
   b. The family life cycle stage.
   c. Where the family lives and their social class.
   d. The composition of the family.

3. Which of the following illustrate the value of the developmental approach when assessing and working with families? (Choose all correct responses.)
   a. Gives cues as to the family's past problems and progress.
   b. Forecasts a given family's future needs.
   c. Views the common experiences of families during each of the life cycle stages.
   d. Highlights critical periods of family and individual growth and development.
   e. Helps to anticipate what to expect in terms of health concerns.
   f. Better able to evaluate the family normatively.

4. The best definition for the family life cycle is:
    a. Predictable stages within the history of the family.
    b. The growth and developmental stages of each family member as he or she progresses throughout life.
    c. Successive phases of growth and development of the family as a unit through its existence.

5. Family developmental tasks have these characteristics (choose all correct answers):
    a. They change in response to cultural imperatives and the family's unique aspirations and values.
    b. They change in response to the developmental needs of its members.
    c. They remain constant throughout the family's existence.
    d. They adapt the family's broad functions to meet the specific tasks of each stage.
    e. They satisfy the biological requirements of the family as a whole.
    f. They avoid clashing with individual needs.
    g. They are growth requirements that must be achieved by the family during each life cycle stage.
    h. Failure to achieve developmental tasks leads to difficulty in achieving later developmental tasks.
    i. Developmental tasks cover only aspects which directly influence psychosocial (interactional) components of family functioning.

6. The developmental approach seeks to explain family dynamics in terms of its:
    a. Unique elements.
    b. Common elements in its history as a family.
    c. Both common and unique elements of family history.

7. The developmental tasks of the family result from a combination of (more than one answer):
    a. Individual developmental tasks of family members.
    b. Sexual norms.
    c. Chronological ages and school placement.
    d. Community pressures for family to conform to societal norms.
    e. General family functions adapted to specific life cycle stages.

8. The stage of the family life cycles are defined in terms of (select one answer):
    a. The age and school placement of the oldest child.
    b. The ages of the parents.
    c. The age of the middle child, if present.
    d. Years of marriage.

Complete the following outlines.
9. In the outline below, list the following:
    —the eight phases in the family life cycle
    —a definition for each phase
    —three basic health concerns (biopsychosocial and health concerns) frequently present and appropriate for intervention by family nurse

Family Life Cycle Stage	Definition of Phase	Health Concerns or Needs
a.		1.
		2.
		3.
b.		1.
		2.
		3.
c.		1.
		2.
		3.
d.		1.
		2.
		3.
e.		1.
		2.
		3.
f.		1.
		2.
		3.
g.		1.
		2.
		3.
h.		1.
		2.
		3.

10. Within each of the eight life cycle stages of the family, identify the developmental tasks of parents as described by Friedman.

Life Cycle Stage	Developmental Task(s) of Parent
a.	1.
b.	1.
	2.
c.	1.
d.	1.
e.	1.
	2.
f.	1.
g.	1.
h.	1.

Choose the correct answer(s) to the following question.

11. When does the marriage relationship, according to studies, appear to be the strongest and most satisfying?
    a. Stage of preschool children.
    b. Stage of childbearing and preschool children.
    c. Stage of marriage.
    d. The postparental period (middle years).
    e. Stage of the contracting family (aging family).
    f. Stage of launching centers.

12. Give the three aspects of the adolescent process that explain the developmental tasks and problems faced in this stage.

13. What is usual impact of adolescent family members on family as a whole?

For each question in this series, select the lettered choice which applies to it. *

     a. Beginning families.
     b. Childbearing families.
     c. Families with preschool children.
     d. Families with school-age children.
     e. Families with teenagers.
     f. Families as launching centers.
     g. Families in the middle years.
     h. Aging families.

14. Beginning of loosening of family ties.

15. Reaching maximum size in number of members and of interrelationships.

16. Being totally responsible for the first time for another human being.

17. Establishing a home base.

18. Releasing members into lives of their own.

19. Rediscovery of couple as husband and wife.

20. Learning to supply adequate space, facilities, and equipment for a rapidly expanding family.

21. Dealing with death of spouse.

STUDY ANSWERS

1. Any three:
     a. Family is seen as long-lived *small group* which changes *over time.*
     b. Families go through *life cycle stages.*
     c. During each life cycle stage certain *developmental tasks* are germane to family's functioning.
     d. Family developmental tasks *are derived from* a combination of individual developmental tasks of each family member and the common family functions.
     e. The developmental approach describes *commonalities* in family experiences through time.

2. b

3. All responses are correct
    (a–f)

---

*This question is from: Borlick M, et al: Nursing Examination Review Book, Volume 9: Community Health Nursing, 2nd ed. Flushing, New York, Medical Examination Publishing Company, 1974.

4. c

5. a, b, d, e, g, and h

6. b

7. a, d, and e

8. a

9.

Family Life Cycle Stage	Definition of Phase	Health Concerns or Needs
a. Married couple	Couple without children.	1. Generating satisfying marriage (communications; sexual counseling). 2. Family planning. 3. Prenatal care.
b. Childbearing	Birth of the firstborn until oldest child is 30 months old.	1. Postpartum care; family planning. 2. Sibling rivalry. 3. Infant supervision and education (also family interactions—parental; marital).
c. Preschool age	Oldest child is 30 months to 5–6 years old (when child starts school).	1. Preschooler's accidents and infectious illnesses. 2. Adequate child care facilities. 3. Marital relationship problems.
d. School age	Oldest child is 6–13 years old.	1. Marital relationship problems. 2. Learning problems of children. 3. Childrearing practices.
e. Teenage	Oldest child is 13–20 years old.	1. Communication problems (parent–teenager). 2. Discipline and power struggles (parent–teenager). 3. Sexual information and family planning services.
f. Launching center	Firstborn through youngest child leave home.	1. Parent–child communication problems. 2. General health promotion. 3. Care of and assistance to aging parents.
g. Middle years	Empty nest (no children home) to retirement.	1. Care of and assistance to aging parents. 2. Emergence of chronic illness—need for wellness life style. 3. Grandparent role.
h. Aging family	Retirement to death of both spouses.	1. Declining health status. 2. Retirement. 3. Death of spouse.

10.

Life Cycle Stage	Developmental Task(s) of Parent
a. Stage of marriage	1. None.
b. Childbearing stage	1. Parents learn cues baby expresses in making needs known. 2. Learning to accept child's growth and development (toddler).
c. Preschool age	1. Learning to separate from child.
d. School age	1. Learning to separate from child continues.
e. Teenage	1. Learning to accept rejection without deserting the child. 2. Learning to build a new life for themselves (marital couple).
f. Launching center	1. Learning to build a new life for themselves (marital couple) continues.
g. Middle years	1. Learning to build a new life for themselves (marital couple) continues.
h. Aging family	1. None.

11. d

12. a. Emancipation.
　　 b. Generation gap.
　　 c. Youth culture.

13. The American family is tremendously affected by the developmental tasks of the adolescent. The turmoil and conflicts between parents and teenagers are inevitable as the teenager's assertion of himself or herself and rebellion is part of becoming independent or emancipated.

14. e　　　　　　　　18. f

15. d　　　　　　　　19. g

16. b　　　　　　　　20. c

17. a　　　　　　　　21. h

THE SYSTEMS APPROACH TO FAMILY ANALYSIS

One of the most salient breakthroughs in science within the last 30 years has been the increasing use of general systems theory in assessing and analyzing areas of concerns as a basis on which to plan and execute logical, comprehensive strategies of action. This theoretical framework is a general structure which has received wide usage in such diverse areas as educational systems, game theory, computer science, systems engineering, cybernetics, and information and communication theories. The growth in the use of systems theory in the health care fields has been especially impressive within the last 10 years, as evidenced by the proliferation of books utilizing this approach to study individuals, the family, nursing and other health professionals, the health care delivery system, and the community. The influence of systems theory has probably stimulated most of the attempts to achieve a systematic understanding of the family itself.[1]

The systems approach is presented in this text as one of the major theoretical frameworks used in analyzing the family. As conceived here, the organizing framework of this text—structural-functional analysis—is viewed as an inherent part of the systems approach. The family system is viewed holistically in the systems approach presented here. In Chapter 7 and in Part II of the text, the structure and functions of the family are further elaborated on so as to furnish the necessary theory and applied guidelines for family health assessment.

GENERAL SYSTEMS THEORY

In looking at human behavior, be it of the individual, the family organization, or a whole community, the systems approach is a valuable "umbrella" under which various theoretical perspectives may be applied. It constitutes a way of explaining a unit, e.g., the family, and how it relates and interacts with both larger and smaller units and of understanding its internal subdivisions (structural-functional dimensions). The basis for this approach is the assumption that matter, in all its forms, living and nonliving, can be regarded as forming systems that have discrete properties capable of being studied. Using a systems theory framework—namely, the organization of knowledge concerning the specific phenomena of interest as a complex system—one focuses on the *interaction among the various parts of the system* rather than describes the function of the parts themselves.[2,3]

In what follows, only the basic definitions and concepts to be used in a systems analysis of the family will be presented. Since these are somewhat simplified and since systems theory is rather abstract and complex, you may need additional sources to sufficiently under-

6

The Systems Approach to Family Analysis

LEARNING OBJECTIVES

1. Define the following general systems theory terms:
   a. Systems.
   b. Social systems.
   c. Open versus closed systems.
   d. Differentiation.
2. Relative to the family system, explain verbally or diagrammatically the family and its internal and external environment (the hierarchy of systems).
3. Apply the energy of exchange and processing model (input-flow-output and feedback components) to the family system.
4. Compare the terms self-regulation, steady state, homeostasis, equilibrium, and adaptation.
5. Identify four prime characteristics of a family system.
6. Explain the significance of the family system and family subsystem boundaries.
7. Identify the three subsystems and explain their function.
8. Explain the term differentiation as it applies to the family system.
9. Name four characteristics of a successfully functioning, healthy family.

stand the general theory. The references at the end of the chapter are suggested as supplementary reading to the discussion presented in this chapter.

Definitions

System

A system is defined as a goal-directed unit made up of interdependent, interacting parts which endure over a period of time. This system, together with its environment, make up a "universe," i.e., the totality of what should be studied in a given situation. Systems and their parts have both functional and structural components. *Structure* pertains to the arrangement and organization among the parts of the system, whereas *function* refers to the purposes or goals of the system, e.g., activities necessary to assure the survival, continuity, and growth of the system.

Social System

A social system is a model of social organization; it is a living system possessing a total unit distinctive from its component parts and distinguishable from its environment by a clearly defined boundary.[4] Parsons defines a social system as composed of two or more persons or social roles tied together by mutual interaction and interdependence.[5]

Open System

Systems are characterized on the basis of their degree of interaction with the surrounding environment. An open system exists in an environment with which it interacts—from which it derives its inputs and to which it gives its outputs. This environmental interaction is necessary for its survival.[6] By definition, it is obvious then that all living systems are open systems.

Closed Systems

Theoretically, a closed system, in contrast to the open system, does not interact with the environment. A closed system would then be a self-contained unit, not dependent on continual environmental interchange for its survival. Since no totally closed system has yet been demonstrated in reality, "closed" denotes a relative lack of energy exchange across a system's boundaries.[7]

Hierarchy of Systems

The universe—the system and its environment—contains a hierarchy of systems. Each higher-level unit contains lower-level systems. For instance, a hierarchy of systems from higher to lower levels might be as fol-

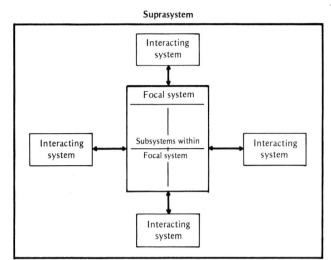

FIGURE 6.1
Schematic representation of the hierarchy of systems.

lows: community → family → parental subsystems → individual organism → organ systems → tissues → cells. When using systems theory as a working framework, one must be clear and specific about what system is being assessed. The system under study at a particular time is called the target or focal system. After specifying the target system, for example, the family, one would examine that system, then the interacting systems within its environment, and finally its suprasystems and subsystems. In the case of the family focus, one would thus study the family *and* both its internal and external environments. The suprasystems are larger environmental systems of which the focal or target system is a part. The subsystems are smaller subunits or subcomponents of the focal system. For example, if the family is the focal system, then a suprasystem would be its sociocultural group and the subsystems would be the sets of family relationships[8] (see Fig. 6.1).

Boundaries

Each system has a discrete boundary which demarcates the system from its environment. Auger explains that

> a boundary may be defined as a more or less open line forming a circle around the system where there is greater interchange of energy within the circle than on the outside. It is helpful to visualize a boundary as a "filter" which permits the constant exchange of elements, information, or energy between the system and its environment.... The more porous the filter, the greater the degree of interaction possible between the system and its environment.[9]

And in contrast, the less porous the boundary, the more isolated the system is from its environment. The ability of a boundary to control the degree of exchange is of great significance, for in regulating the amount of input from the environment at any time, the system can maintain greater equilibrium (stability).

Input

As mentioned above, all open systems must receive input from their environment in order to survive. Input refers to such things as energy, matter, and information that the system receives and processes.

Flow and Transformation

Some input is immediately used by the system in its original state, while other forms of input must be transformed in order to be utilized by the system. In either case, the input must be processed. Whether unaltered or transformed, the processed input flows through the system and is released as output.

Output

The results of processing the input constitute the output. Output in the form of energy, matter, or information is released into the environment.

Feedback

Feedback refers to the process by which a system monitors the internal and environmental responses to its behavior (output) and accommodates or adjusts itself. To describe this more clearly, feedback involves receiving and responding to the return of its own output. The system adjusts both internally by modification of subsystems and externally by controlling its boundaries. Thus it is able to control and modify inputs and outputs. Figure 6.2 describes these last four terms diagrammatically.

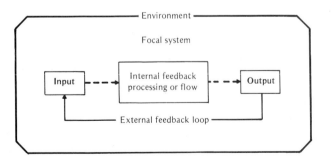

FIGURE 6.2
Model of the energy, matter, and information exchanges and processing of the systems theory. (*Adapted from Hazzard ME: An overview of systems theory. Nurs Clin North Am 6:393, 1971*)

Adaptation

A social, open system must continually adapt or adjust to demands and resources (inputs) from the outer environment and to its internal needs and changes. Adaptation is seen as the second component of feedback, that is, the system's adjustment to input. Adaptation can take two forms: (1) by acceptance or rejection of incoming information or other input without change (assimilation is the acceptance of input without change) or (2) by accommodation (modifying its structure in response to incoming information).

Self-regulation, Homeostasis, Steady State, and Equilibrium

All of these terms are used rather interchangeably in the literature, although there are fine distinctions between terms. Here only two distinctions will be pointed out. Self-regulation is a mechanism within systems that assists in balancing and controlling inputs and outputs, via feedback loops. When the system is in balance the result is homeostasis, a steady state, or equilibrium. This balance is not static, however, but dynamic and always changing within certain degrees of variation. *Adaptation occurs through self-regulatory mechanisms. The outcome of self-regulation and adaptation is equilibrium, a steady state, or homeostasis.*[10]

Differentiation

Another systems concept to be discussed is differentiation. This term denotes a living system's capability and propensity to progressively advance to a higher order of complexity and organization. A social system, if acting normally, has a tendency to "grow." Even in the absence of external stimuli, a social system is actively growing. Energy inputs flowing into the system are utilized for growth in complexity and organization.[11]

Energy

"All dynamic, open systems require continuous supplies of energy in sufficient quantity so that demands for system integrity can be met."[12] The most important factor governing the amount of energy needed is the rate of utilization of energy within the system itself. Systems which have high levels of activity utilize large quantities of energy, and therefore must receive greater amounts of input from the environment in order to meet these energy demands. This, in turn, implies that the system's boundaries would have to be more open, or porous, to allow the greater input of energy.

THE FAMILY SYSTEM

Definitions

Family

The family is defined as a living social system. It is a small group of closely interrelated and interdependent individuals who are organized into a single unit so as to attain specific purposes, namely, family functions or goals. (See Chapter 7, where these functions are more fully discussed.) The interrelationships which are found in this family system are so intricately tied together that a change in any one part inevitably results in changes in the entire system. For example, a 15-year-old daughter has been diagnosed as having a serious chronic illness—rheumatoid arthritis. Because of her health problem, the parents' attention is continually focused on the disabled daughter to the exclusion of the other two children. One child, age 18, spends more time with her friends now. The younger son, age 7, has developed mysterious stomach aches in the morning so that he is unable to go to school and is "allowed" to stay home with mother.

Open System

The family is an *open system*, since it exchanges materials, energy, and information with its environment. Families are in constant interaction with their physical, social, and cultural environment. As with an open system, the family is a dynamic entity ever changing and growing. It is possible to identify degrees of openness in a family and thus to evaluate a family's ability to change.[13] One of the important properties of the family as an open system is called nonsummativity, which means that the family cannot be considered merely as the sum of its parts, but that as a system it is greater than and different from the sum of its parts. In other words, the assessment of the family *unit* cannot be based on the sum of the analysis of each of family members or sets of relationships.[14]

Hierarchy of Systems: Family as Focal System

Figure 6.3 illustrates the relationship of the family to its interacting systems—other societal institutions such as the welfare and educational system—and its suprasystems—e.g., the family's reference group and the community or wider society.

Relative to the family system's environment, generally speaking, the more immediate the environment, the greater the influence on the system and the greater the input to the family. Conversely, more distant environments have lesser influence on the family. Thus systems with which the family continually interacts

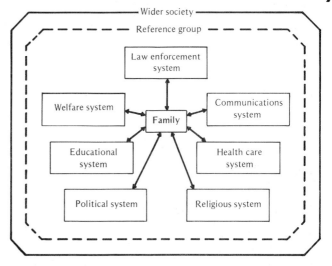

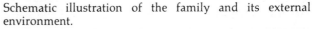

FIGURE 6.3
Schematic illustration of the family and its external environment.

such as the school system generally have a more potent impact on the family than a remote suprasystem.

An example of a family suprasystem—its reference group—is described by Billingsley. In the following quotation he explains how the black family is embedded within a whole network of mutually interdependent institutions and the wider black community:

> The Negro community includes within itself a number of institutions which are also viewed as subsystems. Prominent among these are: schools, churches, taverns, newspapers, neighborhood associations, lodges, fraternities, social clubs, age and sex peer groups, recreation associations and small businesses, including particularly, barber shops, beauty parlors, restaurants, pool halls, funeral societies and various organized systems of hustling.[15]

Family Boundaries

Probably the most crucial means families have of facilitating adaptation to outside demands and internal needs is through the effective use of their semipermeable *family boundaries*. The function of boundaries is to actively expand (or open) and retract (or close) according to need, thus regulating the amount of input from the environment and output to the environment.[16] In other words, the key to successful family adaptation is selective permeability of family boundaries. In healthy functioning, input is screened so that a family takes in what is needed from the environment and assimilates or modifies it to promote its own survival and growth. In addition, the family selectively releases to the environment information, matter, and energy for the same larger purposes of survival and growth.

Satir discusses the importance of families having relatively open boundaries by stating that there are two types of systems—the closed and open. (These two "pure" types are used as a basis for comparison.) Open systems provide for change, whereas closed systems provide for little or no change. She writes that "an open system offers choices and depends on successfully meeting reality for its continuing life. A closed system depends on edict and law and order and operates through force, both physically and psychologically."[17]

Open families welcome new ideas, information, techniques, opportunities, and resources. Moreover, open families take the initiative by actively seeking out new resources and using these resources to solve their problems. Creative solutions to problems are sought and are utilized in response to changing and unique needs. Pratt calls this active coping effort.[18] Open families are those which function optimally, perceive change as normal and desirable, and view people as inherently good and helpful and thus to be sought and needed. Open families reach out to the larger community and interact extensively with it. Thus family boundaries of the open family are much more permeable. Such families are characterized by the continual flow or exchange of energy, matter, information, and services across their boundaries.

In contrast, closed families view change as threatening and are resistant to it. People are perceived as being evil, or at least not to be trusted. They believe that man's negative qualities are a basic fact of life and that people must therefore be under strict control; thus, relationships have to be regulated by force. These types of families are rigid; as a result, things and events in the closed family remain as constant and predictable as possible. Kantor and Lehr describe the situation existing in the closed family:

> Locked doors, careful scrutiny of strangers in the neighborhood, parental control over the media, supervised excursions, and unlisted telephones are all features of a closed-type family. Closed bounding (boundary) goals include the preservation of territoriality, self-protection, privacy, and, in some families, secretiveness. Perimeter traffic control is never relinquished to outsiders or even to anyone within the family not specifically assigned bounding responsibilities.[19]

When families have boundaries which are too rigid and impermeable, important resources are not forthcoming. These families are deprived of the necessary information and support, as well as, perhaps, the physical resources necessary for family wellness.

Family Adaptation

Family adaptation refers to the capacity of the family and its members to modify their behavior to each other and their outer world as the situation demands. In response to internal or external input, the family can adapt by either accepting or rejecting incoming information, energy, or services or by modifying the input to meet its needs.

When forming an open system, the family balances inputs from the external and internal environments by the feedback process. Balanced adequately, this is called *family homeostasis, steady state,* or *equilibrium.* Homeostasis or its synonyms (steady state and equilibrium) should not imply stagnation, however, but the degree of balancing needed while continual change and growth are taking place. Healthy families are flexible, more spontaneous, open to growth and change, responsive to new stimulation, and not status quo oriented.[20]

Since families must change in order to meet both internal and external demands, a sufficient range of behaviors and patterns and the flexibility to mobilize these when needed are essential. Nevertheless, the family system offers resistance to change beyond a certain range and maintains preferred patterns as long as it possibly can. Although alternatives are feasible, the family's threshold of tolerance for change stimulates self-regulatory mechanisms which reestablish the accustomed range. An example of this phenomenon is that when a family crisis appears it is common for a family member to feel that other family members are not "doing their part" and to appeal to group loyalty or use guilt-producing techniques to bring other family members to the aid of the family and restore "normality."

A steady state is achieved internally by balancing family members' roles. Family members help to maintain this internal balance either covertly or overtly. The family's repetitious, circular, and predictable communication patterns will reveal this balancing act.

Failure of Adaptive Strategies

As with individuals, the presence of stress in a family initially aids the family to mobilize its resources and work at solving its problems. Stress causes family homeostasis or its steady state to become precarious, in which case family members will initially exert much effort to regain its balance. However, as initial attempts to resolve problems or to meet demands fail, stress increases. If it initially involved one individual, first one and then the other subsystems are usually called into play in coping with the stress, until finally all components are involved. For instance, problems in the spouse subsystem can be localized for a while. Then as they continue and intensify, other subsystems, especially the parental–child subsystem, also become affected. Although stress is experienced by all the subsystems, each subsystem may tolerate and handle the stress differently.

In time, if no solution is found to reduce the stress, the system eventually reaches its limits to respond adaptively, reaching a point of exhaustion. When important familial resources are depleted, family functioning worsens, and symptoms of family disorganization set in: overt symptoms of an individual family member's distress, economic difficulties, intrafamilial conflicts, or parenting problems. At this point a family crisis is present. If no outside assistance is received, the end result may be a discontinuity in the present family form, such as the separation or loss of a family member. In contrast, a stable system under stress will move in the direction that tends to minimize the stress, e.g., it will seek help from external sources.

Family Subsystems

The family is a system of interacting personalities intricately organized into positions, roles, and norms which are further organized into subsystems within the family. These subsystems become the basis for the family structure or organization. The family system differentiates and carries out its functions through these subsystems, which are made up of sets of relationships involving two or more family members. Each individual belongs to different subsystems, in which he or she has different levels of power and where he or she learns differentiated roles. An adult female, for example, can be a daughter, wife, or older sister. Each of these roles involves different complimentary relationships and the use of a different cluster of behaviors.[21]

The nuclear family has at least three subsystems, each of which serves some unique function in addition to common objectives. These subsystems are the following:

1. *The Spouse Subsystem.* Here two adult members relate to each other as (a) marital partners and (b) parents of their offspring.
2. *The Parent–Child Subsystem.* This subsystem is composed of the parents and their children. The subsystem has parenting functions (socialization) involving the mother–father roles and the children's roles.
3. *The Sibling Subsystem.* This subsystem is characterized by the children's relationships with each other.
4. *Other Subsystems.* These may also exist, as, for example, a grandparent–grandchild subsystem or uncle–nephew subsystem.

Minuchin, a family therapist and the author of several important books in his field, has worked extensively with families using the systems approach in family counseling, and he stresses the need to work with and through the several subsystems of the family to effect positive change within the whole family. His approach is to assist in the strengthening of the subsystems so that they function in an effective manner and do not lose their identity or unique contribution to the whole.

Minuchin suggests that in the same way that the family system has a boundary, so does each subsystem, the purpose of which is to protect the differentiation of the system, i.e., it is through the growth and evolution of subsystems that the whole family differentiates. Each subsystem has specific functions, which in turn lead to special demands on its members. Thus in the spouse system, the parent is given the child-rearing function. Clear and distinct boundaries are required to deter any interference by other subsystems. For example, the spouse subsystem often becomes usurped by the parent–child subsystem because of the overwhelming demands on the adult members (parents) of the parenting role. In another case, the parent–child subsystem cannot function effectively if siblings interfere in the parent–child relationship and compromise the parents' capacity to parent the child with whom they are relating.[22]

A brief explanation of each of the three subsystems will help illuminate their critical functions.

The Spouse Subsystem. The traditional spouse subsystem is formed when two adults of the opposite sex agree to join together for the primary purposes of mutual support and the meeting of each other's affectional and sexual needs. The couple needs to mutually accommodate, in addition to complementing, each other. The spouse subsystem is vital to the couple, since it acts as a refuge from external stresses and constitutes an avenue for contacting other social systems. Utilizing the systems framework, the spouse subsystem boundary needs to be distinct and protected from the demands and needs of other systems. Children especially interfere with the spouse subsystem, creating a situation wherein husband and wife have a relationship based not on their own personal relationship with each other, but one based on their parenting functions.[23]

The Parent–Child Subsystem. With the birth or adoption of a child by the couple, the original dyadic family grows in complexity, since a new subsystem is created. The spouse subsystem now must differentiate itself to perform both mutual support and child-rearing functions. The parent–child subsystem involves both parents and their relationship with each of their children.[24]

The Sibling Subsystem. With the advent of additional children, the sibling subsystem comes into being. As only children will attest, having a sister or brother is important. These relationships serve as the first social-skills laboratory for children. Here they learn to relate in the peer world. They learn to support, become angry, negotiate, cooperate, and imitate each other. In their relating to siblings, children learn to play different roles, which then serve them when they go out into the extrafamilial world. Within these relationships there is an openness and honesty unmatched in outer society; that is, the child obtains constant feedback from siblings concerning his or her behavior.

The significance of the sibling subsystem is underscored by frequent observations made of only-children. Only-children accommodate in the adult world rather than their peer world, often exhibiting precocious development because of extensive parental exposure. Concurrently, they may have difficulty sharing, cooperating, and competing with children of their own age and are usually more dependent in their behavior.[25]

Differentiation

Differentiation refers to the family's propensity to evolve and grow so that as growth takes place the system becomes more complex, articulate, and discriminate. Developmental studies—studies of families throughout their life cycle—have demonstrated this tendency. Families are dynamic systems which are continually differentiating themselves both functionally and structurally. Because of the family's evolution and growth, there is also a concomitant need for increased numbers of specialized roles. This specialization and increased complexity are direct outcomes of differentiation.[26]

In concluding an exploration of the basic concepts and definition of systems theory and how these are applied and illustrated within the family system, it is fitting to draw a "composite picture" of the healthy family. According to Lewis et al., the healthy family is a maximally viable system characterized by complexity of structure; a highly flexible organization capable and tolerant of internal changes; higher autonomous subsystems and considerable internal determination; and an openness with the outer environment that results in a continual flow of a wide variety of information, experience, and input into the family.[27] Pratt elaborates further by saying that healthy families are energized families in which persons are developed in the matrix of the family through freedom and change. Rather than the holding back—conforming to prescribed social patterns through control and stability—the energized family is characterized by the following points:

1. Interaction by all members with each other regularly in a variety of contexts, (tasks or leisure-time activities).
2. Maintenance of varied and active contacts with a wide range of other groups and organizations, including health, educational, political, recreational, and business associations in the community, so as to enhance and fulfill the interests of family members.
3. Active attempts to cope and master their lives by joining groups, seeking out information, discovering options, and making their own decisions.
4. A fluid internal organization, where role relationships are flexible and responsive to changing situations and needs, power is shared, each person participates in the decisions in which he or she is affected, and relationships support personal growth and autonomy.[28]

REFERENCES

1. Buckley W: Sociology and Modern Systems Theory. Englewood Cliffs, NJ, Prentice-Hall, 1967
2. Von Bertalanffy L: General system theory and psychiatry. In Arieti S (ed): American Handbook of Psychiatry, Vol 3. New York, Basic, 1966, pp 705–721
3. Miller, JG: Living systems: Basic concepts. In Gray W, Duhl F, Rizzo N (eds): General Systems Theory and Psychiatry. Boston, Little, Brown, 1969
4. Anderson R, Carter I: Human Behavior in the Social Environment—A Social Systems Approach. Chicago, Aldine, 1974
5. Parsons T, Bales R: Family Socialization and Interaction Process. New York, Free Press, 1955, pp 401–408
6. *Ibid.*, p 162
7. *Ibid.*
8. *Ibid.*, pp 10–11
9. Auger JR: Behavioral Systems and Nursing. Englewood Cliffs, NJ, Prentice-Hall, 1976, p 24
10. Hazzard M: An overview of systems theory. Nurs Clin North Am, 6:385, 1971
11. Bowen M: Family concept of schizophrenia. In Jackson DD (ed): Etiology of Schizophrenia. New York, Basic, 1960, pp 346–372
12. Auger, *op. cit.*, p 26

13. Francis GB, Munjas BA: Manual of Socialpsychologic Assessment. New York, Appleton, 1976, p 27
14. *Ibid.*, p 28
15. Billingsley A: Black Families in White America. Englewood Cliffs, NJ, Prentice-Hall, 1968, p 5
16. Reinhardt A, Quinn M: Current Practices in Family-Centered Community Nursing. St. Louis, Mosby, 1973, pp 90–91
17. Satir V: Peoplemaking. Palo Alto, California, Science and Behavior Book, 1972, p 113
18. Pratt L: Family Structure and Effective Health Behavior. Boston, Houghton Mifflin, 1976, p 86
19. Kantor D, Lehr W: Inside the Family. New York, Harper & Row: Colophon Books, 1975, p 120
20. Lewis J, Beavers WR, Gossett JT, Phillips VA, et al: No Single Thread—Psychological Health in Family Systems. New York, Brunner/Mazel, 1976, pp 10–11
21. Minuchin S: Families and Family Therapy. Cambridge, Mass, Harvard University Press, 1974, pp 60–66
22. *Ibid.*
23. *Ibid.*
24. *Ibid.*
25. *Ibid.*
26. *Ibid.*
27. Lewis J, et al., *op. cit.*
28. Pratt, L: Family Structure and Effective Health Behavior. Boston, Houghton Mifflin, 1976, pp 3–4

STUDY QUESTIONS

Are the following statements True *or* False?

1. A system is defined as a unit with distinctive parts and boundaries, extending over a period of time and with some identified purpose.

2. A social system is either an animate or inanimate system.

3. Open systems depend on the environment for exchange of information, matter, and energy, whereas closed systems do not interact with the environment.

4. Differentiation occurs when a system bifurcates or splits into smaller subunits or systems.

5. With greater energy use, system boundaries need to be more open.

6. Differentiation, particularly as it applies to families, describes the family's tendency to grow and evolve (as time progresses) into a more complex and specialized system.

7. Relative to the family system and its internal and external environments, supply the information asked for.
   a. Name a focal or target system.
   b. Name a suprasystem.
   c. Give three examples of interacting systems.
   d. Give three examples of family subsystems.

8. Draw a diagram of the energy, matter, and information exchange and process model and show a specific example of this energy exchange and processing pertinent to the family system.

9. Match the correct term from the left-hand column with characteristic from the right-hand column.

a. Equilibrium	1.	Synonymous with balancing (used interchangeably)
b. Adaptation		
c. Homeostasis	2.	The result of balancing
d. Steady state	3.	A survival mechanism
e. Feedback loop		
f. Self-regulation		

Choose the correct answer(s) to the following question.

10. The following elements and characteristics are true of the family system. It is a (an):
    a. Open social system
    b. Highly organized system
    c. Highly interdependent system
    d. System with specified purposes
    e. System with necessary processes, e.g., integration, adaptation, and decision making
    f. Independent system
    g. Undifferentiated system
    h. Suprasystem to the spouse, parent–child, and sibling systems
    i. Dynamic system—with little capacity for change and stability

11. What is the significance of the boundaries of the family system and subsystems?

12. Utilizing the systems approach, explain how family boundaries function to maintain family homeostasis.

13. Match the proper function(s) on the left with each of the family subsystems on the right.
    a. A social skills laboratory
    b. Mutual support
    c. Meeting of adult affectional needs
    d. Learning to relate to peers
    e. Socialization function
    f. Disciplining—control and guidance function

    1. Spouse subsystem
    2. Parent–child subsystem
    3. Sibling subsystem

14. Give four characteristics of a successfully functioning, healthy family.

15. Match the advantages/disadvantages and/or characteristics with either "open" or "closed" families (those with open or closed family boundaries).
    a. Open families
    b. Closed families
    c. Does not apply to either

    1. Provide for change
    2. Are stagnated, rigid
    3. Offers choices and flexibility
    4. Change viewed as threatening
    5. Greater structuring and control mechanisms employed
    6. Privacy and territoriality stressed
    7. People seen as good, helpful, and needed
    8. Seek out new resources

16. Sequentially number the events below in terms of their sequencing when a family crisis occurs.
    a. No solution is found to reduce stress, i.e., failure of adaptive strategies exists.

b. Stress and strain are experienced.

c. A change occurs as stressor presents itself.

d. Family homeostasis or its steady state becomes precarious and family exerts additional efforts to maintain balance and reduce stress.

e. Stress spreads from one individual or subsystem to all subsystems of family.

f. System reaches point of exhaustion.

g. Family disorganization results.

STUDY ANSWERS

1. True   4. False

2. False   5. True

3. True   6. True

7. a. Focal system = family
   b. Suprasystem = wider community
   c. Interacting systems = health care system, educational system, law enforcement system, welfare system
   d. Subsystems = spouse, parent–child, and sibling subsystems.

8. See energy, matter, and information exchange and process model (Figure 6.2).

   Various examples could be applied, such as:

   Input (= *Information*): News of risk of inactivity and benefits of exercise program.

   Flow: Spouse subsystem accepts and internalizes this information.

   Output: Spouses begin dance classes weekly for themselves. They also begin hiking with their children on weekends (the energy release—their activity—is the output).

   Feedback: The family members feel better (have more energy, vitality, and strength) plus the parents' figures improve, which then becomes a reinforcer of the exercise program.

9. a. 1
   b. 2
   c. 1
   d. 1
   e. 3
   f. 3

10. a, b, c, d, e, and h

11. *Significance of family boundaries:* Boundaries allow for the exchange processes. By controlling the flow in and out of the system, they prevent overload or underload of the system. *Significance of family subsystem boundaries:* They prevent loss of integrity of the system and interference with their vital functions.

12.   Family boundaries function adaptively by being selectively permeable, i.e., actively expanding (opening up) and retracting (closing down) according to need, thus regulating the amounts of input and output.

13.   a.   3
      b.   1, 2, 3
      c.   1
      d.   3
      e.   2
      f.   2

14.   Four characteristics of a healthy family are:
      a.   Highly organized and differentiated.
      b.   Autonomous subsystems.
      c.   Tolerance and ability to change internally.
      d.   Continual openness to new information and other input.
      (Pratt's characteristics of an energized family are also correct.)

15.   a.   1, 3, 7, and 8
      b.   2, 4, 5, and 6
      c.   None

16.   a.   5
      b.   2
      c.   1
      d.   3 or 4
      e.   3 or 4
      f.   6
      g.   7

THE STRUCTURAL-FUNCTIONAL APPROACH

The structural-functional framework is a major frame of reference used in sociology today,[1] and it is also increasingly mentioned as a theoretical orientation in the health fields relative to family. Applied to the family, the scope of the framework is very broad. Although family structural (organizational dimensions) and family functions are the core of this approach, it can be viewed as an elaboration of the systems approach, where both the focal system (family) and its universe (the subsystems, interacting systems, and suprasystems) are studied each in terms of their structure, functions, and interrelationships.

According to Eshleman, the structural-functional approach has its origin in the functionalist branch of psychology (particularly Gestalt psychology), in social anthropology (as exhibited in the writings of Malinowski and Radcliffe-Brown), and in sociology (particularly as described by social systems theorists such as Parsons). The Gestalt position emphasizes that one must view the whole and its parts, exploring the interrelationship between the whole and its parts. Along the same line of thinking, social anthropologists have concluded that one cannot understand a particular aspect of social life detached from its general environment.[2]

Most of the sociological literature applying the structural-functional approach to the family makes use of a more macroscopic approach, looking at the family as a subsystem of the wider society. The general assumptions made include the following:

1. A family is a social system with functional requirements.
2. A family is a small group possessing certain generic features common to all small groups.
3. Social systems such as the family accomplish functions which serve the individual in addition to those which serve society.[3]

The structural-functional perspective is a very useful framework for assessing family life because it enables the family system to be examined as a relatively autonomous system, looking at it as a whole in addition to its internal processes, yet provides a meaningful way of studying family linkages to other institutions such as the educational and health systems, the family's reference group, and the wider society. This approach has been selected as the text's organizing framework, since its use provides a comprehensive and holistic perspective, and because it is of the essence of family-centered nursing to understand the dynamics of the family and all the forces, both internal and external, which affect it.

7

The Structural-Functional Approach

LEARNING OBJECTIVES

1. Describe the structural-functional approach.
2. Explain the usefulness of the structural-functional approach to family nursing.
3. Analyze the relationship of family structure to family functions and the system's theory approach to the structural-functional approach.
4. List and briefly describe the six basic family functions.

84

CONCEPT OF STRUCTURE

The structural-functional approach primarily analyzes the family's structural characteristics, i.e., the arrangement of the parts which form the whole, and the functions it performs for both society and its subsystems. The structure of the family means how the family is organized, the manner in which units are arranged, and how these units relate to each other. The dimensions, or definitions, of this concept of family structure vary considerably. Some theorists base structure on the type of family form, e.g., nuclear versus extended; type of power structure, e.g., matriarchal versus patriarchal; or marital patterns, e.g., exogamy versus endogamy.[4] Another way of looking at the family's structure is by describing the subsystems as the structural dimension.[5] Taking the family to be a special kind of group, the structural dimensions identified by small-group theory as being relevant for assessing such groups are used in this text. Parad and Caplan, in analyzing a family under stress, have used very similar structural dimensions, which they call the family life style. Family life style refers to "the reasonably stable patterning of family organization, subdivided into three interdependent elements of value system, communication network and role systems."[6] A fourth element or dimension has been added to Parad and Caplan's structural elements—the power structure. To repeat then, the four basic structural dimensions which are subsumed under structure, and which will be elaborated on in separate chapters, are (1) role structure, (2) value systems, (3) communication pattern, and (4) power structure.

These elements are all intimately interrelated and interacting. When one aspect of the internal structure of the family is affected by input from the external environment, the processing of this input within the family system will impact on the other structural dimensions also. The family's high degree of interrelatedness and interdependency is seen when a family health professional observes how certain family behaviors often become indicators of several or all of the major organizing elements within the family. For instance, a husband is observed ordering his wife and children on when and what will be served for dinner in an authoritarian way. The mother is then seen directing the children to each prepare certain assigned parts of the meal. Mother and children carry out father's wishes with no comments or sign of feelings. No other communications are noted. We can see from this one vignette (and this would have to be verified by further observation of the family) that the power figure in this situation is the father; his role is one of a stern, commanding leader of the family, who probably needs and has much control over his family (since even de-

tails are controlled). The communication patterns here are one-way (father to mother and children, mother to children) and completely task centered. No feelings or sharing of thoughts are observed. Again speculating on this situation, the events are more than likely congruent with the family's value system. One of the values central to this family probably would be male dominance, while another related value might be respect for and obedience to elders.

Family structure, or organization, is ultimately evaluated by how well the family is able to fulfill its family functions—the goals important to its members and society. The family's structure serves to facilitate the achievement of family functions, since the conservation and allocation of resources is a prime task for the family structure. Because of this important relationship, functions should be viewed in tandem with family structures.

CONCEPT OF FUNCTION

Family functions can then be defined as outcomes or consequences of the family structure. Although some authors use "function" to mean "consequences of or results of," it is a little easier to think of family functions as being what the family does. Why does it exist? What purposes does it serve? As described in detail in Chapter 1, the family's basic functions meet the needs of both individual family members and wider society. Six family functions are most germane to consider in assessing the family.

1. Affective function (personality maintenance): for stabilization of adult personalities; meeting the psychological needs of family members.
2. Socialization and social placement function: for the primary socialization of children aimed at making them productive members of their society, as well as the conferring of status on family members.
3. Reproduction function: to recruit new members for society.
4. Family coping function: strategies used for the maintenance of order and stability in interacting with inner and outer environment.
5. Economic function: to provide sufficient economic resources and to allocate resources effectively.
6. Provision of physical necessities: food, clothing, shelter, health care (health care function).*

---

* These functions represent an adaptation or modification of several theorists' descriptions of family functions, including those of Murdock,[7] Ogburn,[8] Parsons and Bales,[9] and Hill.[10]

Affective Function

The affective function is a central basis for both the formation and the continuation of the individual family unit, and it thus constitutes one of the most vital functions of families.† Today, when many societal tasks are performed outside the family unit, much of the family's effort is focused on meeting the needs of family members for affection and understanding. The ability to provide for these needs is a key determinant of whether a given family will persist or dissolve. As Duvall[11] says, "Family happiness is gauged by the strength of family love." The family must meet the affectional needs of its members because the affectional responses of one individual to another provide the basic rewards of family life.

Primarily a parental role, this function deals with the family's perception and care of the socioemotional needs of all its members, and it involves tension reduction and morale maintenance. The elevation of this function to a high level of importance within the family is relatively new and found most strongly among more affluent families, where choice is more feasible. In the middle and upper classes, personal happiness in the marital relationship based on companionship and love is critical. The importance of this function still has a decreased emphasis in working-class and lower-class families, largely because more basic functions such as providing the physical necessities of life are paramount.

Socialization and Social Placement Function

Socialization refers to the myriad of learning experiences provided within the family aimed at teaching children how to function and assume adult social roles such as those of husband-father and wife-mother. Since this function is more and more shared with schools, recreational and child-care facilities, and other extrafamilial institutions, the family plays a reduced although still critical role in socialization. Of course, parents still transmit their cultural heritage to their children, the major difference being the greater degree of outside influences.

The family has the primary responsibility of transforming an infant, in a score of years, into a social being capable of full participation in society. Furthermore, socialization should not be thought of as pertaining only to child-rearing patterns during infancy and children, but rather as a lifelong process that includes internalizing the appropriate sets of norms and values for being a teenager at age 14, a bride at age 20,

a parent at 24, an employee on a new job at 30, a grandparent at 50, and a retired person at age 65.[12] Reiss points out that although other functions such as reproduction are listed as necessary for, and performed in, all societies, only the function of nurturant socialization of children is a universal function of the nuclear family structure.[13]

An integral part of socialization involves the inculcation of controls and values—giving the growing child (and adult) a sense of what is right and wrong. Kohlberg[14] has described morality development as a process similar to the stages of emotional and cognitive development as conceived by Erikson and Piaget, respectively. By identifying with parental figures and being consistently reinforced negatively and positively for their behavior, children develop a personal value system that is greatly influenced by the family's value system.

Social placement, or status-conferring, is the other aspect of this vital function. At birth, a child automatically inherits his or her family's status—ethnic, racial, national, religious, economic, political, and educational. The family socializes the child into its social class, instilling in him or her all the relevant aspirations. Additionally, the family has the responsibility of providing necessary socialization and educational experiences that enable an individual to assume a vocation and roles in groups that are consistent with status expectations.

In summary, conferring of status on children refers to passing on of the traditions, values, and privileges of the family, although today tradition no longer dictates life patterns of most adult Americans. Leslie explains: "Indirectly, the family's way of life is still determined somewhat by the husband's occupation and by the value system of his occupation, but the direct participation of the family in defining each member's role in the community is much less than it used to be."[15]

Education in child-rearing patterns and ways of coping with family problems is a major component of family health care, beginning with genetic and reproductive counseling, continuing through prenatal and child care, and extending throughout the life cycle of the family. The common health concerns and family problems in which the family nurse can assist families are outlined in Chapter 5.

Function of Providing Physical Necessities and Care

The physical functions of the family are met by the parents providing food, clothing, shelter, and protection against danger. Health care and health practices (which influence the individual family members' health status) are the most relevant part of this family

---

† See Chapter 13 for a detailed discussion of the affective function.

function for the family health nurse. Chapter 15, The Health Care Function, is devoted entirely to an exploration of this most significant aspect of this function.

Reproductive Function

One of the basic functions of the family is to reproduce and so provide recruits for society. In the past, marriage and the family were designed to regulate and control sexual behavior as well as reproduction. Both these aspects, control of sexual behavior and birth control, are now less important functions of the family, since it is no longer necessary in this society to limit sexual activity or to have children within the confines of the traditional family. Once a child is born, a new family is born—with single parent families becoming increasingly common. The number of illegitimate births, for example, has continued to rise in the United States as greater acceptability and loosening of sexual mores has occurred, with 15 percent of all births in 1977 being illegitimate and more than half of all out-of-wedlock babies born to teenagers.[16]

Along with the having of children outside of the confines of the traditional family is the trend toward greater use of birth control measures, whether or not within the family context. Moreover, the move toward population control and family planning is affecting the importance of parenthood for both women and men. A shift of cultural priorities and personal values continues to deflate motherhood as a woman's central purpose in life* and fatherhood as a man's chief reason to work. Increasingly, public expressions are heard against the bearing of more than two children per couple (as the couple's replacement quota). Maternity may eventually become not an obligation and right, but a privilege for those who have been found to be "qualified." Keller in her discussion of the family's future, states:

---

* The National Center for Health Statistics reported that in 1977 the fertility rate reached a new low for the fifth consecutive year. The rate was 65.8 births per 1,000 women in their childbearing years, compared to the 1957 rate of 122.7 (The Nation's Health, New York, American Public Health Association, June, 1978, p. 5).

this [changing parenthood rights and privileges] along with changing attitudes towards sex, abortion, adoption, illegitimacy, the spread of the Pill, better knowledge of human behavior, and a growing skepticism that the family is the only proper crucible for child-rearing, creates a powerful recipe for change.[17]

Economic Function

The economic function involves the family's provision of sufficient resources—financial, space, and material—and their appropriate allocation by decision-making processes.

An assessment of the family's economic resources provides the nurse with data relevant to the family's ability to allocate resources appropriately to meet family needs such as adequate clothing, food, shelter, and health care. By gaining an understanding of how a family distributes its resources, the family-centered nurse can also obtain a clearer perspective on the family's value system, i.e., what is important to them.

This function is difficult for most poor families to fulfill satisfactorily. All health personnel must accept the responsibility of assisting families to obtain appropriate community resources where they can secure needed information, employment, vocational counseling, and financial assistance.

Family Coping Function

Families are continually being faced with demands and expectations from the outside environment (community pressures, economic needs, stressors such as a loss in the extended family or the loss of a job) and the inner environment (from the subsystems and individual family members). Inner demands are usually created by the emergence of new developmental tasks of family members. Confronted with these demands and inputs, the family must have adaptive patterns or problem-solving mechanisms for insuring its survival, continuity, and growth. Chapter 16 covers this function in depth.

REFERENCES

1. Eshleman JR: The Family: An Introduction. Boston, Allyn and Bacon, 1974, p 38
2. *Ibid.*, pp 38–39
3. *Ibid.*, p 40
4. *Ibid.*, p 41
5. Minuchin S: Families and Family Therapy. Cambridge, Mass, Harvard, 1974
6. Parad HJ, Caplan G: A framework for studying families in crisis. In Parad HJ (ed): Crisis Intervention: Selected Readings. New York Family Service of America, 1965, pp 55–58
7. Murdock GP: Social Structure. New York, Macmillan, 1949
8. Ogburn WF: The family and its function. Recent Social Trends in the United States. New York, McGraw-Hill, 1933

9. Parsons T, Bales RF: Family Socialization and Interaction Process. New York, Free Press, 1955
10. Hill R: Challenges and resources for family development. Family Mobility in Our Dynamic Society. Ames, Iowa, Iowa State, 1965
11. Duvall EM: Marriage and Family Relationships, 5th ed. Philadelphia, Lippincott, 1977, p 114
12. Eshleman, *op. cit.*, p 68
13. Reiss IL: The universality of the family: A conceptual analysis. J Marriage Family 27:443, 1965
14. Kohlberg, L: Education for justice: A modern statement of the platonic view. Moral Education: Five Lectures. Cambridge, Mass, Harvard, 1970
15. Leslie ER: The Family in Social Context, 3rd ed. New York, Oxford, 1976, p 247
16. Woodward KL, Lord M, Maier F, Foote DM, Malamud P: Saving the family. Newsweek, May 15, 1978, p 67
17. Keller, S: Does the family have a future? In Coser RL (ed): The Family: Its Structure and Functions, 2nd ed. New York, St. Martin's, 1974, p 587

STUDY QUESTIONS

1. The interactionist approach analyzes internal family dynamics. The structural-functional approach, which is broader in focus, analyzes what?

Choose the correct answers to the following questions.

2. The following are reasons for selecting the structural-functional approach over other frameworks for assessing and working with families. Select the most accurate and inclusive reason:
   a. Since it is a microscopic approach, it centers on inner dynamics and provides information for transactional-based diagnoses.
   b. It consists of a comprehensive, holistic perspective by which not only the family can be assessed, but also the family's universe (its inner and outer environments).
   c. It provides the family health worker with an understanding of the forces from within and without that impinge on the family.
   d. Using this framework the common health problems are recognized as the family progresses through the life cycle.

3. The relationship of the family structure to family function is that (select one answer):
   a. The structure provides the organization for family functions to be accomplished.
   b. The functions mandate the family structure.
   c. Structure and function are separate entities and have no direct relationship to each other.

4. The structural-functional approach compares to the systems approach in what way? (Select the *best*, most inclusive answer.)
   a. They are two separate frameworks.
   b. The structural-functional approach is in opposition to the systems approach.
   c. The systems theory approach is a variation of the structural-functional approach.
   d. The structural-functional approach emanated from theories in psychology (Gestalt), social anthropology (Malinowski), and social systems theory (Parsons).

5. Indicate whether the four descriptions in the left-hand column are structural dimensions or family functions.

   a. Roles of two adult family members

   b. Reproduction

   c. Communication patterns

   d. The provision of adequate economic support

   1. Structure
   2. Function

6. Using the following case study for data, list and then describe how this family is fulfilling each of the six basic family functions.

FAMILY CASE STUDY

Family Composition:

Name	Relationship	Age
Emma	Wife	40
Arthur	Husband	44
Danny	Son	17
Ronny	Son	14
Leonard	Son	11
Sammy	Son	7
Cindy	Daughter	5
Arlie	Son	4
Iris	Daughter	2

All the children appeared in good health and were dressed adequately. Arthur and Emma were rather short and obese.

The house was located in a suburban area, in a neighborhood full of children and pets. The house has three bedrooms, one-and-a-half bathrooms, attached garage, with small front and back yards. The interior is reasonably clean and orderly with bare floors and sparse furniture. The TV is in the front room; there are no pictures, books, or decorations.

This is a Mexican-American family. All the members are bilingual. Arthur completed the 10th grade and served in the Army. He has since worked as a maintenance man on refrigeration units of food trucks. He has medical insurance through his company.

Emma has been a housewife since her marriage at 19. She has devoted most of her energies to the family and their care. She spends time cooking and provides hearty, nutritious meals, although overabundant in carbohydrates.

The children are in school with the exception of Iris. They do passable work. The older two boys are involved in athletics, which is a source of pride for the parents.

This is the only marriage for Arthur and Emma. There has been significant marital discord the past 11 years.

From Emma's description of home life, she "wears the pants in the family." She describes her husband as a meek, passive man who takes no responsibility in the household. He brings home the check, eats and sleeps there. She states she finds him "sexually unattractive," difficult to be "close" to. Emma says she wants to be with her children but that she has no love for her husband.

Arthur says he works and makes a living. The house is a woman's responsibility which he has left to his wife.

Emma does all of the disciplining and is the parent children go to for permissions. Emma states that when Arthur tells the children to do something and they disobey, their excuse is they didn't think that he really meant it. The children verified that Emma does the greater part of the discipling and that when she is home, they really watch their behavior.

Emma prefers her children to her husband. They are the apparent reason the marriage holds together. She seems very fond of all her children, but she mentions Leonard and Iris the most. She seems to favor Leonard because other children tease him for being fat. She tries to give him special attention. She talks about Iris as being her baby.

Arthur appears to love all the children, but makes extra comments about the oldest sons. Arthur says his wife is a wonderful mother and good housekeeper but makes no comments about their personal relationship.

Danny and Ronny seem to pair because of their ages. Leonard and Iris prefer mother's company, while Sammy cares for and plays with Arlie. Cindy, age five, appears withdrawn and a loner.

STUDY ANSWERS

1. Both internal family dynamics (structure) and other internal dimensions (functions and subsystems). The systems interface with other systems and suprasystems, e.g., reference groups and wider society, which are also assessed.

2. b

3. a

4. d

5. 1. a
   2. b
   1. c
   2. d

6. *Affective function:* Not being adequately fulfilled for all family members. Minimal data on children, although mother seems quite involved and enjoys her children. Mother is feeling unfulfilled emotionally in her relationship with her husband. No concrete data on husband's feelings, although it appears he has withdrawn from family affectively.

   Family coping patterns: Spouse subsystem is nonfunctional. How does family cope with this situation? It appears that mother and children have formed an unhealthy coalition against husband-father and have shut him out of the family's life to a large extent. This would be termed emotional neglect, although active exploitation or scapegoating may also be occurring.

   Provision of physical necessities: Food: mother cooks and provides nutritional meals, although excessive carbohydrates; shelter: adequate home provided; clothing: family adequately dressed; health care: children appear in good health. Would need to assess further this area, as it is inadequately described.

   Reproductive function: Family has seven children. All living with the family.

   Socialization: Emma's central family concern is childrearing; father participates minimally in disciplining and guidance. Family actively fulfills this function via the mother. Social placement: Society will identify family as members of working class.

Economic function: Father employed and provides family with basic necessities for independent living.

Part I dealt with the basic information on the family, the major approaches used to analyze families, and the prime goals and germane roles of the family-centered nurse. The process of providing family health care and the family life cycle was also explored. From this broad perspective we now move into a specific framework for assessing families. The framework on which the assessment tool and process is built is the structural-functional approach, modified to meet the special needs of family health care. There are four basic areas subsumed under this comprehensive approach: (1) identifying data, (2) environmental data, (3) structural dimensions, and (4) family functions.

Chapter 8 covers the identifying and environmental data regarding the family. The four dimensions of family structure will be discussed in Chapters 9 to 12. Four of the most critical family functions (affective, coping patterns, socialization, and the health care) are elaborated on in Chapters 13 to 16. Chapter 17 deals exclusively with cultural theory and assessment. In each of the chapters, assessment areas related to and part of the broad assessment topic give sufficient detail, in terms of both theory and application, for collecting and interpreting assessment data pertaining to families in a multitude of settings and throughout the family's life cycle. The actual family assessment tool, along with a suggested care plan form, is included as Appendixes A and C. Appendix B presents a hypothetical family situation, which is followed by an analysis of the family in Appendix D.

II

FAMILY HEALTH ASSESSMENT

IDENTIFYING DATA

Composition of the Family

As with all assessment tools, it is important to begin by obtaining broad identifying information about the client (in this case the family).* As discussed in Chapter 3, during the initial home visit (or client contact in another setting) it is vital to attempt to meet the immediate needs of the family, coupled with getting to know the family and all its members. By completing the family composition roster, an excellent opportunity is afforded for learning about the family. Duvall says that with information about who lives in the home and their relationships, along with knowledge of the time (family life cycle and season, day, and hour) and the family's social and cultural status, one can generally predict what is going on in the family.[1] Beginning with family composition also lets the members know of your interest in the whole family, not just the individual for whom the visit was ostensibly made.

The nurse should obtain the following information:

Family name
Address
Telephone number
Family composition: In the form given in Fig. 8.1, the adult family members are recorded first, followed by the children in order of their birth beginning with the oldest. Include any other related or nonrelated members of household next. If there are extended family members or friends who act as family members, although not living in household, include them also at end of listing. The relationship of each family member, as well as birth date, birthplace, occupation, and education needs to be specified.

When working with a family whose structure is not that of the traditional nuclear family (father, mother, and children in the same household), it is customary to list the adult male first. If the family is a single-parent family, the missing parent is deleted or his or her name inserted with brackets placed around it. Second marriages, adoptions, and so on are included under the "relationship" column. The children's last names should also be included because of the large proportion of second marriages or serial unions.

Type of Family Form

After the composition of the family, it is helpful to include the "type of family form" which the family represents, as discussed in the latter part of Chapter 1.

---

* The discussion in this chapter correlates with and enlarges on the information contained in the Guidelines for Assessment and Care Plan for the Family (see Appendixes A and C).

Identifying and Environmental Data

LEARNING OBJECTIVES

1. Define and describe the following family identifying data, applying content to written case example:
   a. Composition of family.
   b. Type of family form.
   c. Religious and cultural (ethnic) orientation.
   d. Social class status, including occupational, income, and educational data.
   e. Social class mobility.
   f. Developmental history of family.
   g. Recreational activities.
2. Define and describe the following environmental data and apply content to written case example:
   a. Physical setting: home (characteristics, safety hazards, spatial adequacy, provision of privacy).
   b. Physical setting: Neighborhood and community, including geographic mobility patterns.
   c. Associations and transactions of the family with the community and their perception and feelings regarding their neighborhood and community.
   d. Family's support system.
3. Explicate territorial concept and apply to case example.
4. Discuss housing and the family's habitat relative to its effects on:
   a. Self-perception.
   b. Stress.
   c. Health.
   d. Life satisfaction.
5. Describe the impact crowding has on health.

Name (Last, First)	Sex	Relationship	Date/Place of birth	Occupation	Education
1. (father)					
2. (mother)					
3. (oldest child)					
4.					
5.					
6.					
7.					
8.					

FIGURE 8.1
Family composition form.

Noting the family form provides an encapsulated view of the family and its overall, larger structure.

Cultural or Ethnic Orientation

A family's cultural orientation or background may be by far the most pertinent variable in understanding the family's behavior, value system, and functions. Culture includes both racial and religious dimensions. The degree of influence the family's cultural background has on the family's life style and functions depends on the family's identity with its ethnic subculture. For example, does a particular family still identify with its Italian cultural heritage, or does it now see itself as being American? Putting the question this way seems to suggest that identifying with the old culture or new culture is a matter of choice. In many cases, however, we know that language, color, prejudice, and oppression make it impossible to assimilate successfully and find acceptance in the new culture. Moreover, this illustration is overly simplistic, since a person's cultural identification is not a matter of all or nothing. When we speak of acculturation or assimilation, all degrees of accommodating to the new culture exist.

Since understanding the family's cultural background is so critical in working with families, familial differences among two major ethnic groups are explored in Chapter 17, in addition to a discussion of acculturation. Chapter 12 on the family's value system will also help the family nurse look at cultural patterns, since family values are often a reflection of the value system of their reference group and the ethnic subculture with whom the family identifies, as well as wider society.

Degree of Acculturation

Acculturation refers to the assimilation process, that is, the replacement of the values, beliefs, practices of one's traditional culture by those of the dominant culture into which a family has moved or now resides. The assessment question posed here is, "To what extent has the family being assessed retained its ethnicity or cultural heritage?" Or posed in the reverse way, "To what extent has the family assimilated to the dominant white, Anglo-Saxon Protestant (WASP) value orientation?" Has the family recently migrated from another country or region and retained much ethnic-cultural tradition? Or has the family been in the area many years, retaining ethnic identification because of strong identification and/or residential patterns within a predominantly ethnic neighborhood? Obviously the family's degree of acculturation is more dependent on the amount and concentration of exposure to WASP culture and the meaningfulness of their ethnic background than to the time factor.

What are some of the signs which indicate that a family still retains traditional (ethnic) practices, values, and beliefs? Some of the important behavioral clues are as follows:

1. The family's friends are of the same ethnic group.
2. Family lives in an ethnically homogeneous neighborhood.
3. Religious, social, cultural, recreational, and/or educational activities are within the family's cultural group.
4. Dietary habits and dress are traditional.
5. Traditional family roles are carried out.
6. Home decorations, art, and other visual representations evidence the cultural background.
7. Native language is spoken exclusively or frequently in the home.
8. The territorial complex—the wider community the family frequents—is within the ethnic community primarily.
9. The family uses folk medicine or traditional healers, or perhaps a community health worker in whom the ethnic neighborhood has confidence.

Again, not all members of the family may have the same emotional ties to their ethnic background. The older person and parents who are in the life cycle stages of raising children are usually more traditional than the children and young adults without children.

Within immigrant groups the degree of acculturation into the new culture has generally increased with each succeeding generation. An illustration of this phenomenon is the Japanese acculturation pattern. The first generation Japanese-Americans, the Issei, who came here from Japan between 1890 and 1920, retained almost all of their former traditions. The second generation Japanese-Americans, the Nisei, occupied an intermediate position on the assimilation continuum, while the third generation, the Sansei, are quite Westernized. Interestingly enough, as with other groups, there is a resurgence of interest in ethnic "roots," particularly among the fourth generation Japanese-Americans, the Yonsei, with whom the learning of the Japanese language and culture has become increasingly popular.[2]

Religious Status

The family's religious practices should be noted, taking into account how individuals within the family differ in their religious beliefs and practices. How actively involved is the family in a particular church, temple, or other religious organization? Is the religious background of the family usual for family's ethnic and social class background? If not, some further stress may be or may have been experienced by the family. Take the case of a working-class Episcopalian black family that moves into a new community and finds there is only one Episcopalian church in the area, which has an upper-middle class membership. When this family joins the church they will probably experience some degree of social discomfort and alienation due to social class differences.

Social Class Status

Every society differentiates and ranks people, styles of life, automobiles, dress, and work in accordance with what it views as most valuable and important. No society is classless, and although Americans believe theirs is an open society with equal opportunity, where people can pull themselves up by their own boot straps, American society is stratified into classes. Status consciousness is present even among children who begin very early to recognize their "place" and also the "place" of others in their little world.

In our society we generally base social class status on the man's occupational status (and increasingly so on the woman's occupation and joint income level). Generally the work which is deemed to be of the greatest value to the society receives the greatest rewards, which include not only money, but also power, prestige, and autonomy. Income level and educational level

of parents are the other two criteria used generally in social class determination. And lastly, family background can also be a factor for determining social class status, especially among the upper classes.

Family life style, structural and functional characteristics, and associations with the external environment of home, neighborhood, and community vary tremendously from social class to social class. Partially this variance results from differences in preferences and perspectives. More importantly, these variations originate in the different conditions of and demands placed on the families of the several social classes. Social class probably more than any other factor exerts the greatest overall influence on family life, influencing our early socialization, the role expectations we hold, the values we stress, the types of behavior we consider acceptable or deviant, and the world experiences we have. A description of each of the social classes and a discussion of how the family's class position influences its life style and value system are given in Chapter 12. By identifying a family's social class we can better anticipate the family's resources and some of its stressors.

Since educational and occupational data were included along with the composition of the family, the only remaining information needed to evaluate social class is the family's economic status.

Economic Status

Economic status, for the purpose of social class determination, refers to the family's income level. Of course, asking how much the husband or wife earns can be an invasive question—since income is considered a private matter among most families. A specific question should be asked only if there is an important reason to do so, such as in determining eligibility for assistance or services. Questions relevant to this area include the following:

Who is (are) the breadwinner(s) of the family?
Does the family receive any supplementary funds or assistance? If so, from where, e.g., retirement fund, Social Security, food stamps?

From this information, plus information on occupations, one can estimate weekly or monthly income or ask a question regarding approximate income.

Does the family consider their income adequate? How do they see themselves managing financially?
What financial resources does the family or could the family have (for example, medical insurance, disability insurance, dental insurance, workman's compensation, food stamps, unemployment insurance, crippled children's services, reduced transportation fares)?

Geismar and La Sorte[3] developed criteria and descriptions for assessing the economically adequate, marginal, and inadequate family. Income which is sufficient to meet a family's needs is generally derived from the work of family members or from private sources such as pensions and support payments (nonpublic), while income derived partially from general relief or unemployment is generally marginal, unstable, or barely adequate. The family that is functioning inadequately in this area exhibits these characteristics: (1) income derived entirely from general relief because of failure or inability of adult(s) in the family to work; (2) income derived from welfare by fraudulent means; (3) amount of income so low or unstable that basic necessities are lacking. Families receiving income from programs such as Aid to the Totally Disabled, Aid to the Blind, Aid to Families of Dependent Children, and Old Age Assistance, although in most cases based on legitimate need, would fall under the marginal or inadequate criteria, since the level of funding is so low that basic necessities are barely or inadequately provided for.

One of the basic family functions is the provision of adequate economic support and allocation of resources. Hence not only income level should be estimated but also expenditures, focusing on the allocation of resources. Assessing expenditures, again a sensitive subject which should be discussed specifically only when needed, consists of asking about regular financial obligations: rent or mortgage payments, insurance, transportation costs or car payments, phone and utility bills, food expenses, and so on, as well as any special bills the family may have incurred.

Again paraphrasing Geismar and La Sorte's description of the economic levels of the family, adequate refers to monies spent on the basis of an understanding that finances are the responsibility of one or both of the parents. The family budgets and realistically manages expenditures. At the marginal level, there is disagreement and conflict over who controls income and expenditures; the family is unable to live within its means, and poor money management resulting in luxuries sometimes taking precedence over basic necessities. The poor money management, however, may or may not endanger the children's welfare. Very poor money management, however, involves impulsive spending and accumulation of excessive debts, and does result in the lack of providing for basic family needs.[4]

Social Class Mobility

Another family assessment area related to social class is social class mobility. This refers to vertical mobility upward or downward through the social class strata and is included here because a change in either di-

rection produces considerable stress. Holmes and Rahe, in their social readjustment scale, identify changes of position, status, or prestige, whether positive or negative, as stress producing.[5] Although upward mobility is seen as desirable by most persons, and does often result in new recognition and social prestige, it may also result in rejection and social isolation. The cohesiveness of the extended family most likely decreases, in addition to lower levels of family participation.[6] Interpersonal relationships and the degree of personal comfort are also often compromised.

In America, people expect a move upward as a natural state of affairs. Social mobility seems to be increasing recently but was probably never as widespread as generally believed.[7] Cavan reports as follows: "A number of studies indicate that about 30 percent of people occupy a different class position than that of their parents, as judged primarily by differences in the occupational rankings of the fathers and sons."[8] The remaining 70 percent of families remain in the same social class, and this stability of social class placement can be seen through a number of generations. Examples of the stability of social class status are found among upper-class families, where their wealth or prestige has continued through several generations. A similar continuity is also observed in the lower classes.[9] In the well-known social class study by Hollingshead, he showed that the lower-lower social class of "Elmstown" had held this position since before the Civil War.[10] Mobility occurs most frequently in the lower-middle and upper-lower classes. The majority of the vertical mobility in America has been upward, as evidenced by our growing middle class. In some cases, widespread mobility may result for entire communities or regions as a consequence, for instance, of a prolonged economic depression—producing downward mobility. This process occurred in some East Coast textile communities when the textile industry moved its plants to the South. At the other end of the continuum, the full employment and prosperity experienced generally in the 1960s may have carried many families upward.

Developmental History of the Family

The family's developmental history pertains to assessing the family's common and unique experiences, feelings, and perceptions as they progress through the family life cycle. It also includes assessing the parent's family of origin. Before completing this portion of family assessment, it is suggested that Chapter 5, Developmental Approach to Family Assessment, be read, since that chapter covers the family developmental tasks and common health concerns observed during each of the eight stages of the family's life cycle.

It may be more significant to elicit the developmental history from some families than others. Make sure the family you are working with is open to exploring their past and that your collecting historical data in any of the suggested areas has a meaningful purpose.

Developmental or historical data on a family can be gleaned by (1) asking about common experiences and tasks and how these were accomplished and perceived, and (2) asking about special or unique family problems or experiences. It may be important to learn about both common and unique past experiences. The latter include divorces, deaths in nuclear or extended family, separations due to illness or military service, unemployment, and so forth. Asking parents about their present and past relationships with their family of orientation and what life in the original family was like gives the family-centered nurse a better appreciation and understanding of the parents during their formative years.

In order to elicit a family history, Satir, in *Conjoint Family Therapy*, begins by having parents first talk about their own marital relationship, focusing on this relationship since the parents are the family architects. Satir and the parents, though including the children when appropriate, discuss the following areas:

First meeting of the couple, their relationship prior to marriage, and how they decided to get married.

Any obstacles to their marriage. Their responses to getting married.

Marriage without the children; how they established tasks and roles.

Picture of what life was like in both original family environments, including both parents' families of orientation.

Any other persons who live or have lived with the family.

Relationships with in-laws.

Description of each mate's parents and their relationship with them.

Plans for and arrival of each new child. Were children planned, what was the impact of the arrival of each child?

How much time does family spend together?

Daily routine of family life.[11]

Smoyak, in her nursing practice as a family therapist, stresses the significance of assessing the parents' respective families of orientation:

It is important to know how each present parent was reared and what lessons in childrearing were learned. How the two present parents put together their different backgrounds in childrearing is easier to understand when the background of each has been described. For instance, a German-Jew married to an English Protestant who live

as a nuclear unit produce a very different set of mutual expectations than do two Catholics ... Mexican-Americans living in an extended family.[12]

She also inquires into each parent's ordinal position among their siblings, quoting Toman's work on family constellation, which showed that this position greatly influences the type of interactions and relationships one is likely to have with others, as well as one's personality development.[13] For instance, Toman found that first-born children were more apt to be leaders than followers, while the reverse was more common among the last-born child.[14] Another point of inquiry related to the couple's families of origin involves the state of health and marriage of their own parents. Are they still alive, well, married, living together, residing nearby or geographically distant?[15]

Family Recreational Activities

Each family member has his or her own special leisure-time activities, depending on their individual needs and interests, age, and available time. In addition to individual needs, the family unit will also, hopefully, have regular family-centered activities in which all members can share, and enhance their life together. These activities may be religious, educational, recreational, civic, or cultural.

Recreation refers to activities apart from the obligations of work, family, and society to which the individual and family turn at will for either relaxation, diversion, self-development, or social participation.

Although recreation, as a basic family function, has in some ways declined in importance in the modern nuclear family, other factors are responsible for its continued significance as a family activity: longer paid vacations, shorter working hours, more three-day weekends, and greater accessibility to recreational facilities, at least for the more affluent social classes. Nye reports that there is considerable evidence that recreation is highly valued among families and that the spouses feel a sense of duty to provide for such activities for the family.[16] "Normatively it appears to be a shared role among the parents."[17]

Research on family recreation has focused on its effect on marital satisfaction. Gerson,[18] in studying college student couples, found a positive relationship between a number of leisure-time factors and marital satisfaction. West and Merriam[19] also found a positive correlation between outdoor recreation and family solidarity. Kelly concluded that the family is "a central social context of leisure.... The home is the most common locale and family members are the usual companions for most kinds of weekday, weekend and vacation leisure."[20]

Leisure activities are thus a vital aspect of marriage

and are probably not sufficiently underscored by family health workers. Kelly explains that

> leisure may be or become the most significant social area of marriage development.... Family counselors and those seeking to better understand their own family patterns may need to give greater attention to leisure satisfactions and expectations, to the opportunities and strains of parenthood, and to escalating standards for leisure companionship. Leisure is not necessarily secondary to task and role performance in assessing marriage viability or in developing approaches to marriage enhancement.[21]

Assessment Areas: Recreation

Suggested assessment areas pertaining to the family recreational or leisure-time activities include the following:

1. Identifying the family's activities—what types and how often do these activities occur?
2. Listing the leisure-time activities of family subsystems (spouse subsystem, parent–child subsystems, and sibling subsystems). Keeping the family subsystems strong and functioning effectively is crucial to family health. Thus recreational activities involving the subsystems should be counted as an important family strength.

ENVIRONMENTAL DATA

Housing: Family's Home

Provision of a healthy environment in the form of adequate shelter is an aspect of family functioning which is of special concern to the family-centered community nurse. Through home visits the nurse is able to observe the physical setting of the home and the particular arrangement of family life space, observations which otherwise would be impossible. Such assessment of the home environment provides a most valuable aid in understanding the family and its life cycle. Because it is their territory, the family behaves more naturally and comfortably, and one is able to assess more accurately the particular dimensions of a family's life.

Before describing actual assessment areas relative to the home environment, a review of some of the current literature on housing and its effect on families, as well as a review of the concept of territoriality and the impact of crowding on families, will be given.

Housing and Its Effects

The placement of houses and apartments in relation to one another and to the larger urban environment clearly influences family and social relationships. In particular, extremely poor housing conditions percep-

tibly, and adversely, influence behavior and attitudes.[22] The effects of housing and neighborhood can be seen in two major areas. First, there are psychological aspects which affect self-perception and life satisfaction; if these are negative, they can serve as stressors and illness-producing factors. Second are the effects of space—the house's state of repair, its facilities, and its arrangement. Such physical conditions may influence privacy, child-rearing practices, and housekeeping or study habits.

Psychological Effects: Self-Perception. Residents of deteriorating neighborhoods who resist being moved from one location to another make it plain that they do not view their surroundings with contempt. In fact, such neighborhoods may serve functions that are useful to residents, if only that of satisfying territorial need (see below), of having a place to call one's own. Since house and neighborhood are generally felt to be extensions of one's self, housing is usually a subject of highly charged emotional content, a matter of strong feeling. These feelings about one's habitat are significant factors in determining how individuals and family perceive themselves and are perceived by others. Thus, one evaluates his or her surroundings far from objectively. If one then calls a house a slum, the tenant is likely to hear that he or she is being called a slum dweller![23]

To the middle-class resident, the social elements that are involved in self-identification with his or her housing may be evident. The following questions are common to the process of deciding where to live: Who is accepted there? Are they my kind of people? Is it a step up or down? What will it do for me and my children? Whom shall I meet?

Hence living in poor housing influences self-evaluation and motivation. A good deal has been written about the pessimism that is common to the poor, their readiness to seize the present satisfaction and let the future care for itself, and their feeling that one is controlled *by* rather than in control *of* events. Although there is considerable variability in attitudes, not to say aspiration, among even the very poor, studies of families living in deteriorated neighborhoods make the same point: pessimism and passivity present the most difficult barriers to rehabilitating neighborhoods or relocating families. In any case, where vigorous effort has gone into the upgrading of neighborhoods, some families have improved their housing and, as a consequence, feel they have improved their situation and status.

Psychological Effects: Stress. It has been proposed that migration from a rural to an urban setting places "excessive adjustive burdens" on migrants. How housing affects families and individuals is a special form of the same general question, and stress has been suggested as the common denominator. That is, housing may affect behavior by contributing to or dissipating stress. Some people have more effective adjustive mechanisms than others—patently a factor that influences reactions.

Almost any characteristic of housing that negatively affects individuals may be interpreted as stressful—crowding, dilapidation, vermin infestations, or high noise levels are examples. Two further stressful factors are social isolation and inadequate space. There is some evidence that aged people who live alone are more likely to require psychiatric hospitalization than those living with families. Any environment which tends to isolate an individual from others offers a stress that will lead to distinguishable personality changes. It is significant that the amount of space per person and the way space is arranged to promote or interfere with privacy have been related to stress.[24]

Effects on Health. Substantial evidence links poor housing with poor health. It is well understood that the following diseases are correlated with poor housing:

1. Acute respiratory infections related to the multiple use of toilet and water facilities, inadequate heating or ventilation, and inadequate and crowded sleeping arrangements.
2. Certain infectious diseases of childhood.
3. Minor digestive diseases and enteritis, related to poor facilities for the cold storage of food and to inadequate washing and toilet facilities and sharing of food and drink.
4. Injuries resulting from home accidents related to crowded or inadequate kitchens, poor electrical wiring, and poorly lighted and unstable stairs.
5. Infectious and noninfectious diseases of the skin related to crowding and shared or inadequate facilities for washing.

Another disease that results from poor housing is the lead poisoning in children who eat scaling paint.[25] The large number of family pets in homes today also causes health problems, either directly of animal bites or through animal-transmitted infections (salmonella from dogs, psittacosis from pet birds, fleas from dogs and cats, allergies—eczema and asthma—from the fur of hairy pets).

Life Satisfaction. In 1976 Campbell and co-workers found that in spite of the conflicting findings in this area, no clear association could be found between family satisfaction and the kind of housing, neighborhood, and/or community in which people lived.[26] However, Chilman reported that the quality of interpersonal family relationships, as perceived by both men and women, was the central, pervasive factor in overall satisfaction with life.[27] In considering these conflicting findings, one must remember that family housing is only one area on the total list of family needs, especially among the poor. Poverty, racism, mental and physical illness and handicaps, family disorganization, unemployment, and poor community services are some of the other pressing family needs demanding attention.

Territoriality

We recognize that animals, as part of their innate repertoire of behaviors, lay claim to a specific area and defend this area against intruders, while other animals in turn tend to respect this claim. A similar type of instinctual characteristic applies to man and family. The human desire to possess and occupy specified areas is very pervasive, even though overt expression of infringement by others is attenuated by socialization. It has been noted that the most sacred prerogative in Western civilization is that of ownership of private property and especially of the individual home.

The first home visit by a student community health nurse may therefore seem quite threatening to him or her partially due to the feeling of intruding into someone's "territory." Families may also feel aggression and/or hostility regarding this intrusion, especially when health workers have not been specifically invited into the home.

Home territory is an area where the family has relatively much more freedom of behavior and a sense of control and power over both the area and its members. When a family member leaves home, personal space becomes important. Stea defines personal space as a small circle in physical space, with the individual in its center and a culturally determined radius around the individual.[28] The following territorial typology has been developed by Stea.[29]

1. *Unit.* The territorial unit is the smallest component. The person lives in this part of the total territory. Regardless of who is the legal owner, the individual considers that this space is *his* or *hers.* For example, a child may consider a desk, dresser drawer, chair, bed to be his or her own.
2. *Cluster.* The territorial cluster is peripheral to the unit, enclosing those people frequently visited and/or the paths taken to reach them. Most families and individuals will stay within their territorial cluster when leaving home territory.
3. *Complex.* This is the largest territorial space. It consists of units and clusters and involves the neighborhoods and communities where the family moves and relates to others.

In public health, one will often observe families who are constricted in their movement due to feelings of fear, discomfort, and/or poverty. They are essentially home-bound and uncomfortable moving from their neighborhood. Other families may be much more at ease moving through a wider geographic complex. The territorial complex of a family may in part be a function of income, physical mobility, cultural or personal values, or a result of socialization. In the Los Angeles area, for example, there are many Mexican nationals who are more comfortable visiting Mexico and receiving health care there than attending a local Anglo health agency.

Within families there are both spatial (physical) and behavioral dimensions of territoriality. The feelings of belonging and cohesiveness among family members make up the behavioral component, while the actual physical space of home, yard, family name and address, and frequently visited community systems—school, work, shopping centers, churches, and community agencies with which the family interacts—are the spatial aspects of territoriality.[30]

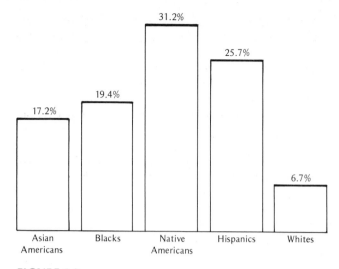

FIGURE 8.2
Crowded housing conditions by ethnic/racial group (percent of households with more than one person per room) for 1970. *(From: United States Department of Health, Education, and Welfare, Health Resources Administration: Health of the Disadvantaged Chartbook, September 1977. Washington D.C., Government Printing Office).*

Impact of Crowding

In 1970 Schorr summarized the results of "crowding studies" and commented that fatigue and too little sleep may be consequences of seriously inadequate, crowded housing. The effect of crowding on intrafamily friction has also been observed in various connections. One of the results of seriously inadequate space appears very often to be that family members spend their time outside the home. This tendency may be a particularly serious matter in relation to children. It has been observed that these children do not study sufficiently and are not within reach of parental control.[31]

In 1976 a well-controlled study analyzing the impact of crowding on health was undertaken by Booth and Cowell. They concluded that crowded household and neighborhood conditions generally have little or no effect on people's health,[32] although some types of crowding may have a small adverse affect on health under certain conditions.[33]

From Figure 8.2 it can be seen that the percent of racial and ethnic minorities who live in crowded conditions in 1970 was more than three times that of whites.

Assessment Areas: Home

1. Describe the dwelling type (home, apartment, or rooming house). Does family own or rent their home?
2. Describe the home's condition (both the interior and exterior of house). House interior would include number of rooms and types of rooms (living room, bedrooms, etc.), their use, and how they are furnished. What is the condition and adequacy of the furniture? Is there adequate heating, ventilation, and lighting? Are the floors, stairs, railings, and other structures in good repair?
3. In kitchen, observe water supply, sanitation, and the adequacy of refrigeration.
4. In bathrooms, observe sanitation, water supply, toilet facilities, presence of towels and soap.
5. Assess the sleeping arrangements in the house. Are they adequate for family members, considering their age, relationships, and special needs?
6. Observe for infestations of vermin (interior especially).
7. Assess family's subjective feelings about home. Does the family consider its home adequate for its needs?
8. Identify the family's territorial unit.
9. Evaluate the privacy arrangements and how the family feels about the adequacy of their privacy.

Privacy functions to protect and maintain an individual's need for personal autonomy; to serve as an emotional release; and to provide an opportunity for self-appraisal and protected communication. Having one's own room, bed, possessions, clothes, toys, and pets is an asset. Privacy for an adolescent is especially significant in assisting him or her to achieve the developmental needs of independence, and marital privacy is critical in most families.

Homes reflect the influence of a family's life style,

culture, interests, values, and income, and an evaluation of the degree of privacy and living space, or lack of privacy, may clearly suggest stress level. Territorial assignments, too, may indicate the dominance or the subordination of family members. In a healthy state, a family will attempt to create a sheltered, protective, and satisfying environment.

Safety Appraisal of Home

One of the most valuable assessment areas relative to the home is the assessment of safety conditions and potential or real hazards, both inside and outside the house. This assessment forms the basis for the suggestions of appropriate safety measures.

Home accidents kill about 27,000 and injure more than 4.2 million persons in the United States each year. Of the above deaths, 9,800 result after falls; 5,700 result from fires; and 2,500 are the consequence of poisoning. Furthermore, home accidents kill more children between the ages of 1 and 14 years than all the next six causes of death combined. Nearly all of these deaths and injuries could be prevented by proper protection and safety education.[34]

The following are some of the safety education tips that we should be sharing with families after our initial assessment.

1. How to prevent falls by: arranging furniture to avoid obstacles; installing handrails on all stairs; placing cords for electrical equipment away from walking areas; having adequate lighting for all traffic areas, especially the stairs; keeping scatter rugs away from head and foot of stairs; installing handrails for shower and bathtub; using nonskid mats for bathtub and bathroom floor; and placing lights so that they can be turned on from bed and groping in dark can be avoided.
2. How to prevent fires by: removing rubbish like old newspapers, wastebaskets, trash cans; never emptying ashtrays or tossing matches into wastebaskets unless one is sure they are out; never smoking in bed; and checking the chimney, fireplace and furnace and keeping safe from fire dangers.
3. How to avoid lifting accidents by: using good body mechanics in lifting, reaching, and carrying heavy items.
4. How to avoid poisoning accidents: most poisonings are due to carelessness, so keep medicines locked and away from food if small children are in family; give medicine only as prescribed (never give leftovers to other family members); keep medicines in their original containers (label contains vital information); make sure medicine bottles have safety caps; and store and use

household cleaners with the utmost care (they can be killers if swallowed by children).

5. Make sure the house is tailored to the safety needs of the age(s) of the children and adults in family. Both the very young and the old have special safety needs. The very young, for instance infants, should never be left unattended on table or in tub and should be kept away from stove. The older person requires excellent lighting, handgrips in bathroom (by toilet, shower, or bath), and stairs that have nonskid surfaces and good, sturdy handrails.[35]
6. Last, but not least, point out to families that they should have an emergency plan, so that if an emergency does arise, they will be fully prepared. This includes posting a list of important telephone numbers on a wall by the phone; keeping a first-aid chart accessible and becoming familiar with its instructions; and having on hand in the medicine cabinet the items needed to treat common emergencies.

Physical Setting: The Neighborhood and Community

The neighborhood and community in which the family lives exerts a tremendous influence on the family. Using the social systems and structural-functional frameworks for assessing families, the family nurse needs to examine "the family and its universe." Its universe consists of the inner and outer environments of the family. The outer environment includes the territorial concepts previously described. The territorial unit includes the small "home" circle, while territorial cluster and complex pertain to the family's neighborhood and community.

Neighborhood Effects on Families

Most researchers, in describing the effects of neighborhood on families, have looked at the type of social interaction which occurs in different types of neighborhoods. Substantial social and economic homogeneity has existed in most of the communities that have been studied. Since the families' behavior patterns, values, and interests are alike, they naturally tend to form friendships with one another. Homogeneity is found to be more significant in creating a large number of friendships than is proximity.[36]

In working-class neighborhoods, family membership is concentrated in the locality, and the most active ties are with other members of the family. Proximity makes for frequent contacts with relatives and other neighbors, casually in passing and less casually on the sidewalk or in the corner tavern or shop. Neighbors tend to be deeply involved in one another's family life.

There is considerable attachment to the place itself. Relationships are identified with locality.

Working-class neighborhoods have a mood of warmth, security, and identity. It is evident that when these working-class families move, many find it difficult to maintain their neighbor- and extended family-centered patterns of relationships. This necessitates a complex series of adjustments by the family.[37]

It has been noted that urban communities have drastically different effects on individuals and families than do rural areas. Rural areas lend themselves to more personalized social contact, while in urban areas social contact is more impersonal and inhibited.

In summarizing social interaction patterns in communities and neighborhoods, it has been consistently found that social class homogeneity, and frequently age, ethnic, racial, and religious similarity, fosters social interaction, whereas social class disparity discourages it. People want to live and mix with their neighbors (other families) who share the same, or similar, values and life styles.[38]

Assessment Areas: Neighborhood and Community

1. What are the level and physical characteristics of the immediate neighborhood and the larger community?
    Types of dwellings (residential, industrial, combined residential and light industry, agrarian).
    Condition of dwellings and streets (well kept up, deteriorating, dilapidated, being revitalized).
    Sanitation of streets and home (clean, trash and garbage collected, etc.).
    Incidence of crime in neighborhood or other safety problems.
    Presence and types of industry in neighborhood (air or noise pollution problems?).
2. What are the demographic characteristics of the neighborhood and community?
    Social class and ethnic characteristics of residents.
    Occupations and interests of families.
    Density of population.
3. What health and other basic services and facilities are available in neighborhood and community?
    Marketing (food, clothing, drug stores, etc.).
    Health agencies.
    Social service agencies (welfare, counseling, employment).
    Family's church or temple.
    Schools. What is the accessibility and condition of the neighborhood school? Are there busing and integration conflicts which affect the family?
    Recreational.
    Availability of public transportation. How accessible (in terms of distance, suitability, and hours) are these services and facilities to family?

4. How long has the family lived there? What has been their history of geographic mobility? From where did they move or migrate?
    Many middle-class Americans have few geographic roots and move from city to city and region to region as their jobs and personal preferences dictate. Mobility is highest among young adults and at middle-income levels. Hence their support systems within the community are lacking. Families of migrating workers are also on the move constantly.
5. What is the incidence of crime in the neighborhood and community? Are there serious safety problems?
    The rates of certain crimes—robbery, aggravated assault, larceny (pickpocketing), and purse snatching—are much more frequent problems for persons over 65 years of age. More than 60 percent of the elderly live in metropolitan areas, and most of these reside in the central city. For cultural, emotional, and economic reasons, many of the elderly have lived in the same areas for decades. Many cannot afford alternative housing, and they are often dependent on public transportation. Consequently, these urban elderly are close to those most likely to victimize them—the unemployed, drug addicts, and teenage school dropouts.
    The psychological impact of fear of crime is very great. The 1974 Louis Harris and Associates national survey of the problems of the elderly found that they rank crime as their most serious problem—above health, money, and loneliness. Persons with low income and the black elderly were found to experience a higher rate of crime than the nonpoor white oldster.[39]

Associations and Transactions of Family with the Community

Healthy families are those who are active and reach out in self-initiating ways to relate to various community groups.[40] Hence the family that is functioning in a healthy way perceives itself as being related to and part of the larger community. Part of a family's successful coping is its ability to secure compliance from the environment, meaning that within the community the family is able to seek out, receive, and/or accept the appropriate resources to meet their needs for food, services, and information.[41] Passive acceptance of community services, however delivered, may be an indication of an isolated, estranged family or a family functioning on a much lower level of health.

Assessment Areas: Community Associations

1. *Who* in family uses *what* community services or is known to which agencies? For example, the family with school-age children might be involved with

public school system, church group, the welfare department, or scouting organization.

2. How frequently or to what extent do they use these services or facilities?

3. What is the family's territorial cluster and complex?

4. Is the family aware of community services relevant to their needs, such as transportation? Is the family aware of availability of lower transportation fees (monthly card, discount cards for transportation for children and senior citizens) and direct route to health clinics and community resources?

5. How does family feel about groups or persons from whom it receives assistance or with whom it relates? Assess the family's perceptions and feelings regarding association with above community groups and agencies. If the experiences in using community or the neighborhood agencies have been positive, these are resources which can be used again and with greater success or use.

6. How does the family view the community? For example, is it a community where the family is worried about having children play outside during the day because of high crime and personal attack rate in the neighborhood? Satisfaction with neighborhood and community have been found to be closely associated with satisfaction with life in general.[42] It is also true that expectations of neighborhood and communities by people differ, depending on social class status: the higher the social class, the greater the expectations of the community.[43] These same differences in expectations are noted in all community agencies. The poor demand little, while the affluent have high demands and expectations. The lower expectations are correlated with and result from feelings of powerlessness and fatalism.

Social Support Systems

"The provisions of support systems are the powerful means people have found for maintaining health, despite the pressures of society, and nurses can strengthen and augment their care by understanding support systems."[44] A support system for the family refers to all the family and family members' friends and all helping persons who stand ready to serve the family, and the linkages or relationships among those people. They assist by providing both emotional support and task-oriented assistance.[45] More detail on support systems is included in Chapter 16.

Assessment Questions: Social Support Systems

Does the family have meaningful ties with friends, relatives, social groups which provide satisfaction and assistance when needed?

Who are they and what is the nature of their relationship?

Or does the family have little or no contacts with neighbors, relatives, social groups and is dissatisfied or hostile toward community?

Hogue suggests that these types of questions be asked to elicit information on the family's support system. She says that it is more acceptable with clients to move from life events already identified and ask:

"Who helps you with . . . ?" "If you had any problems about . . . who would you talk to, get help from?" Asking general, then more specific questions is helpful. For example, "Who helped you through retiring from your job?" (general), "Who or what kind of help have you had with the financial concerns most people have when they retire?" (specific). Another useful question is, "Who has helped you through tough situations in the past?"[46]

REFERENCES

1. Duvall E: Marriage and Family Development. Philadelphia, Lippincott, 1977, p 137
2. Peterson W: Japanese Americans. New York, Random House, 1971, pp 196–210
3. Geismar LL, La Sorte B: Understanding the Multiproblem Family. New York, Association Press, 1964, p 216
4. Ibid., p 217
5. Holmes TH, Rahe RH: The social readjustment rating scale. J Psychosom Res 11:213, 1967
6. Eshleman JR: The Family: An Introduction. Boston, Allyn and Bacon, 1974, p 273
7. Ibid.
8. Cavan RS: The American Family. New York, Crowell, 1969, p 181
9. Ibid.
10. Hollingshead AB: Elmstown's Youth. New York, Wiley, 1949
11. Satir V: Conjoint Family Therapy. Palo Alto, Calif, Science and Behavior Books, 1967, pp 115–135
12. Smoyak S: Introducing families to family therapy. In Smoyak S (ed): The Psychiatric Nurse as a Family Therapist. New York, Wiley, 1975, p 8
13. Ibid.
14. Toman W: Family Constellation. New York, Springer, 1961
15. Smoyak, op. cit., p 9
16. Carlsen J: The recreational role. In Nye FI (ed): Role Structure and Analysis of the Family, Vol 24. Beverly Hills, Calif, Sage Publications, 1976, p 136
17. Ibid., p 146
18. Gerson WM: Leisure and marital satisfaction of college married couples. Marriage and Family Living. 22:360–361, 1960.
19. West P, Merriam LE: Camping and cohesiveness: A soci-

ological study of the effect of outdoor recreation on family solidarity. Minnesota Forestry Research Notes 201, 1969

20. Kelly JR: Family leisure in three communities. J Leisure Res 10(1):47–48, 1978

21. *Ibid.,* pp 59–60

22. Schorr AL: Housing and its effects. In Proshansky HM, et al (eds): Environmental Psychology. New York, Holt, Rinehart, and Winston, 1970, p 320

23. *Ibid.,* pp 320–321

24. *Ibid.,* p 322

25. *Ibid.,* pp 322–323

26. Campbell A, et al: The Quality of American Life. New York, Russell Sage, 1976

27. Chilman CS: Habitat and American families: A social-psychological overview. Family Coordinator, April, 1978, p 106

28. Stea D: Space, territory, and human movement. Landscape, Autumn, 1965, p 14

29. Stea D: Space, territory and human movements. In Proshansky HM et al: Environmental Psychology. New York, Holt, Rinehart, and Winston, 1970, pp 37–42

30. Anderson RE, Carter IE: Human Behavior in the Social Environment. Chicago, Aldine, 1974, pp 108–110

31. Schorr, *op. cit.,* pp 324–328

32. Booth A, Cowell J: Crowding and health. J Health Soc Behav 17:218, September, 1976

33. *Ibid.,* p 216

34. Bete C: Don't Worry About Home Accidents. Greenfield, Mass, Channing Bete Co., 1976, pp 2–3

35. *Ibid.,* pp 1–15

36. Schorr, *op. cit.,* p 329

37. *Ibid.,* pp 329–330

38. Chilman, *op. cit.,* p 108

39. Mallinchak AA, Wright D: Older Americans and crime: The scope of victimization. Aging 281–282, March–April 1978, p 16

40. Lewis JM: No Single Thread. New York, Brunner, 1976, p 209

41. Hall J, Weaver B: Crisis: A conceptual approach to family nursing. In Hall J, Weaver B: Nursing of Families in Crisis. Philadelphia, Lippincott, 1974, p 5

42. Chilman, *op. cit.,* p 107

43. Rainwater L: Fear and house as haven in the lower class. In Gutman R (ed): People and Buildings. New York, Basic Books, 1972

44. Hogue CC: Support systems for health promotion. In Hall J, Weaver B: Distributive Nursing Practice: A Systems Approach to Community Health. Philadelphia, Lippincott, 1977, p 67

45. Caplan G: Support Systems and Community Mental Health. New York, Behavioral Publications, 1974

46. Hogue, *op. cit.,* p 77

STUDY QUESTIONS

1. "Housing affects a person's self-perception." Discuss in what way this occurs.

2. Housing may affect behavior by contributing to or dissipating stress. Several aspects of housing have been identified as frequently stress producing. Name four.

3. Substantial evidence of linkage between extremely poor housing and physical health exists. Identify three health problems associated with poor housing.

Choose the correct answers to the following questions.

4. Choose the correct qualification(s) in relation to the statement, "Satisfaction influences housing."
   a. Satisfaction is related to where the person lived previously and is living presently.
   b. Satisfaction is linked with "practicality of the home."
   c. General life satisfaction is positively correlated with satisfaction with one's housing arrangements.

5. Which effect(s) of severe crowding have been described?
   a. Increased intrafamilial tension.
   b. Too little sleep.
   c. Fatigue.
   d. Excessive amount of time spent inside home for children of all age groups.

6. Social interaction in neighborhoods is *more* a function of:
   a. Physical proximity rather than homogeneity.
   b. Homogeneity rather than physical proximity.
   c. Satisfaction with community and neighborhood rather than dissatisfaction with habitat.

Are the following statements True *or* False?

7. Where families live close to each other in working-class neighborhoods, the most active social ties are with other members of the family.

8. In working-class neighborhoods there is considerable attachment to the neighborhood itself.

9. Working-class neighborhoods have been described as being warm and as providing security and identity.

10. Territoriality as a concept refers to a person's possession of physical land and the resources on that land.

11. Territorial complex is defined as the person's exclusive and private space at home or in the work setting.

12. A family that displays a wide and dynamic territorial complex is one that feels comfortable relating to the wider community.

13. Please read the following case study and answer the study questions following this hypothetical case.

FAMILY CASE STUDY

One year ago, the Juarez family moved to Los Angeles from their birthplace, a small agricultural area in northern Mexico. The husband and wife both worked as migrant workers on a large cooperative farm in Mexico and stated life was "hard" (basic necessities—food and shelter—were a struggle to obtain). Mr.J., age 30, and Mrs.J., age 25, now live with their three children, Maria, age 8, José, age 6, and Pedro, age 5, in an older small wooden house in a low-income Mexican-American district in Los Angeles. The district has a paucity of health and social services, although there is a market and shopping center within walking distance.

Their housing is minimally adequate. There are two bedrooms, with parents sleeping in the larger bedroom, two boys sharing the other, and Maria sleeping on a cot in small room off the kitchen. The living room is small, with two chairs. The family owns a large old-fashioned radio, an older stove, a refrigerator, and washing machine. The rooms are clean, have no carpeting, few lights, and electrical wall heating in living room and hallway which is minimal, but functions. The electric wall heater had a protective screen which has been torn off.

Since the family arrived they have pretty much stayed within their immediate vicinity. Mr. J. is employed in a steady job as a dishwasher for a local Mexican restaurant. Mrs. J. has a part-time janitorial job in a small business nearby.

Because both parents speak very little English and are embarrassed because they did not go beyond the third grade, they have not been to school to talk with the teachers, although the children appear to be having learning problems. The parents and children belong to no community groups except for attending mass at the Spanish-speaking Catholic church in their neighborhood. They have no family recreational activities, except that Mrs. J. occasionally takes the children to a neighborhood park.

In spite of isolation from their extended family, which still resides in Mexico, and their language barrier, they like the community, feel they are starting to get ahead, and that the neighborhood is friendly and its people helpful. They are, however, worried about their children's associations (are they associating with "good" children?) and with the high crime rate in the neighborhood.

Only a limited amount of information was gained about the family's history. Mr. and Mrs. J. were neighbors as children and Mrs. J.'s brother and her husband were friends. Both families felt they would be happy together, so they married when Mr. J. was 20 and she was 15. Maria was conceived six months later; both parents were very pleased. Each new child was positively accepted as a natural part of the family life. They seem to be quite content in their relationship together, with well-delineated (traditional) roles and functions. Mrs. J. is in the home except for her part-time work; Mr. J. is the breadwinner and "leader" of the family.

Describe the identifying data and appropriate information under these broad headings from the family case study cited.

Identifying Data

13.1   Composition of family.
13.2   Type of family form.
13.3   Religious and cultural orientation.
13.4   Social class status.
13.5   Social class mobility.
13.6   Developmental history of family.
13.7   Recreational activities.

Environmental Data

13.8   Home.
13.9   Neighborhood and community, including geographic mobility.
13.10   Associations and transactions of family with community.
13.11   Family's perceptions and feelings about neighborhood and community.
13.12   Family's support system.
13.13   Family's territorial hierarchy.

STUDY ANSWERS

1. Housing is the symbol of status, of achievement, and of social acceptance. It controls, to a large extent, the way in which the individual and family perceives himself/itself and is perceived by others.

2. a. Crowding.
    b. Dilapidation.
    c. Cockroaches, insect infestation.
    d. High noise level.

Also acceptable answers:

e. Social isolation.

f. Inadequate space (inadequate internal space of home and arrangement of space in home).

3. a. Acute respiratory infections.

b. Certain infectious childhood diseases.

c. Infectious gastrointestinal diseases.

Also acceptable:

d. Home accidents.

e. Infectious and noninfectious skin diseases.

4. c   9. True

5. a, b, and c   10. False

6. b   11. False

7. True   12. True

8. True

Identifying Data—

13.1 Composition of family:

Name	Sex	Relationship	Date/Place of Birth	Occupation	Education
Juarez, Mr.	M	Husband/father	1948 Mexico	Dishwasher (full-time)	3rd grade (Mexico)
Juarez, Mrs.	F	Wife/mother	1953 Mexico	Janitorial work (part-time)	3rd grade (Mexico)
Juarez, Maria	F	Daughter	1970 Mexico	Student	?
Juarez, Jose	M	Son	1972 Mexico	Student	?
Juarez, Pedro	M	Son	1973 Mexico	Student	?

13.2 Type of family form: nuclear.

13.3 Religious and cultural orientation: Religion—Roman Catholic; attend mass regularly. Cultural—Ethnicity is Mexican. Family is not acculturated to WASP culture; evidence—stay within small ethnically based neighborhood territorial complex. Language is Spanish. Family has no community association except for Spanish-speaking Catholic church. Live within Mexican-American neighborhood; friendly with neighbors. Couple has traditional family structure (patriarchal).

13.4 Social class status: Upper-lower social class. Economically independent. Both parents work in unskilled jobs. Father is primary breadwinner. Parents' education limited to third grade. Income very marginal, but steady work.

13.5 Social class mobility: Have moved upward from state of dire poverty, where basic necessities—food and shelter—were difficult to obtain to upper-lower class, where family not only has adequate food, but has rented house and both parents have jobs. They are still poor, but relative to their past they have moved upward.

13.6 Developmental history of family: Parents were neighbors as children and their families encouraged their marriage. Early marriage (husband was 20; wife 15). They conceived first child six months after marriage and felt positive about pregnancy and birth. All of the children were welcomed additions to the family; they were seen as a natural event in family life. Marital relationship—both partners seem content. Family roles are well-delineated along traditional lines.

13.7 Recreational activities: Very limited. The mother occasionally takes children to the neighborhood park. No books or toys seen.

13.8 Home: Noted to be "minimally adequate." Two-bedroom, old, small wooden house; no carpeting, paucity of furniture, clean. Have a stove, refrigerator, washing machine, and radio. Heating is adequate (electric wall heating). Only unsafe condition mentioned was screen off electric wall heater. Inadequate lighting may be safety problem.

Types of privacy available: Parents share one bedroom. Have privacy. Boys share another bedroom. Maria does not have the privacy she needs nor a place of her own to play. Family may not perceive themselves as being crowded, since former housing was probably much less spacious.

13.9 Neighborhood and community: Neighborhood is low-income Mexican-American district in Los Angeles. Neighborhood is part of wider Los Angeles community (a large metropolitan, heterogeneous city).

Geographic mobility: Moved one year ago from northern agrarian area in Mexico to the Los Angeles area.

13.10 Association and transactions with community: No association in community except children in school and family attends mass at local Spanish-speaking Catholic church.

13.11 Family's perceptions and feelings about the community: "Neighbors have been friendly." Family likes community, although worried about childrens' friends and high crime rate.

13.12 Family's support system: Each other (nuclear family members). May have persons at church or neighbors who serve as supports; however, no information available in this area.

13.13 Family's territorial hierarchy: Territorial units were not mentioned. Territorial clusters—the family; no close social relationships, extended family, or pathways mentioned. Territorial complex—the immediate Mexican-American neighborhood. They do not journey from this neighborhood to any extent. Do not associate with community groups other than Spanish-speaking church.

Before beginning to discuss the areas within family structure and how they are assessed, it is helpful to look at the larger picture, i.e., the family system structurally and functionally, and to identify the components subsumed under the structural and the functional dimensions. The structural–functional approach analyzes the family's structural characteristics, i.e., the arrangement of the parts that form the whole, and the functions which the family performs for society and its subsystems. The structure of the family refers to how the family is organized, the manner in which the units are arranged, and how they relate to each other. The four basic structural dimensions of the family elaborated on in this text are (1) role structure; (2) power structure; (3) communication patterns; and (4) value system. These elements are all intimately interrelated and interdependent. Because the family is a social system, there is continual interaction and feedback between its internal and external environments. A change in one part of the family system is generally followed by a compensatory change in the other internal structural dimensions. Hence, although these dimensions are not separable in real life, they will be individually dealt with in the text for heuristic purposes. The family system may be conceptualized as being structurally organized as shown in Fig. 9.1.

In addition to having an organized scheme, i.e., structure, the family must have "system" functions—its reasons for being. Family structure or organization is ultimately evaluated by how well the family is able to fulfill its general functions (the goals important to its members and society). The family's structure, especially its communication structure, serves to facilitate the achievement of family functions, since the conservation and allocation of resources is a prime task for the family structure to handle.

The systems approach to family analysis, as described in Chapter 6, will be used as the organizing framework for this chapter. Four basic sections are included here: elements of communication, functional communication, dysfunctional communication patterns, and assessment questions.

Families function to meet both societal needs and the needs of their family members. One of the prime tasks the family assumes relative to assisting its members to grow and become socialized is to provide the nurturing environment in which they may develop self-esteem. Clear and functional communication among family members is the crucial vehicle through which the necessary feelings regarding self-worth develop and become internalized.

Chapter 9 was coauthored by De Ann Young, R.N., M.S., Associate Professor, Department of Nursing, California State University, Los Angeles, Los Angeles, California and Barbara E. Bailey, R.N., M.S., Instructor, Department of Nursing, California State University, Los Angeles, Los Angeles, California, and Marilyn Friedman.

9

Family Communication Patterns

LEARNING OBJECTIVES

1. Define the following information-processing terms: information, channels, and negative feedback.
2. Identify the content and instructional levels of messages.
3. Compare the effects of underloading and overloading of channels.
4. Compare the effects of loose and tight negative feedback.
5. Describe the effects of overflow and underflow of information in boundary maintenance.
6. Discuss briefly the four basic components of functional communication.
7. Name the four primary characteristics of the functional sender.
8. Describe the manner in which listening, feedback, and validation facilitate the receiver's comprehension and response to a message.
9. Give specific illustrations of the use of assumptions, unclear expressions of feelings, judgmental expressions, inability to define needs, and incongruent communication.
10. Given a family case example, utilize the assessment questions included in this chapter to assess family communication patterns.

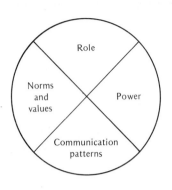

FIGURE 9.1
The structural dimensions of the family.

Satir aptly describes the importance of communication:

> I see communication as a huge umbrella that covers and affects all that goes on between human beings. Once a human being has arrived on this earth, *communication is the largest single factor determining what kinds of relationships he makes with others and what happens to him in the world about him.*[1]

ELEMENTS OF COMMUNICATION

As a consequence of making use of a general systems framework, family communication patterns will be treated here as an aspect of the broader concept of information processing. According to Miller,[2] information is the degree of freedom that exists in a given situation to choose among various units that contain enough energy or matter to enable a person to make a decision. Thus in our focal system, information passing from one member of a family to the other is used to make either present or future decisions in relationships with others. Communication is then defined in this chapter as the processing of information. Within the family it is a key element in the fulfillment of family functions, as well as a critical vehicle in binding the subsystems together to form a cohesive whole and maintain the entire system.

In the language of information processing, communication entails a sender, a channel, a receiver, and some interaction of the sender and the receiver. The sender is the person who is attempting to transmit a message to another person; the receiver is the target of the sender's message; channels are the routes of the message. They extend from the cognitions (the thoughts) of the sender, through space, to the cognitions of the receiver. Interaction is a broader term referring to the sending and receiving of messages, including the response the message causes in the receiver *and* the sender. Interaction encompasses the dy-

namic, constantly changing process of communication between people.

Information is carried on "markers," which may be words, gestures, body posture, or shared symbols.[3] The manner in which the markers are sent adds meaning and significance to the message for the sender and/or the receiver. Meaning may add or decrease security or anxiety, clarify or cloud issues being discussed.

Level of Communication

Messages always contain two levels of communication: content and instruction.[4] Content is the literal definition or what actually is being said (verbal message), while instruction or "metamessage" conveys the intent of the message.[5] The content of a message may be a simple statement, but the metamessage or instruction depends on variables such as emotion, intent, and context, and may be expressed nonverbally by the rate and flow of speech, gestures, body position, and tone of voice. If "I am bored" is whispered in a theater to another member of the family, it may be a comment on the quality of the movie. If the "I am bored" message is sent in an emphatic manner during prolonged family discussion, the meaning differs. In this instance, it probably signifies anger, frustration, and heightened emotionality. Hence emotion, intent, and context have produced very different meanings although coming from the identical content. In the presence of disparity between the two levels of communication, the receiver usually "tunes in" more to the instructional level.

Channels of Communication

Channels of information flow are the routes that information may take to reach the receiver. In the family, these involve the flow of information between the various sets of relationships. Families have usual channels of information flow, which reveal the family power structure, the closeness of relationships, family roles, and the popularity of individuals within the family. The popularity or centrality of individual members is indicated by a convergence of many channels of information to one person. This person serves as intermediary or "go-between" in families. In contrast, a relative absence of channels to a family member may reveal unpopularity, fear, or rejection. Chapter 10, Family Power Structure, further explains this process.

Messages initiated by the sender are always somewhat distorted—either by the sender, through the interaction between sender and receiver, or by the receiver. One primary cause of distortion is anxiety of either interactant, and the greater the level of anxiety, the greater the possibility of misunderstanding. Another common cause of message distortion is a difference in the frames of reference of the interactants, as either the result of sociocultural or idiosyncratic dissimilarity. In their daily interactions, family members usually assume that the other members have a similar frame of reference; since this is untrue in many cases, misunderstandings inevitably arise.

At certain times in most families, and on a more continual basis in others, channels may become under- or overloaded with information flow. The overloading of channels is frequently due to environmental variables such as the number of people present in the home, the intensity of sound, excessive movement and crowding, or other distracting stimuli. On the individual level, internal variables of defensiveness, preoccupation, demands on time, drugs, and illness all may cause under- or overloading of channels, with consequent distortion of communication.

Commands are a particular type of communication which overloads the channels. According to MacKay,[6] commands penetrate and usurp the work of the receiving system. When there is a continual use of commands, the functioning and autonomy of the receiving person is compromised, resulting in pathological dependency. The negative effects of commands are an important concept for nurses to consider in their work with families, especially in the area of parent education and counseling.

The underloading of channels, as may occur during sensory deprivation, occurs at various times, with consequent distortion of messages. For instance, a family member who is deprived of a particular sensory input such as of vision or hearing will generate unique types of communication patterns in his or her family. In general, communication patterns are developed which create alternative channels of sensory input to the deprived member. Thus the family interacting with a member with vision impairment learns to decrease gestures and increase explicit verbal input; conversely, those families with hearing-impaired members learn to increase gestures and decrease verbal input.

Underloading of channels also creates other types of communication patterns. When an impasse has been reached in a discussion and a period of time passes before the discussion is reopened, the first message sent is likely to be highly distorted, by either the sender or the receiver. Underloading of channels, especially of physical and/or verbal affective messages, creates a state of deprivation of cognitive input; and this deprivation may result in poor thought processes and a blunting of emotional response.[7]

Feedback Loops

Communication is an organizing, purposeful, and self-regulating process in families. Self-regulating processes in a system are dependent on two-way commu-

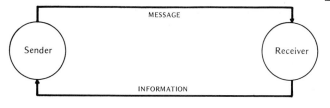

FIGURE 9.2
Negative feedback loop. (Adapted from von Bertalanffy L: General system theory: A critical review. In Buckley W (ed): Modern Systems Research for the Behavioral Scientist. Chicago, Aldine, 1968, p 16)

nication, termed feedback loops. According to von Bertalanffy,[8] feedback loops are "circular, causal chains." As Figure 9.2 indicates, feedback loops in communication provide opportunities for adjustment, adaptation, and growth in a relationship and in the larger family system.

Negative feedback is the most productive type of feedback. "Negative" is not a judgmental term, but is simply a reference to the direction in which the information flows (see Fig. 9.2). Self-regulating negative feedback is present when a sender initiates an interaction by sending a message and then, because of new input received, modifies the message before a reply is possible or expected.

Problem solving and decision making depend on negative feedback. The former begins when a problem arises and is identified. In the family problem-solving situation, the sender or initiator of the interaction usually identifies the problem, family members then explore the problem, various solutions are discussed, and a decision is finally made through one of the processes described fully in the next chapter.

"Loose negative" feedback refers to interactions that do not deal with issue at hand, leading to disequilibrium within the family. If, for instance, a parent's intoxicated behavior is explained to the children as the result of some physical illness, loose feedback is occurring, with resultant changes in family equilibrium. Such disequilibrium can be expected to continue to increase until feedback is "tightened," i.e., the situation and important issues are confronted and dealt with.

"Tight" feedback corrects and modifies deviations from equilibrium promptly. For example, if a teenager begins to stay out late, is seclusive, and acts in an unusual manner, the family with a tight feedback system will request an explanation, followed by the negotiation of new family rules which consider the changing developmental needs of family members.

Family Boundaries

Family boundary maintenance in information processing determines the openness of the system to exchange information with the external environment.

The amount of information a family can handle adequately is limited, and an excess of information or conflicting information from the outer environment amplifies and creates family disequilibrium. Conversely, too little information can also threaten family stability. In the healthy family, boundaries adequately screen information input and output—when an excessive amount of information flows into the family, the boundaries are closed, and when an underflow of information occurs, the boundaries are opened.[9]

The family with an underflow of information from the environment creates a greater reliance upon inner familial resources. Relatively closed families may exhibit more energy than they can discharge in constructive ways, and disorganization results. The abused child is frequently found in families that are isolated and have closed boundaries with society. In healthier isolated families, the members tend to believe that all or most of the needs of the members can be met within the family or the family's reference group. Family self-sufficiency may be overemphasized, however, causing family members to view wider society in a distorted or negative way. The children of such families often experience great problems when forced to interact with the wider society.

On the other hand, families that are indiscriminately open to information tend to become disorganized and chaotic. In this case, ineffective boundary regulation allows information to flow constantly into the family system, with resultant distortion and high levels of anxiety being generated and manifested among family members. The children and adults of these families are forced into the extrafamilial environment of neighbors, community organizations, and state agencies in order to meet their needs. Relationships are generally shallow, nonrewarding, and frustrating to all concerned, both inside and outside the family.

FUNCTIONAL COMMUNICATION IN THE FAMILY

Functional communication is viewed as the cornerstone of a successful, healthy family and as such is defined as the clear transmission and reception of both the content and instructional level of any message.[10] When the family utilizes functional communication patterns, the responsibilities of socializing children, meeting the emotional needs of the members, maintaining the spousal relationship, and participating in society can be accomplished.

The family system and the communication patterns within this system have a major impact on the individual members. Individualization, learning about other people, the development and maintenance of self-esteem, and the ability to make choices are all dependent on the information that is passed between members in the family.

Functional communication in the family setting requires that the intention or meaning of the sender be sent through relatively clear channels and that the receiver of the message have an understanding of its meaning that is similar to that of the sender.[11] Effective communication means matching meaning, gaining consistency, and attaining congruence between the intended message and the received message. Thus effective communication in the family is a process of constant definition and redefinition that will achieve a matching of the content and instructional levels of messages. Both the sender and the receiver must be actively involved and capable of interchanging positions by becoming either sender or receiver during the process.

Interactional Characteristics of a Functional Family

Functional families have certain characteristics which are revealed in the communication patterns they utilize. A functional family uses communication to create and maintain mutually beneficial relationships. Their interaction reveals a tolerance for error, as well as an understanding of the member's imperfections and individuality. Differentness,[12] acknowledgment of the individuality and uniqueness of each mate, is encouraged to the degree that is reciprocally beneficial to the family system and each individual. A sufficient amount of overt openness and honesty exists to enable members to recognize the needs and emotions of one another.

The communication patterns in a functional family demonstrate acceptance of differentness, as well as a minimum of judgments and unrealistic criticism of each other. Adjustments in individual behavior which have been necessitated by the stress of external social demands or the needs of the family system or of personal development generate healthy adjustments in the whole family; one person is not expected to do all of the changing necessary for the family to continue in a stable manner, and sufficient cohesiveness and flexibility exist for the family to adapt effectively.

Communication in families is an extremely dynamic, at least two-way process. Messages are not simply sent and received by a sender and a receiver. For instance, as the sender begins a message, the receiver may show an expression that will, through "negative" feedback, change the sender's message. As a result, the sender might change the wording of a message in the middle of the sending action so that the receiver will have a similar frame of reference. The dynamic nature of communication makes functional interaction complex and unpredictable. So complex and tenuous is functional communication, that even in the well-functioning family clear communication occurs only about one-third of the time.

The Functional Sender

Satir states the sender who communicates in a functional way can:

1. Firmly state his case,
2. yet at the same time clarify and qualify what he says,
3. as well as ask for feedback,
4. and be receptive to feedback when he gets it.[13]

Each of these four elements is vital in understanding healthy communication.

Firmly States Case

Congruent Levels. One of the foundations for firmly stating one's case is the use of communication which is congruent on both the content and instruction levels. For example, when a person is angry not only should the literal message denote anger, but the tone of voice, body position, and gestures should also reflect the same message.

Intensity and Explicitness. When a person communicates, the sender is asking something of the receiver. Such requests include various degrees of intensity and explicitness, both of which involve how firmly the sender states his case. Intensity will be defined as the ability of the sender to effectively communicate internal perceptions of feelings, desires, and needs at the same intensity he is experiencing these perceptions internally. Normally there will be a fluctuation of intensity in the expression of feelings, desires, and needs, instead of a monotone presentation or "reasonableness" of expression. In other words, the functional sender conveys an accurate appraisal of his or her perceptions.

To be explicit, the sender should inform the receiver of how serious the message is by stating how the receiver should respond to the message. An example illustrating a high degree of explicitness is: "I want to sit in that chair."

Clarifies and Qualifies Statements

A second dimension which Satir identified as an essential characteristic of the functional sender is the use of clarifying and qualifying statements in his or her communication. The use of such statements enables the sender to be specific and to check out his or her perception of reality against that of the other person.

Specific types of clarifying and qualifying statements include those described below.

"I Want" Statements. A statement that clearly states what the sender wants.[14] Example: "Stop contradicting me when I'm disciplining the children."

"I Feel" Statements. Sender directly states his or her internal perceptions of a specific feeling. These feelings may be internally triggered or may be a reaction to another person's behavior.[15] Example of internally triggered expression: "I sometimes feel frustrated when my hands ache and I'm unable to do the chores around the house" (a patient with arthritis); externally triggered expression: "When you call me stupid in front of the children, I feel embarrassed and irritated."

"I Intend" Statements. This type of statement implies a concrete independent action will be initiated by the sender. Example: "I'm still experiencing weakness after my surgery and plan to take a nap this afternoon."

"I Like" and "I Don't Like" Statements. These are statements in which the sender states precisely what gives him or her pleasure and/or displeasure, or what the receiver does or does not do that bothers the sender.[16] Examples: "I like it when you clean up your room" and "I don't like it when I have to stay in my room by myself when I am sick."

Self-disclosure Statements. A self-disclosure statement by an individual refers to an open and honest revelation of an intention, a desire, a past action or a fallibility that is considered private or personal to that individual. Examples: "I'm concerned about my biopsy because my mother died from cancer of the breast" and "I'm scared to show my anger because my husband may leave me."

Direct Questions. This involves asking concrete questions to elicit specific information. Example: "Are your stitches causing you any pain?"

Open-ended Questions. Open-ended questions focus on a general area of interest and encourage the receiver to select his own response, i.e., open-ended questions do not structure the receiver's response. Example: "Tell me more about your reluctance to have the surgery."

Elicits Feedback

A third element of the functional sender is the use of asking for feedback, which enables him or her to verify whether the message was received accurately, as well as enabling the sender to gain information needed to clarify his or her intent. In the following examples the sender seeks feedback to obtain the receiver's perception or reaction to what the sender has communicated: "I keep asking myself, should we tell the children that I have cancer? What do you think?" "Since you're still on limited activities because of your heart condition, I think your parents should visit at another time. What's your reaction?"

Receptivity of Sender to Feedback

When the sender is receptive to feedback, he or she will exhibit a willingness to listen, react nondefensively, and attempt to understand. In order to understand, the sender must not have so narrow a perspective that he or she is unable to comprehend the validity of the receiver's point of view. Thus by asking for more specific criticism or "checking out" statements, the sender demonstrates his or her receptivity and interest in feedback.[17] Examples: George's wife has criticized his lack of sexual responsiveness. To gain further information he asks, "What things bother you when we're making love?" Or JoAnn states, "I just bought the children some new clothing for school." Don reacts, "I'm really angry you did that." And JoAnn replies, "Are you angry because of the amount of money I spent, the type of clothing I purchased, or did you want to shop for the children?"

Functional Receiver

Persons receiving messages generally tune in to the metamessage level of communication, but in the case of the functional receiver there would be an even greater ability to make an accurate assessment of the intent of a message. Therefore, he or she would be better able to weigh correctly message's meaning and would be able to assess more precisely the sender's attitudes, intentions, and feelings as expressed in the metacommunication. According to Anderson, the functional receiver tries to comprehend the material fully before attempting to evaluate.[18] This means that motivations and metacommunication, as well as content, are analyzed. The new information is checked with that which is already known, and the decision to act is carefully weighed. Each of the communication techniques discussed below facilitate and enable the receiver to comprehend and respond more fully to the sender's message.

Listening

The ability to listen is perhaps the most important quality of a functional receiver. Listening effectively means focusing one's full attention on what is being communicated, thus blocking out all extraneous "noise." The receiver attends to the sender's complete message rather than prejudging the meaning of the communication. Sells explains:

> To listen is
> to be still
> to expect
> to wait for a response
> to practice restraint.[19]

Many people are passive listeners, responding with blank expressions and a seemingly "couldn't care less" attitude. An active listener responds with gestures that communicate actively listening. Asking questions is a vital part of active listening.[20] It is as if the receiver were a student learning a new subject, and as a good student, he or she would ask questions and explore the facts. To actively listen means to be empathetic, to think of the other person's needs and desires, and to not disrupt the sender's flow of communication.

Feedback

The second major characteristic of the functional receiver involves feedback, that is feeding information back to the sender that tells him or her how the message was interpreted by the receiver. The following are examples of eliciting feedback.

Asking Sender to Clarify and Qualify. These statements encourage the sender to elaborate more fully. Example: "What do you mean when you say I get frustrated too easily with the children?"

Associating. In the process of associating, the receiver makes a relationship between previous personal experiences[21] or past related incidents and the sender's communication at both content and instructional levels. Example: During her last trimester of pregnancy, Susie comments to family nurse, "I have been getting upset quite easily and feel more dependent upon my husband. I never felt this way until I got pregnant."

The nurse responds, "I remember when I was pregnant having the same type of feelings. I would frequently ask my husband to do little things for me which I always did for myself before I was pregnant. In the families I visit the women have often shared these same types of feelings with me."

Paraphrasing and Checking Perceptions. The receiver, by using either a question or a statement, summarizes the sender's message.[22] He or she does this by restating the sender's message in his or her own words.

The central purpose of paraphrasing is to clarify the sender's message. Examples: "So you're saying . . ." and "What I understand is . . . ."

Validation

Another major technique for facilitating communication is validation. In utilizing validation the receiver conveys the following: "I can see how you think and feel that way" or "It makes sense and is reasonable to feel that way." Validation does not imply that the receiver agrees with the sender's communication, but demonstrates an acceptance of the merit and/or worth of the message.[23] Examples:

1. *Validation of thoughts.* "You're saying that you're spending too much money on food and medication and want help with budgeting?"
2. *Validation of feelings.* "Sounds like you were hurt when I complained about your mother's behavior." Or, "I sense that you're really frightened that your tumor might be malignant."
3. *Validation plus statement of own point of view.* "I feel you're really angry with me, although I'm still feeling that your punishment of Tommy was too excessive."

FUNCTIONAL INTERACTIONAL PATTERNS

As distinguished from the discussion of functional communication, this section covers family interaction more broadly or macroscopically, dealing with patterns of communication rather than specific or discrete interactional exchanges.

Family interaction patterns are the characteristic on-going communication patterns of the family, which in addition to influencing and organizing the members of the family, produces the meaning of transactions between family members.[24] Most importantly, it is through interaction that the affective needs of family members are fulfilled.

Interaction in families is affected by the roles and tasks of the members as prescribed by the culture. For instance, in some cultures direct sexual assertiveness by women is subject to disapproval; in other cultures, affectional interaction between fathers and children is discouraged. Other types of interactions, such as conflict resolution and decision-making techniques, are also culturally prescribed.

Communication patterns in families may take several forms, on both verbal and nonverbal levels. Moreover, the degree of verbal behavior is dependent on the culture and socioeconomic level of the family members.

Affective Communication

Affectional communication patterns are composed of verbal messages of caring and nonverbal, physical gestures of touching, caressing, holding and looking. As Bowlby et al. demonstrated,[25] physical expressions of affection in early childhood are essential in the development of normal affectional responses. Later in life, verbal affectional communication patterns become more important, if not predominant, in relaying affectional messages. Most functional communication patterns contain both physical and verbal affectional messages, with the predominance of one form or the other depending on the needs of the family members and the particular situation.

As part of healthy affective communications, the family members need to be able to enjoy themselves and other family members. When their responses to each other are fresh and spontaneous, rather than controlled, repetitious, and predictable, this enjoyment can be realized.

Open Areas of Communication

Functional families, that is, those with functional communication patterns, value openness; a mutual respect for each other's feelings, thoughts, and concerns; spontaneity; authenticity; and self-disclosure. It follows then that these families would also be able to discuss most areas of life—both personal and social issues and concerns. These areas are referred to as "open areas of communication." The more functional the family, generally the fewer areas of closed communication exist and vice versa. Consideration of a family's culture is crucial here, however, since cultural norms concerning modesty, privacy, and sexual roles play a very large part in influencing areas of open and closed communication.

Power Hierarchy and Family Rules

Family systems are based on power hierarchies or "pecking orders" wherein communication generally flows downward. *Functional* interaction in the power hierarchy occurs when power is distributed according to the developmental needs of the family members, or when power is assigned according to the abilities and resources of family members and is consonant with the family's cultural prescriptions of family power relationships. (See Chap. 10 for a complete discussion of family power structures.)

Power communications have characteristics that are readily apparent. The communication, "Joan, I want you to go upstairs and clean your room now or I will not take you to the show this afternoon" is typical of a coercive power communication. It is a command type message, specifying the action the receiver is to carry out and negatively reinforcing alternatives.[26]

Family Conflict Resolution

Interactional conflicts occur when two or more contradictory, equally compelling messages are conveyed, and when the family decision makers fail to resolve the conflict. In other words, conflict occurs in families when the course of action for solving a problem or meeting needs of family members cannot be agreed on—when there is no consensus. The disagreeing members of the family become emotionally invested in a specific solution and are unwilling to yield entirely to another person's wishes.

Conflict resolution is a vital task of interaction in the family. Functional conflict resolution occurs when the conflict is openly discussed and strategies to solve the conflict are employed, or when parents appropriately utilize their authority to make a decision (see Chap. 10).

DYSFUNCTIONAL COMMUNICATION IN THE FAMILY

In this chapter functional and dysfunctional communication have been separated for discussion purposes. In reality, however, this demarcation does not exist, and the communication patterns in families are not all totally healthy or unhealthy. Rather, they should be viewed on a continuum from functional to dysfunctional, with all but a small percentage of families falling somewhere between these poles. In contrast to the definition of functional communication, dysfunctional communication is defined as the unclear transmission and reception of either or both the content and instruction (intent) of a message.

Characteristics and Values

One of the primary factors which generate dysfunctional communication patterns is the presence of low esteem of both the family and its members.[27] Three interrelated values which perpetuate low esteem are self-centeredness, total agreement, and lack of empathy.

Self-centeredness

Self-centeredness is characterized by focusing on one's own needs to the exclusion of the other person's needs, feelings, or perspectives. In other words, self-centered individuals seek to get something from the other to meet his or her own needs. When these individuals must give, they do so reluctantly and then in a hostile, defensive, or self-sacrificing manner. Thus bargaining or negotiating effectively is difficult, because the self-centered persons believe they cannot afford to lose what little they have to give.[28]

Value of Total Agreement

The family's value of total agreement begins when the marital partners discover that each is different in a unique way, although what these differences are exactly may be difficult to explain. Differentness—as expressed in opinions, habits, preferences, or expectations—may be seen as a threat because it can and does lead to disagreements and the awareness that they are both separate individuals. If these partners feel that it is absolutely necessary to be loved and approved at all times, and so must constantly please the other, then they can neither communicate openly when displeased nor acknowledge disagreement. The couple perceives that expressions of their own unique thoughts and feelings might lead to conflicts that could then result in a "catastrophe."[29]

Thus unwritten rules come into being which forbid open expression of one's own individuality and differentness as a means of staving off this threat. These rules are often rigid and elude negotiation, so that there is no consideration of alternatives which would enable each mate to interact differently and yet be accepted. As part of the socialization process, the children learn these same values and ways of relating and thus have difficulty in recognizing and interpreting a variety of feelings and experiences. These values and resultant communication patterns constrict the growth of all family members.

Lack of Empathy

Family members who are self-centered and cannot tolerate differentness also cannot recognize the effect of their own thoughts, feelings, and behavior on other family members; neither can they understand other family members' thoughts, feelings, and behavior. They are so consumed with meeting their own needs that they do not have the ability to role take or be empathetic. Underneath a facade of unconcern, these individuals may suffer feelings of powerlessness. Not only do they devalue themselves, they also devalue each other. This leads to an atmosphere of tension, fearfulness, and/or blame.

The stage is therefore set for a style of communication which is confusing, vague, indirect, and covert, with defensiveness rather than openness, clarity, and honesty prevailing. The more dysfunctional the communication, the more dysfunctional the family.[30]

Dysfunctional Sender

The dysfunctional sender's communication is often ineffective in one or more of the four basic characteristics of the functional sender: in stating case, in clarifying and qualifying, in eliciting, and in being receptive to feedback. The receiver is often left confused and has to guess what the sender is thinking or feeling. The communication of the dysfunctional sender is either actively or passively defensive and often negates the possibility of seeking any clear feedback from the receiver. "Unhealthy" communication in the sender will be discussed under five major categories: assumptions, the unclear expression of feelings, judgmental expressions, inability to define needs, and incongruent communication.

Assumptions

When assumptions are made, the sender takes for granted what the receiver is feeling or thinking about an event or person without validating his or her perceptions. The dysfunctional sender is usually not aware of these assumptions. He or she rarely clarifies content or intent, thus serving to obscure and distort meaning. When this dysfunction in communication occurs, it elicits anger in the receiver since he or she is being given the message that his or her own opinions and feelings do not matter much. As a result, the responses of the receiver indicate a "fight back" or "give up" attitude, rather than one of taking responsibility for his or her behavior. The following illustrations represent various forms of the use of assumptions.

Speaking for the Other. The sender acts as a spokesman for another person by telling someone else what that person is thinking or feeling.[31] Example: Without checking with spouse, the husband comments to the children, "It is perfectly obvious that your mother never wants to go on walks with us."

What Is Perceived or Evaluated Cannot Be Altered. The individual assumes that what he or she has perceived or evaluated cannot be changed. Examples: "Jim has always been messy. I've just had to learn to live with that fact." Or, "Joey's so accident prone, but that's life."

Incomplete Messages. The sender does not finish the sentence or message but assumes that the receiver will complete it. Example: "He said we couldn't agree on . . . you see what I mean?"

Assumes Others Share Same Perceptions, Thoughts, and Feelings. The sender automatically takes for granted that other people share his same perceptions,

thoughts, and feelings.[32] Example: "I dislike going to the free clinic; I know you feel the same way."

Generalizations. The content of the message describes behavior or events in general terms instead of citing specific behaviors and observations. The sender assumes that the receiver will fill in the specifics. Example: "You're such a poor father," as opposed to, "I wish you would discipline Sarah when she doesn't put away her toys."

One Instance Exemplifies All Instances. The individual, in failing to learn that thoughts, actions, and sentiments change, falls into the error of overgeneralizing and makes an assumption that one situation is an example of all similar situations to follow.[33] Example: "The nurse at the free clinic was impatient and blunt with me. I'm not going there again to get this same treatment from her and the rest of the staff."

Unclear Expression of Feelings

Another type of dysfunctional communication by the sender is unclear expression of feelings. Due to fear of rejection, the sender's expressions of feelings must go underground or be uttered in such a covert manner that the feelings are not recognizable. In another instance, the sender may express his or her feelings but does so without the same intensity as the feelings were perceived internally, the usual situation being that feelings are understated. Various types of unclear expression of feelings will be presented.

Sarcasm. Sarcasm denotes the use of humorous or witty statements which enable the sender of a message to avoid taking responsibility for his or her hostile feelings. If he or she is confronted, the sender can always reply that he or she was just being humorous.[34] Example: "Fathers were made to play with their sons while mothers were made to take all the responsibility for raising them."

Silent Resentment. In the case of unclear expression of feeling, the sender feels irritated with the receiver but does not express the anger overtly and/or may displace the resentment onto another person or thing.[35] Example: The children have broken a second window in the period of a week. Joan is infuriated but remains silent. When her husband comes home from work, she coldly stares at him and then leaves the room (displacement of anger).

Expression of Hurt as Anger. The sender expresses anger as a defensive maneuver to cover up feelings of hurt, rather than expressing the more basic emotion of hurt. Example: Eileen takes great pride in creating various artistic items for her home. She has just completed a new floral arrangement and some new drapes for the living room. When her husband comes home from work she proudly shows him the items, at which he only nods his head and seems preoccupied and disinterested. Eileen angrily states, "I'm sick and tired of trying to share my interests with you."

Judgmental Expressions

This category of dysfunctional communication by the sender is characterized by a tendency to constantly evaluate messages in terms of the sender's own value system. Judgmental statements always carry moral overtones in that the sender is evaluating the worth of the other person's message as being "right" or "wrong," "good" or "bad," "normal" or "abnormal," and so on. It is not only the message which is being evaluated or judged, of course, but the sender of the message is also being indirectly evaluated or judged. Two types of judgmental expression are put-down statements or questions and "you should" statements.

Put-down Statements or Questions. These are statements or questions that carry a negative connotation and value judgment. These judgmental expressions may also involve a covert unmet need or an unexpressed dissatisfaction with the other interactant. Examples: "You are really clumsy." (As opposed to, "I want you to be more careful when carrying a glass of milk.") And, "When are you going to amount to something?" (As opposed to, "I want you to spend more effort doing your homework").

"You Should" Statements. The words "should" or "ought to" imply that the sender is an authority figure who knows what is "good" or "bad." If the sender is a parent and the receiver the child, this type of communication may be functional and necessary in the socialization process, but must generally be held to be a dysfunctional mode of communication. Example: Family health nurse to mother, "Johnny's too fat! You should feed him less."

Inability to Express Needs

The dysfunctional sender is not only unable to express his or her needs, but due to fear of rejection is incapable of defining the behaviors he or she expects from the receiver to fulfill them. Often the dysfunctional sender unconsciously feels unworthy, with no right to express needs or to expect that personal needs will be met. Various examples of the sender's inability to express needs will be discussed.

Silent Need for Nurturance. The silent need for nurturance is defined as an unexpressed need for help,

empathy, or some aspect of "being taken care of." This may also include an expectation that others should be able to anticipate the sender's needs and that asking for nurturance or assistance renders the response to such requests inauthentic and unsatisfying.[36] Example: After her radiation therapy, Jane sometimes experiences nausea. Amnon, not realizing his wife's discomfort, does not offer to prepare dinner. When Jane finally asks for Amnon's assistance, she feels angry even though he agrees to prepare dinner.

Covert Requests. These types of requests are made without acknowledging "ownership" (the sender does not overtly admit his or her wishes).[37] Example: "It would do you good to spend more time with the children." (The sender does not directly ask the other to spend time with the children.)

Complaints. In this case the sender appears unable or unwilling to describe the desired behavior needed from the receiver, and the sender expresses these needs in terms of a dissatisfaction. Example: The Smiths, a couple in their seventies, typically complain to their children, "You never visit us." (As opposed to, "Please come over for dinner Wednesday evening.")

Incongruent Communication

In this type of dysfunctional communication, two or more simultaneous and contradictory messages are sent. The receiver is left with the conflict of attempting to respond.

Verbal–Verbal Incongruency. In this case two or more literal messages are sent simultaneously which oppose each other. Examples: "Jimmy's such a well-behaved child. Did I tell you last week he had another fight at school?" And, "I don't mind being alone so much when I'm sick; of course, it would be nice if the children would visit me more often."

Verbal–Nonverbal Incongruency. The sender communicates a message verbally, but the accompanying nonverbal metacommunication contradicts the verbal message.[38] Example: "I'm not angry with you!" spoken in a loud, gruff tone of voice with fists clenched.

Dysfunctional Receiver

In the dysfunctional receiver, the breakdown in communication occurs when the message is not received as intended either due to the failure to listen or message distortion, misinterpretation, or misunderstanding. Two additional causative factors creating dysfunctional reception are the use of disqualification and responding offensively, both of which are defensive in nature.

Failure to Listen

In the case of failure to listen, a message is sent, but the receiver does not attend to or hear the message. There may be many reasons for failure to listen, ranging from willful inattention to a wish but an inability to listen. This is commonly due to concomitant distraction, e.g., noise, improper timing, or high anxiety.[39] A frequently used way in which individuals do not listen is by ignoring messages.

Client: I keep wondering if I will always be this limited in my activities because of my heart condition.

Nurse: Has the swelling in your ankles decreased?

Disqualification

A disqualification is an indirect response which allows the receiver to disagree with a message without really disagreeing.

"Yes-butting." The dysfunctional receiver partially agrees with the intent of the message, yet at the same time finds something wrong with the sender's opinion, feeling, or suggestion.[40]

Nurse: When Bobby has temper tantrums, why don't you try going in to see that he's all right, and then leave him alone until he calms down.

Bobby's mother: Yes, that's a fine idea, but I'm afraid he would hurt himself.

Evasion. The receiver disqualifies the message by avoiding the crucial issue.

Nurse: Well, how effective was leaving the room when Bobby had a temper tantrum?

Husband: Wouldn't you say it worked, Jean, because the number of tantrums decreased this week?

Wife: Bobby's constant requests are driving me crazy.

Tangentialization. Here the receiver responds to a peripheral aspect of a message and ignores the central intention or content of the message.

Husband (hospitalized for a myocardial infarction six weeks prior to the visiting nurse's visit): All of my recreational interests were of a strenuous nature, so all I do now is complain to my wife that I have nothing to do all day.

Wife: I love strenuous activities myself and have always been interested in tennis.

Offensiveness

Offensiveness in communication denotes that the receiver of a message reacts negatively, as if being threatened. The receiver seems to react defensively to the message by assuming an oppositional posture and an attacking position.

Attacking with a Different Issue. Before any progress is made on a threatening issue introduced by the sender, the person receiving the message responds with an extraneous issue that hurts or threatens the sender (i.e., the receiver utilizes a "counterattack").

Wife: I very rarely see you set any limits on the children.

Husband: After five years I keep wondering when you're going to learn to cook a decent meal.

Insulting. The receiver attributes a negative or insulting characteristic to the sender. In other words, the receiver attacks the sender, not the issue.[41]

Child: Dad, you never play baseball with me anymore.

Father: You're so uncoordinated that you can't even catch the ball.

Rebuff. In response to requests to clarify or qualify, the receiver conveys disgust by refusing to elaborate or to comply with the sender's request. Examples: "How many times do I have to repeat myself?" And, "You heard me the first time."

Lack of Exploration

In order to clarify the intent of a message, the responder often has to explore to seek the correct meaning. When the receiver is unclear as to the meaning of a message, the functional receiver seeks further explanation, whereas the dysfunctional receiver will use responses which negate exploration, such as making assumptions (as discussed previously), giving premature advice, or cutting off communication.

Premature Advice. Premature advice is defined as the offering of a suggestion or solution to a problem before exploring it sufficiently or requesting additional feedback.

Patient: This diagnosis of multiple sclerosis has really been a shock.

Nurse: I'd suggest rest periods during the day, and don't overtire yourself by engaging in strenuous activities.

(A functional response would have been to explore the emotional impact of the diagnosis on the patient.)

Cutoffs in Communication. When the receiver does not want to continue discussing the issue at hand, he or she makes a statement or uses an action that curtails any further discussion of that issue. This technique is often used to avoid dealing with unpleasant or negative feelings.[42] Examples: "Let's just forget it" and "It's not that important." In addition, physical actions are another way of cutting off communication. For example, the receiver could leave the room, engage in busywork, or turn away from the sender.

Lack of Validation

As stated previously, the receiver in an interaction often has the difficult task of attempting to correctly interpret both the content and the intent of the message. Validation, as previously defined, refers to the receiver's conveyance of acceptance. Therefore, lack of validation implies that the receiver either responds neutrally (shows neither acceptance nor nonacceptance) or distorts and misinterprets the message. Assuming rather than clarifying the thoughts of the sender is one example of a lack of validation.

New mother: My mother has just come to stay with us for three weeks to take care of the new baby while I get my strength back.

Family nurse: How wonderful! I'm sure that your mother will be a tremendous help to you during this time.

This interaction is dysfunctional because the nurse assumes that the client has positive feelings about her mother's assistance.

DYSFUNCTIONAL INTERACTIONAL PATTERNS

In this type of patterned interaction, two or more family members have established repetitive networks and strategies of dysfunctional communication which attempt to maintain the integration of the family unit. These dysfunctional processes are often subtle, and the intent of the communication is covert or hidden. Thus accurate assessment of this type of unhealthy communication becomes more difficult. In this section, four dysfunctional interactional communication processes which are less difficult to assess have been selected.

Self-perpetuating Syndrome

Each individual in the interaction constantly restates his or her own issue without really listening to the other's point of view or acknowledging the other's needs.

Wife: To discipline the children, I have them spend fifteen minutes in their room. I'm not a believer of severe punishment.

Husband: I believe in stern limits. Last week I took Jody's allowance away for a month and refused to let him play outside for a week.

Wife: Yes, fifteen minutes in their room gets the point across.

Husband: If you dish out stern punishment, the children really listen.

In this situation, each partner continued to restate his or her own viewpoint and did not acknowledge that of the other.

Inability to Focus on One Issue

Each of the individuals in the interaction rambles from one issue to another instead of resolving any one problem discussed or obtaining closure.

Husband: I'm tired of your mother visiting without calling first.

Wife: When are you going to take Jack shopping?

Husband: Soon as you balance the checking account correctly.

Notice how each partner introduces a new problem without any attempts of a discussion of one problem at a time.

Chitchat Over Daily Events

A common interactional pattern utilized in families to avoid discussing meaningful issues and/or expressing salient feelings is termed "chitchat." The family, in using "chitchat" consistently, talks about superficial daily occurrences and avoids the meaningful issues of family life.

For example, mother has been taking her child to a pediatric clinic because of recurrent convulsions. At the clinic the diagnosis of epilepsy was recently confirmed. Since hearing of the diagnosis, the family has never discussed their thoughts or feelings about the diagnosis; their only conversation in this area has dealt with the inconvenient hospital parking arrangements and the long travel time to the clinic.

Closed Areas of Communication

While more functional families have more open areas of communication, less functional families displaying dysfunctional interactional patterns will demonstrate more closed areas of communication. Families have unwritten rules and negative sanctions forbidding certain discussion areas. These restrictions may be limited to certain family subsystems: for example, discussion of sexual habits in front of the children or a parent's alcoholism. Moreover, an area may be closed in terms of expression of feelings but open in terms of expression of thoughts.

As mentioned previously, cultural norms of modesty, privacy, and sexual roles probably play as large a part in influencing the areas of closed and open communication in some of the areas of communication as the status of the family's mental health.

Negativity as a Communication Pattern

According to Harris, negativity refers to statements or requests that are repeatedly made in a negative manner or with a negative expectation.[43] The family member receiving the negative pattern of communication learns to respond with similar statements or behavior. The focus of the interaction is on the forbidden instead of what is desired.

Mother (to son): If you don't spend your allowance wisely, then you'll never get that baseball glove that you want.

Mother (to son): Look at how you neglect to take care of your toys and sports equipment.

Note that the child only learns what he is expected not to do. The parent offers no clear expectations or explanations about behavior they desire from the child.

ASSESSMENT QUESTIONS

The following assessment questions should be considered when analyzing a family's communication patterns.

1. In observing the family as a whole and/or the family's set of relationships, how extensively is functional and dysfunctional communication used? Give examples of recurring patterns.
   a. How firmly and clearly do members state their needs and feelings?
   b. To what extent do members use clarification and qualification in interaction?
   c. Do members elicit and respond favorably to feedback or do they generally discourage feedback and exploration of an issue?
   d. How well do members listen and attend when communicating?
   e. Do members seek validation from one another?
   f. To what degree do members use assumptions and judgmental statements in interaction?
   g. Do members interact in an offensive manner to messages?
   h. How frequently is disqualification utilized?
2. How are emotional (affective) messages conveyed in the family and within the family subsystems?

   a. How frequently are these emotional messages conveyed?
   b. What types of emotions are transmitted within the family subsystems? Are negative, positive, or both types of emotions transmitted?
3. What is the frequency and quality of communication within the communication network and familial sets of relationships?
   a. Who talks to whom and in what usual manner?
   b. What is the usual pattern of transmitting important messages? Does an intermediary exist?
   c. Are messages appropriate to the developmental age of the members?
4. Are the majority of messages of family members congruent in content and instruction (including observations of nonverbal messages)? If not, who manifests incongruency?
5. What types of dysfunctional processes are evident in the family communication patterns?
6. What important issues to the family's wellness or adequate functioning are closed to discussion?
7. What internal (familial) and external (environmental, socioeconomic, and cultural) influences are affecting communication patterns?

REFERENCES

1. Satir V: Peoplemaking. Palo Alto, California, Science and Behavior Books, 1972, p 30
2. Miller JG: Living systems: basic concepts. Behav Sci 10:194, July 1965
3. *Ibid.*, p 194
4. Friedman M: Assessment of Family Communication Patterns. Los Angeles, California, California State University, Los Angeles Intercampus Nursing Project, 1976, p 6
5. MacKay D: The informational analysis of questions and commands. In Buckley W (ed): Modern Systems Research for the Behavioral Scientist. Chicago, Aldine, 1968, p 205
6. *Ibid.*

7. Harlow H, Harlow M: Social deprivation in monkeys. Sci Am pp 154–161, November 1962

8. von Bertalanffy L: General systems theory—a critical review. In Buckley W (ed): Modern Systems Research for the Behavioral Scientist. Chicago, Aldine, 1968, p 160

9. Reinhardt A, Quinn M: Current Practices in Family-Centered Community Nursing. St. Louis, Mosby, 1973, pp 90–91

10. Sells JW: Seven Steps to Effective Communication. Atlanta, Georgia, Forum House, 1973, p 1

11. *Ibid.*

12. Satir V: Conjoint Family Therapy, Palo Alto, California, Science and Behavior Books, 1967

13. Satir, *op. cit.*, p 70

14. Strayhorn JM Jr: Talking It Out: A Guide to Effective Communication. Champagne, Illinois, Research Press, 1977, p 15

15. *Ibid.*, pp 16–17

16. *Ibid.*, p 18

17. *Ibid.*, p 27

18. Anderson KE: Introduction to Communication Theory and Practice. San Jose, California, Cummings, 1972, p 71

19. Sells, *op. cit.*, p 23

20. Gottman J, Notarius C, Gonso J, Markman H: A Couples Guide to Communication. Champagne, Illinois, Research Press, 1977, p 148

21. *Ibid.*, p 150

22. *Ibid.*, p 151

23. *Ibid.*, p 17

24. Peters LR: The family and family therapy. In Hall JE, Weaver BR: Nursing of Families in Crisis. Philadelphia, Lippincott, 1974, p 36

25. Bowlby J: Maternal Care and Mental Health, New York, Shocken, 1966

26. Miller, *op. cit.*

27. Anderson, *op. cit.*, p 73

28. Satir, *op. cit.*, pp 11–19

29. Gottman, *op. cit.*, p 14

30. Satir, *op. cit.*

31. Gottman, *op. cit.*, p 10

32. Satir, *op. cit.*, p 66

33. *Ibid.*, p 65

34. Strayhorn, *op. cit.*, p 64

35. *Ibid.*, p 80

36. *Ibid.*, p 83

37. *Ibid.*, p 86

38. Satir, *op. cit.*, p 83

39. Sells, *op. cit.*, p 31

40. Gottman, *op. cit.*, p 12

41. *Ibid.*, p 36

42. Strayhorn, *op. cit.*, p 53

43. Harris SE: Negativity as a major communication pattern in a family. In Smoyak S (ed): The Psychiatric Nurse as a Family Therapist. New York, Wiley, 1975, pp 210–211

STUDY QUESTIONS

1. From the list below select the four primary characteristics of the functional sender.
   a. Listens.
   b. Receptive to feedback.
   c. Elicits feedback.
   d. Assumptions.
   e. Firmly states case.
   f. Validates.
   g. Clarifies and qualifies.

2. Name the four basic components of functional communication.

3. Match the five major categories of dysfunctional communication in left column with the specific illustrations given at the right.

Category	*Example*
a. Assumptions.	1. "I'm not mad at you," spoken in loud, sharp tone.
b. Unclear expression of feelings.	
c. Judgmental expressions.	2. "I dislike patients who are constantly complaining."
d. Inability to define needs.	3. "I don't understand how you can be so dumb."
e. Incongruent communication	4. "I just love it when you don't come home for dinner, then I have only a few dishes to wash."
	5. "If you would like to go out for dinner, so would I."

4. Which of the following situations *best* demonstrates that information has been received from a sender?
   a. A parent tells a child to stop playing with his food and the child continues to play.
   b. A parent shows a child how to use a fork and the child stops eating.
   c. A parent tells a child to drink his milk and the child looks at the parent.
   d. A parent shows a child how to butter bread and the child eats the bread.

5. Which of the above situations (in question 4) *best* indicates that interaction has not occurred and the receiver needs more information to make a decision?

6. Select the statement below which *best* describes channels of information flow.
   a. Overloading and underloading of channels of information flow may cause an impasse in interaction depending on the sensory modalities that are utilized.
   b. Channels of information flow extend from the sender to the cognitions of the receiver depending on the sensory modality that is utilized.
   c. Distortion of information occurs as a result of anxiety in the receiver which is independent of the utilization of a particular sensory mode.
   d. Channels of information flow include all sensory modalities as well as cognitions of the receiver and sender.

7. Negative feedback is a nonjudgmental term used in systems theory to describe the organizing and self-regulating process of information flow (answer *True* or *False*).

8. In the following situations describe *both* the content and instructional level of the message.
   a. A newlywed couple is watching a movie. The woman caresses the man's arm and hugs it to her while she whispers, "I'm really not interested in this movie."
   b. A child starts to crawl on his parent's lap. The parent pushes the child away and says, "You know I love you, go play with your new toy."
   c. A child is throwing cereal with a spoon. The mother grabs the spoon and cereal bowl and emphatically states, "Stop it! You may not play with your food!"

9. Illustrate the difference in development of channels of information flow in a family with a blind 8-year-old as opposed to a family with a retarded child of the same age.

10. A mother, while cleaning her 14-year-old daughter's room, finds a small, plastic bag of greenish dry leaves. The mother had noted that the girl had been doing poorly in school after breaking up with her boyfriend and has not been participating actively in family activities.
    a. In a family with "loose" negative feedback, how would this problem be approached?
    b. In a family with "tight" negative feedback, how would this problem be approached?

11. How does the underflow of information through family boundaries affect the family members?

12. How does the overflow of information through family boundaries affect the family members?

FAMILY CASE STUDY

During the reading of this family case example, jot down your interpretation of the interactions (using the theory presented in chapter), in addition to completing assessment questions at the end of the case description.

A member of the Visiting Nurses' Association is going out to visit Mr. Herman Katz, a Jewish male, age 68, who has suffered a myocardial infarction and has just recently returned home after four weeks of hospitalization. The doctor has requested that the visiting nurse review his dietary and exercise regimen and report back her appraisal of his diet and tolerance to the progressive exercise regime.

The nurse's notes on the interagency referral form from the hospital states: Mr. Katz was alert, very conscientious about his care, but was quite reluctant to do any of the activities—and thus was somewhat demanding and dependent on the nurses. He ate poorly and got up to go to the bathroom by himself. During the last week he has had no pain or dyspnea during self-care activities.

The visiting nurse on her first visit learned that Mr. K. had been a business manager for many years and that he retired three years ago. This was his second heart attack according to his wife (the first occurring six months postretirement). Past recreational interests had been heavy gardening and remodeling of his home prior to his first heart attack.

Mrs. Sylvia Katz is 65 years old and also Jewish. She has been in fairly good health except for being overweight and having osteoarthritis which has made walking much more difficult for her. She prepares rich Jewish foods for herself, and her single daughter Marian (age 40), who also lives with her and her husband. She or her daughter constantly answers for Mr. K. when the nurse asks questions. Mrs. K. is very talkative and complains of being very tired herself.

The Katz family lives in a nicely furnished three-bedroom house. Mr. K. has a college education and is a certified public accountant. They have two grown sons, who live nearby, and an unmarried daughter, Marian, who is temporarily living with them to help her father out.

On the second visit a week later, the nurse observed the following: Mr. K. continued to be unwilling and afraid to do things for himself and had not increased his level of activity. He appeared short of breath and uncomfortable (as though in pain) when talking about his illness and symptoms, but when distracted he appeared to have no dyspnea or pain. Mr. K. has seen none of his social or work friends since he has been home according to Mrs. K. He has not been getting dressed or taking care of his personal hygiene adequately.

The following interactional vignettes were extracted as the nurse began to discuss Mr. K.'s rehabilitation program:

NURSE (question directed at Mr. K.): What activities did the doctor recommend for you to do this week?

SYLVIA (interceding): I told Herman that he should take it easy because after all this is his second heart attack and the next one will be his last!

MARIAN: Yes, mother's right. He should be taking it easy. Isn't that right? (Looks at mother for agreement.)

NURSE: I understand both of your concerns for your husband's and father's welfare. But, Mr. Katz, I want to know your understanding and feelings about what activities and the amount of exercise your doctor wants you to get.

HERMAN: Well, my understanding is that I shouldn't do anything that upsets or fatigues me. And up to now I haven't felt like doing anything much.

NURSE (again looking at Herman): What specifically did the doctor say you should do?

Herman looks at his daughter and then wife, and Marian immediately jumps up to get his written directions on exercises and diet guidelines. Nurse reads these guidelines and explains the concept and importance of the recommended progressive exercise program. As this is being carefully explained, Mrs. K. looks over to the kitchen as if she is disinterested and then walks out to begin lunch preparations.

As the exercise program continued to be discussed, Herman remarked:

HERMAN: These activities don't use up much of my time and I'm tired of watching TV. I feel restless 'cause I have nothing to do.

NURSE: But, Herman, I understand that you have been refusing to get out of bed or dress yourself every day. We discussed last week that you could go outside and sit on the front porch, socialize, play cards and quiet table games, but you have not been interested in doing any of these things.

MARIAN: Dad, you're just stubborn and unwilling to do anything the doctor says!

MOTHER (looking over at her daughter): Oh, Marian, you're always attacking your father. He's just scared to death to move too much for fear of hurting his heart again.

MARIAN: But you don't help him any by cooking him that rich Jewish food and caring for his every need.

MOTHER: Let's drop it.

From the family case example, answer the following assessment questions involving family communication.

13. How extensively does family use functional and/or dysfunctional communication?

14. How well do members state feelings and needs?

15. Are qualification, clarification, or feedback techniques used?

16. How well do members listen to each other?

17. Are judgmental statements or assumptions used?

18. What values underlie the family's communication?

19. Are affective messages communicated?

20. Describe the family communication network.

21. What variables influence the family's interactions?

1. b, c, e, and g

2. *Sender.*
   a. Intention or meaning sent through clear channels.
   Receiver. Intended message and the received message is:
   b. Consistent.
   c. Congruent.
   d. Matches in meaning.

3. a. 2
   b. 4
   c. 2 or 3
   d. 5
   e. 1

4. b   6. d

5. c   7. True

8. a. *Content level.* Disinterest expressed in movie.
      Instructional level. Expression of warmth, sexual attraction and interest.
   b. *Content level.* Statement of love and demand that child play with toy.
      Instructional level. Expression of rejection of child's request for closeness and attention.
   c. *Content and instructional level.* Both consonant: Demand to stop behavior.

9. *Blind:* Channels will have a larger component of hearing-related interactions.
   Retarded: All sensory modalities will be used, but at a lower than age-related intellectual level.

10. a. Topic and problem would not be approached. The mother would wait to see if daughter shows further changes in behavior before she approaches the problem.
    b. Mother would show the bag with its contents to daughter, state she is concerned about substance and about her daughter's recent behavior. Some negotiation about how family members might accommodate one another's needs at this time would probably occur. In essence, the parent would not wait until further changes occurred.

11. Insufficient information and resources are brought in, which result in members' greater reliance on each other and family, and pose problems to family members in their interactions with the wider community.

12. The members become chaotic and disorganized, their needs are unmet, and they must meet needs through resources outside the family.

FAMILY CASE STUDY

The following interactional vignettes are followed by interpretations in the brackets:

NURSE (question directed at husband): What activities did the doctor recommend for you to do this week?

SYLVIA (interceding): I told Herman that he should take it easy because after all this is his second heart attack and the next one will be his last!
[Speaks for other person; tangentialization and "you should" statement.)

MARIAN: Yes, mother's right. He should be taking it easy. Isn't that right? (Looks at mother for agreement.)
[Short-term, issue-oriented coalition; assumption that father shares their same feelings—lack of exploration or validation with the father.]

NURSE: I understand both of your concerns for your husband's and father's welfare. But, Mr. Katz, I want to know your understanding and feelings about what activities and the amount of exercise your doctor wants you to get.
[Nurse refocuses and paraphrases her question by utilizing an "I want" statement.]

HERMAN: Well, my understanding is that I shouldn't do anything that upsets or fatigues me. And up to now I haven't felt like doing anything much.

NURSE (again looking at Herman): What specifically did the doctor say you should do?

Herman looks at his daughter and then wife, and daughter immediately jumps up to get his written directions on exercises and diet guidelines. Nurse reads these guidelines and explains the concept and importance of the recommended progressive exercise program. As this is being carefully explained, Mrs. K. looks over to the kitchen as if she is disinterested and then walks out to begin lunch preparations.
[Silent disagreement by wife. Perhaps this program violates her need to care for her husband, or maybe she feels it might be too much and is quite concerned over his possible future death. Also, culturally there is a tendency for family to greatly assist patients in Jewish families and this often runs counter to "pushing" a patient to be more self-sufficient.]

As the exercise program continued to be discussed, Herman remarked:

HERMAN: These activities don't use up much of my time and I'm tired of watching TV. I feel restless 'cause I have nothing to do.
[This is a case of incongruent behavior—between what he is now saying and what he has been doing and saying.]

NURSE: But, Herman, I understand that you have been refusing to get out of bed or dress yourself every day. We discussed last week that you could go outside and sit on the front porch, socialize, play cards and quiet table games, but you have not been interested in doing any of these things.
[Nurse points out the incongruency.]

MARIAN: Dad, you're just stubborn and unwilling to do anything the doctor says!
[Insulting, judgmental remark.]

MOTHER (looking over at her daughter): Oh, Marian, you're always attacking your father. He's just scared to death to move too much for fear of hurting his heart again.
[She interprets his behavior for him, but neglects to ask for feedback or even to look at him for his reaction.]

MARIAN: But you don't help him any by cooking him that rich Jewish food and caring for his every need.
[Attacks with new issue, as well as changing issues—failure to focus on one problem until closure is reached.]

MOTHER: Let's drop it.
[Cutoff in communication.]

13. Extensive use of dysfunctional communication (from short vignette). Most dysfunctional recurring patterns entail: (a) speaking for Mr. K. and daughter and mother assuming that they know his thoughts and feelings; (b) not completing one subject or issue; and (c) not asking for feedback from other family members.

14. They do state some of their fears for and feelings about Mr. K., although they do so indirectly. But none of them state their obvious reticence about the medical regimen.

15. Qualification, clarification, or feedback techniques are not shown in this vignette.

16. The family members sometimes listen to each other. When they agree, they show they are listening particularly. Mother walks away when she doesn't want to hear.

17. Judgmental statements or assumptions are made in speaking for Mr. K.; daughter commenting on father's stubbornness and mother's cooking.

18. The values underlying the family's communication involve concern over the father and spontaneity of response.

19. Affective are messages communicated, as in Mrs. K.'s concern for her husband (caring response). However, it was indirectly stated.

20. Nurse asks questions of Mr. K. Both the daughter and the wife speak to nurse for him and interact among each other. Herman is passive in interaction except for one interaction where he initiated complaint.

21. *Internal variables.* Family role relationships and power structure (roles of husband-father, wife-mother, and daughter). *External variables.* Cultural influence, as described in the vignette. Home environment is an important variable, since nurse does not have the same influence over the situation. Wife and daughter are the dominant ones here.

Numerous authors in the fields of family sociology and family conseling have written of the importance of the power dimension within the family. Cromwell and Olson, specialists in this aspect of the family system, write that "power is one of the most fundamental aspects of all social interaction. . . . Power has been used as a causal explanation of everything from conflict between nations to conflict between couples."[1]

All social systems, including the family, have structures which determine who wields power and what the hierarchy or "pecking order" is expected to be. Power, as viewed in this text, is one of the four interdependent structural dimensions of the family and, as such, is a reflection of family's underlying value system. In addition, it is of significance in understanding the interpersonal dynamics of all the types of family relationships—parent–child, sibling–sibling, and spouse–spouse—as well as the family's relationship to health professionals and outside agencies. Power and status dimensions are crucial in the establishment and maintenance of communication channels and networks. Blood and Wolfe go even further, asserting that "the most important aspect of the family structure is the power position of the members."[2] Furthermore, the close interrelationship with family roles is apparent in that a person's roles and positions are basic to his or her capacity to influence others.[3]

Power structures vary greatly from family to family, with differences positively related to the overall health status of the family. Moreover, decision making, as one measure of family power, has been a central concern in family therapy. Satir has noted that "there is probably nothing so vital to maintaining and developing a love relationship (or to killing it) as the decision-making process."[4]

Contemporary changes in the family have created an even greater need for family-centered health professionals to assess the power dimension. As part of the rapid changes in family life, families are not rigidly bound by tradition to relationships as they once were. Decision making and family power are generally more shared in families. Blood and Wolfe underscore the significance of this: "No change in the American family is mentioned more often than the shift from one-sided male authority to the sharing of power by the husband and wife. . . . The balance of power between the husband and wife is a sensitive reflection of the roles they play in marriage."[5] One of the outcomes of all these changes, choices, and blending of roles and decision-making in the family is the confusion, turmoil, and conflict observed in many families today.[6]

Knowledge and an appreciation of a family's power structure may be crucial in providing effective health care, especially when there are problems in assisting families to comply to a health regimen or obtain needed health services. The family member who acts as health leader, making the decisions and having the recognized authority in the área of health or in the

10

Family Power Structure

LEARNING OBJECTIVES

1. Describe the importance of understanding the family power structure.
2. Define the following concepts: power, authority, and family power.
3. Distinguish between the various bases for power and recognize some of the major sexual, ethnic, age, educational, and socioeconomic differences in the use of power sources.
4. Differentiate between the three decision-making techniques and the three processes utilized in family governance.
5. Identify and explain the role which each of the following variables plays in influencing family power: family communication network, control over implementation, interpersonal resources, coalition formation, social class, and developmental or life cycle changes.
6. Describe the most commonly used typology or classification for family and/or conjugal power.
7. Explain briefly how the overall power structure and marital satisfaction are associated.
8. Discuss the major contemporary change in the family power structure.
9. Using the family power continuum, identify where the "healthy" family usually lies.
10. Apply the following assessment areas in a written case history:
    a. Who makes which decisions?
    b. What are the decision-making techniques utilized?
    c. On what bases of power are decisions made?
    d. What are the significant variables affecting family power?
11. From your assessment of the above areas in a case situation, classify whether the family is dominated by a family member (and if so, who), is egalitarian (syncratic or autonomic), or is leaderless and chaotic.

family more generally, must be identified, acknowledged, and consulted. For instance, although the mother may be the person with whom the nurse is usually in contact, some channel of communication with the father must be found if he, in fact, has the final decision-making powers.

Following a presentation of basic definitions, this chapter discusses the following basic areas in the assessment of family power: (1) the bases for power; (2) decision-making (areas, outcomes, and process); and (3) the variables affecting power. A family power typology is then suggested, followed by a description of the attributes of healthy and unhealthy families.

FAMILY POWER: DEFINITIONS AND CONCEPTS

Power has numerous meanings, including influence, control, and dominance. For the purposes of the discussion to follow, *power* will be denoted as the ability—potential or actual—of an individual(s) to control or influence another person's behavior. *Family power*, as a characteristic of the family system, is the ability—potential or actual—of individual members to change the behavior of other family members.[7] Major components of family power are influence and decision making. The term *influence* is practically synonymous with power, being defined as the degree to which formal and informal pressure exerted by one member on the other(s) is successful in imposing that person's point of view, despite initial opposition.[8] *Dominance* is also used in the same context. In this chapter power, dominance, and influence will be used interchangeably. *Authority* is another closely associated term referring to the shared beliefs of family members which are culturally and normatively based, and which designate a family member as the rightful person to make decisions and assume the leadership position. In other words, authority is present when the individuals involved feel that it is proper for power to be held by a particular member of the group. Traditional beliefs and values, and their concomitant roles, are largely the basis for such feelings. *Legitimate power* is a synonymous term.

A word of caution is necessary at this point: power and authority do not always go hand in hand. A family member who has the authority to decide or act may not exercise this power for a variety of reasons. Thus there may be an incongruency between the power and authority elements in a family. Comparing the family to a larger social system, one could equate authority with the formal power structure and power with the informal power structure of a bureaucracy. It has long been recognized that within an organization the formal and informal power structures may be quite different from each other. The same situation applies to families.

Power is an abstract, complex, and multidimensional phenomenon and as such is not directly observable. It must then be inferred from observable behaviors in combination with self-reporting of family members, conducted through goal-directed interviews.

Power is a dimension of the family *system*, not a characteristic of a family member apart from that social system. Thus family power can be assessed only within the context of this system, and more specifically, within the context of the circular process of family interaction. Communication patterns reveal the family role and power dimensions. Family power can be seen in family processes ranging from daily routine exchanges to negotiation of complicated conflictual issues involving, for example, decision making, problem solving, conflict resolution, and crisis management. Moreover, family power applies to all of the following situations: the various dyadic, triadic, and larger sets of relationships within families; the functioning of the family as a total system; and the family system's relationship with the external social systems.[9]

MEASURING FAMILY POWER

How does one measure or assess power in a family? This is the key question, and one for which there is no consensus concerning the appropriate methodology and focus.

Relationship of Task Allocation to Family Power

Starting with Blood and Wolfe's large study of 900 families, which was completed in 1955 and reported on in 1960, researchers have examined task allocation on the assumption that there existed a positive relationship between whoever was in charge of carrying out a particular task and power in that area.[10] But later investigations of family differences in the allocation of responsibilites for the various decision areas and tasks indicated that such division of responsibility seldom reflected the dominant authority pattern. Reiss explains:

We must keep in mind that division of labor does not indicate in any direct way who has power or how a decision was arrived at regarding such division of labor. Rather, such a division of labor indicates that these are the traditional ways that tasks are allocated because of reasons that used to, and in some cases still do, have roots in the differences between the sexes in physical and cultural training. Males are still often trained to be more handy with mechanical tasks and tasks that take muscle power, and females are still trained to know more about cooking and cleaning, and those cultural traditions seem the essential basis of the division of tasks in the family.[11]

Johnson[12] verified this difference between family power and task and responsibility allocation. She interviewed 104 Japanese-American wives in Honolulu, including specific questions about who was responsible for and made decisions in the major areas of family life. She then asked questions to determine the wives' overall freedom to pursue individual interests, counter to wishes of their husbands.

Interestingly enough, Johnson discovered that only questioning about specific areas often distorted the real source of overall power, since one partner can be delegated responsibility, but ultimate power may lie with the other partner. When wives were queried about specific responsibilities and task allocation, they appeared more responsible than the husbands. But when asked broadly stated questions pertaining to the wife's evaluation of her power vis-à-vis her husbands' power, the data elicited contradicted the responses to the more specific questions. Relative to their husbands' power, most of these wives placed themselves in a subordinate position, largely attributing this fact to their Japanese heritage and its norms regarding male–female roles. Power here was defined as authority (legitimate power).

Thus while Japanese-American wives played active roles in decision making, they did so by virtue of a delegation of power from their husbands. In this instance, the husband assigns responsibilities while retaining final authority and orchestrates the power structure according to his preferences and wishes.

Focusing on Decision-making Outcomes

From Blood and Wolfe's large and influential work came further studies and questions about what constitute the important and valid measures of family power. Family power has primarily been researched by focusing on decision making. But is power identified by determining the outcome of a decision, i.e., what was the decision and who decided it, or is the decision-making process itself more significant? Current thinking prevails on the side of process. When we look at power as a process rather than the outcome of a decision, our concern shifts to an emphasis on family interaction rather than independent and isolated events,[13] an approach much more appropriate when working with families.

Studies of family power have been under criticism because of methodological limitations. Researchers have relied heavily on the survey and structured interview schedule, with little direct observation to validate the data so derived. When information has been gathered by interviewing families, a strong tendency has been discovered for couples to report an egalitarian relationship with each other, a characterization which is later not verified by observational study.[14] Hence it is suggested that the most accurate way to assess family power is to combine observation of marital, parent–child, sibling, and family interaction with self-reporting by all family members if possible.[15]

ASSESSMENT AREAS

To determine whether a dominant or mixed pattern of power exists, data on several facets of family life need to be collected to provide a sufficiently broad perspective for accurate appraisal. These assessment areas include (1) the bases for power, (2) the process and outcomes of decision making, and (3) the major variables or determinants of power. Using a systems approach, the target system is the family, but in addition, the conjugal (marital), parent–child, and sibling subsystems and their inherent sets of power relationships must not be forgotten.

Bases for Power

One salient aspect of family power concerns the bases for power within the family and its subsystems, that is, the source from which a family member's power is derived. Again this information often has to be inferred from observed behavior and by asking relevant questions. The importance of making this determination lies in the fact that the nature of the particular power base significantly affects interpersonal relationships, marital satisfaction, and family stability.

Raven et al. conducted a significant study of family power bases. Using their own data and that of previous studies, they generated a comprehensive list of the various types of power bases commonly observed in families.[16] A brief description of each type follows.

Legitimate Power or Authority

Legitimate power (sometimes called primary authority) refers to the shared belief and perceptions of family members that one person has the right to control another member's behavior. By virtue of the roles and positions a person occupies, certain rights and privileges exist which are associated with these roles and positions. An example would be the "rightness" of parental control or dominance over children. This is a traditionally based authority. Where the husband is traditionally in control of the whole family, a patriarchal pattern exists. The husband and wife would both accept the husband's dominant role as being "right" and "best" (indicative of role acceptance). Primary authority has remained a basic and significant base for power in many families. Turner underscores this by stating that "the fundamental determinant of family dominance (power) is authority or the belief in the propriety of unequal dominance."[17] Hence for authority to be effective, the whole family must accept and support this ideology.

In addition to tradition as a form of legitimate power is the often overlooked "power of the powerless," an important form of legitimate power that is based on the generally accepted right of those in need or the helpless to expect assistance from those in a position to render. it. *Helpless power* may be very effective in families. A spouse or a disabled family member may control the family on the basis of his or her frailty or helplessness. This is a commonly seen base for power and, unfortunately, a situation which makes it difficult for other family members' needs to be adequately met.

Referent Power

A second source for power is termed referent power and applies to the type of power persons have over others because of positive identification with them, as in a child's identification with a parent. Imitative behaviors and role modeling are the outcome of the existence of this type of power.

Expert Power

Expert power is in effect when the person being "influenced" perceives that another person (the "expert") has some special knowledge, skill, or expertise that gives him or her power. This notion of expert power corresponds well with the "resource theory" first expounded by Blood and Wolfe. When power is defined as an ability to influence or pressure, resources such as any attributes, circumstances, or possessions are seen as primary determinants of that ability.[18] The most important resources which serve to increase family power are education, occupation, income, social participation, and role competence (adequate performance of various roles).[19] The greater resources of one spouse over the other are viewed as the chief alternative source of family power to traditionally based authority.[20] For example, the husband may be dominant because he controls the purse strings, or the wife may be dominant because she is more practical and goal directed than the husband.

Reward Power

This base of power stems from the expectation that the influencing, dominant person will do something posi-tive in return if the other person complies. Overt bargaining may accompany the use of reward power.

Coercive Power

The effective use of this source of power is based on the perception and belief that the person with power might or will punish other individuals if they do not comply. Coercive power is used with coercive decision making (see below).

Informational Power

This power base stems from the content of the persuasive message. An individual is convinced of the "rightness" of the sender's message due to a careful and successful explanation of the necessity for change.[21]

A variation of this direct informational power is "indirect" informational power. This occurs when a more subtle dropping of hints, suggestions, and information influences a person to act without the obvious indication of persuasion (a common doctor–nurse game tactic).[22]

The Process and Outcomes of Decision Making

It is agreed that decision making is a principal index of power. Blood and Wolfe explain the relationship of power to decision making: "Power is manifested in the ability to make decisions affecting the life of the family."[23] Turner speaks of decision making as central to the fulfillment of family functions and tasks, and that power or dominance patterns are the primary by-product of decision making.[24]

In assessing family decision making, one can analyze the decision making process (felt to be the most important by those working with families in the helping professions[25]) or the areas and outcomes of decisions. Of course, a consideration of both aspects adds to the comprehensiveness of any assessment of this dimension of family power.

Relative to areas and outcomes of decision making, the focus would be on who makes what kinds of decisions. Specific questions can be asked of the family to elicit this information. For instance, one might ask who is responsible for making decisions about and takes responsibility for the areas of major importance in family life. In conjugal relationships power can vary from one domain to the next, with role definitions determining who had power in a given area. For example, the wife might have more power in regard to social and kin relationships and household matters, while the husband has more control over the finances. In other families power may be more equally divided, with a pattern of shared power prevailing.

As described previously, though, it must be remembered that specific areas of responsibility and of decision making do not often coincide with the more general and dominant power pattern in a family. What pattern actually exists could be determined by asking more general questions, supplemented with observation, of family members concerning who they feel in the family is most powerful overall and why.

The second area calling for assessment is the actual outcome of decisions—not only who proposes ideas and solutions to problems, but also whose idea or suggestion is finally adopted (who "wins"). In families where decisions are shared and represent the outcome of mutual discussion and exploration, this kind of information is difficult for family members to recall. But despite the difficulty involved in accurately describing the outcome (people remember what decision was made but find it harder to remember who had the last say or made the ultimate decision), assessment of the outcome of an issue, conflict, or argument is helpful in ascertaining the source of power and in whom this resides. Komarovsky notes that "power is most visible in contested decisions ending in victory of one partner. But it exists irrespective of conflict because the powerful partner may so influence the wishes and preferences of his mate that a contest of wills does not even arise."[26]

In regard to decisions and their outcomes, discerning what kinds of problems or issues are involved and how important they are to the family is helpful. Does a decision cut across all the major areas of family life or is it limited to a specific area? Komarovsky underscores the significance of ascertaining the centrality of the issue by observing that "general decision-making in one or two areas of family life may not be a good index of general power. It depends upon the importance of such areas for each partner."[27]

To the question of who makes the decisions, one must question who decides who is to make decisions. Recalling Johnson's findings of power within Japanese-American families, the significance of discovering this information becomes apparent. An assessor can easily be misled by the obvious responsibilities and decisions of one mate rather than realize that these are actually delegated, or relegated, to the weaker partner by the dominant member of the couple. Thus on the surface it may appear that the wife is responsible for grocery shopping, cooking, and child rearing. But these tasks may only be relegated to her by her husband, and should her actions incur his displeasure, her power may be withdrawn. This is the usual case in authoritarian or patriarchal families. The husband's power may derive not only from a traditional value structure, but through effective control of economic resources and access to transportation and by opposition to family planning with resultant pregnancies and child-care responsibilities that keep the wife at home.

Male dominance is commonly seen in unacculturated immigrant families from Europe, Asia, and Latin America. Moreover, an older matriarch is sometimes present in these families. On the surface, the wife-mother may seem to be the locus of initiative and decision making, but in this instance, the male head of the family or the aging matriarch usually only concedes this authority, ready to take it back whenever he or she wishes. Thus a distinction again needs to be made between everyday decisions and negative authority—the right to prevent others from doing as they wish.[28]

As previously mentioned, another covert source of power which can be quite misleading to the observer-history taker is the family member who utilizes "helpless power." Here a family member unconsciously controls the family by using illness or debility as a control mechanism.

The process used in arriving at family decisions is also crucial in the assessment of family power. Family decision making in this context refers to a process directed toward gaining the assent and commitment of family members to carry out a course of action or to maintain the status quo. In assessing this area, the central focus is how decisions are made. By understanding the techniques used in family decision making, the assessor will be better able to identify who makes decisions and, more important, the relative power of each family member and his or her participation in family affairs and decisions. The family's decision-making process is also reflective of one's cultural and socioeconomic background, as well as how well a family meets the individualized needs of its members.

Families tend to make use of one particular method of decision making although the secondary use of the other basic techniques of decision making will also be observed. Analysis of the power structure and decision-making process reveals the tremendous interrelationship of these features with the other structural dimensions of the family. The family which extensively uses democratic methods of decision making (consensus decision making), for example, will generally have an egalitarian structure and value system, in which role sharing and open, functional communications exist.

Decision Making by Consensus

The first technique of decision making is termed consensus. According to American ideals, this is the healthy way to make decisions. Here a particular course of action is mutually agreed on by all involved. There is equal commitment to the decision, as well as satisfaction, by the family members or mates. Consensus decisions are agreed on through discussion.

Since a substantial degree of interdependence and egalitarianism among family members is needed to utilize this method, as well as an ability to discuss and problem solve, this kind of decision making is not as frequently used by real-life families as television would perhaps have us believe.

What happens when consensual decision making is utilized by a family after an initial disagreement? A change takes place in the opinions or views of some or all of the family members. This occurs during the decision-making process when those in disagreement eventually perceive that action to be taken corresponds with their personal or shared values.[29]

Decision Making by Accommodation

A second type of decision making is termed accommodation. Here the family members' initial feelings about an issue are discordant. One or more of the family members make concessions, either willingly or unwillingly. Some member(s) assent in order to allow a decision to be reached. Hence it may involve voluntary compromising in which concessions may involve all persons concerned or may involve a sacrifice by one so that others may have their way. Privately or publicly the conceding member(s) will not be convinced, however, that the decision in question is best.[30]

Accommodative decisions are made somewhere on a continuum from coercion to bargaining, marked by differences of degrees in attitudes of participants towards their commitment and in their relationship under which the forms of accommodation take place. There are several ways in which accommodation occurs: by use of compromising, bargaining, and coercion.

Compromising, as stated above, refers to the making of concessions by all the family members involved so that the decision reached is not reflective of either partner's original choices, but has some acceptable elements for all concerned.

Ideally, bargaining leads to a willing agreement to which each interactant is committed because of the benefits he or she is to derive from the agreement. Concessions that members make to each other are expected to be reciprocated, so that ultimately the sacrifices of each will balance out. The use of bargaining in family negotiations demonstrates that a trust exists among the members along with a belief that others will be fair and honest in keeping up their ends of the bargain.

Coercion is the least functional technique along the accommodation continuum since it results in an unwilling agreement to which commitment is assured only by the continuance of coercive power. The existence of coercion shows the dominance of one member over others.

To summarize, an accommodation is always an agreement to disagree, to adopt a common decision in the face of irreconcilable differences.[31]

De Facto Decision Making

Family members may also arrive at decisions by using a de facto route. In this case, things are allowed "to just happen" without planning. A decision is forced by events in the absence of active, voluntary, or effective decision making. De facto decisions may also be made when arguments occur to which there was no resolution or when issues were not brought up and discussed. These decisions, then, are made in fact rather than by planning.

De facto decision making is seen in many disorganized, multiproblem families, many of whom believe in fate and feel powerless to control their own destiny. Moreover, de facto decision making may be situationally limited or occur when problems in communication exist, as when significant problems or issues are not discussed. Cultural norms are important to consider here, since obstacles to communication and active decision making may also have a cultural or ethnic basis. For example, among Latino couples, family planning may be an area of closed communication, and pregnancies therefore become the outcome of de facto decision making.

Variables Affecting Family Power

In addition to power bases and decision making, Turner has identified some of the major variables affecting dominance or power. He calls these the "determinants of dominance." These factors consist of (1) the family communication network, (2) control over implementation, (3) interpersonal resources, and (4) formation of coalitions. In addition, social class and developmental variables, as well as cultural influences on family power (discussed at length in Chap. 16), are important considerations.

Family Communication Network

Communication is seldom of equal intensity within each of the pairs of relationships in the family. The husband and wife may communicate frequently, intensely, and over a wide area of topics, while the father and youngest son may have very little communication with each other. Two siblings may have a close, confidential type of relationship. Age and sex characteristics, as well as personality attributes of family members, influence the nature of the family communication network.

When there is unequal communication between family members, intermediaries ("go-betweens") usually exist. The person in the family who serves as an intermediary in communications between others (in many instances the mother), but who is able to interact directly with all family members, holds a central position in the communication network.

Communication networks are mentioned here because of their correlation with the power structure. The greater the centrality of the family member, the greater his or her dominance, due to his or her control over the outcome of the decision-making process. Since the intermediary understands the attitudes and opinions of most of the family members, he or she can use this information to influence family members. The go-between is also able to censor or screen information from the sender to the other family members. This censorship function and ability to alter messages as seen fit gives the intermediary extensive power, at least in some areas. In larger families one may find a secondary intermediary—such as an older son or daughter—who acts as a link between other children and the mother.[32]

Implementation Control

A second factor affecting the power structure in a family is who has control over implementation. The family's organization gives some family members unequal control over the means of carrying out family decisions. When a family member, the husband, for example, exerts his influence or control and convinces his nonworking wife that she should maintain more discipline of the children, he depends on the wife's commitment to carry out his wishes, since he is typically not in a position to supervise. In this case, the wife, in her central position, has substantial power, since she will decide how and what to implement. In many families, where the mother is home most of the time and the father is working long hours, the mother is firmly in control of family life.[33]

Interpersonal Resources

In addition to the family communication network and control over implementation, each person in the family has certain resources that contribute to his or her ability to wield power over the others. One important resource is the use of interpersonal techniques. "It is not uncommon to find one family member who has few of the objective resources that ordinarily facilitate dominance actually controlling much of family life through his masterful use of a broad repertoire of interpersonal techniques."[34]

It is also commonly observed that individuals who have a good repertoire of interpersonal skills frequently do not use them effectively within the family. Turner identifies some of the primary reasons for the ineffectual use or lack of use of these interpersonal skills as being (1) a person's lack of self-confidence in a relationship with other members of the family, (2) the unimportance of the issue, (3) norms restricting the use of certain interpersonal techniques, (4) negative attitudes toward conflict, and (5) the unequal importance of the relationship to one or more family members.

Self-confidence. Lack of self-confidence or a sense of inferiority in a relationship with another member of the family is a pervasive problem. When persons in authority do not use their "rights" effectively, this is usually the consequence of lack of self-confidence or, more generally, a low self-concept.

Importance of Issue. The extent to which family members utilize effective interpersonal skills depends on the significance of the issue being discussed, i.e., the more meaningful the issue to an individual, the greater expenditure of energy to effect a decision favorable to the person involved.

Restrictive Norms. Another reason for ineffectual use of interpersonal resources involves the constraints imposed by the set of norms that regulate the techniques which are acceptable in a particular family and within specific relationships (brother–sister, husband–wife, parent–child). For instance, there are normative gender differences in relationships of siblings. It is usually acceptable for a young daughter to use "helpless power" by crying when hit by her brother, whereas the reverse situation might result in parental irritation at their son's "sissy" behavior.

Attitudes Toward Conflict. Another factor leading to nonuse of interpersonal skills is the family member's aversion to conflict. Those who fear rejection or regard expression of anger as a serious threat to a relationship will feel constrained in their use of communication that might result in open conflict. In contrast, persons who do not become disturbed by conflict and who are able to recover quickly from confrontations have much greater interpersonal skills.[35]

Importance of Relationship. The last variable affecting the use of interpersonal skills in family communication has to do with the strengths and the unequal nature of the family relationships.[36] Waller explains this case by what he calls "the principle of less interest."[37] This principle explains that exploitation is likely to occur in a relationship where the differences in levels of involvement are great. For instance, the principle of less interest states that within a dyadic relationship, the person who cares least about whether the relationship continues or not has the greatest power over the relationship. He or she usually has less interest and involvement in maintaining the relationship because he or she has many more alternatives or resources. With decreased involvement, the less interested person can use manipulative or coercive techniques at the expense of the other. A commonly seen example may help elucidate this principle. In a marital situation, one member may be quite valued and independent, while the other individual feels dependent and inferior. Decisions are then made by the dominant mate, since he or she has many more options open and there is less involvement in the relationship. In middle-class America this principle still probably operates in favor of the man.

Formation of Coalitions

A fourth factor affecting family power is the formation of coalitions. Coalitions are either temporary, means-oriented alliances or long-term alliances made to offset the dominance of one or more other family members. Subgroups within a family band together to support each other and to increase their power position vis-à-vis other members of the family. Obviously then, coalitions generate more power for the members who join together.

Coalitions in families are most healthy when they exist within the appropriate power levels.[38] It is pointed out by family therapists[39-41] that a sustaining parental coalition is a healthy and a virtually necessary phenomenon to effectively parent children. In contrast, long-term parent–child coalitions are unhealthy, since they disrupt the intact functioning of the parent–child and spouse subsystems. Nevertheless, mother–child coalitions are especially common in patriarchal families, where the father's power is great and together the mother and child can to some degree dilute his power. The child in this case can also expect special favors from the mother. Sibling coalitions are also common. Children join forces to more efficaciously oppose or evade the rules parents establish.[42]

One of the difficulties in a single-parent family is the obvious inability to form a parental coalition. Two-parent families tend to have significantly more resources and alternatives available to them than do one-parent families, since couples in the former can support each other and form a coalition. In one-parent families, the strength of authority may be a dominant and necessary factor in controlling the family situation.[43]

Social Class Differences in Family Power

Lower-Class Families

Besmer summarizes the frequently seen power characteristics of poor families. The husband is more likely to proclaim authority simply because he is a male, although actually having to concede more authority to the wife due to the paucity of his resources. The father most generally loses influence in the family at the lower levels as a consequence of his social and occupational inadequacy. The authoritarian theme is a strong underlying factor in the interpersonal relationships of the poor. There is a strong belief in the validity of strength as the source of power and on the rightness of existing patterns. An individual's dominance, rather than expertise and the merit of his or her suggestions, is relied on as the common source of decisions.[44]

The lower-class wife has relatively more duties than either the middle- or upper-class wife or the lower-class husband and thus frequently has more influence in the family decision making than housewives of the other classes. This is especially true in the financial area, where the lower-class wife may feel that "earning money is the man's responsibility, spending it wisely is the woman's."

Komarovsky, who studied a group of working-class* families, found that there was extensive variation of dominance patterns within this large group. She reports that the husbands are dominant in 45% of the marriages, the wives in 21%, and in 27% a balance of power exists. Education was found to be the important determinant as to how authoritarian the family power structure was—the higher the education, the more flexible and "middle class" certain ideals and protocols in marriage became. The incidence of dominance by the husband declined with better education of the husband, and in contrast, partriarchal attributes were more prevalent among the less educated.[45]

Middle-Class Families

According to Kanter, the most egalitarian or companion-based marriages seem to be found among the lower middle-class, white-collar workers, perhaps as a result of the greater availability of husband's time to share chores and act as a companion to his wife. "In other occupational groups, such as professors or executives, the spillover of work into leisure time can generate irritability and lack of attention at home."[46]

Changes in Family Power through the Family's Life Cycle

The decisions a family makes about an individual member or about the family are also closely associated with the family's life cycle, as is the distribution of power among the family members. Thus during the

---

* Working class is defined as the upper-lower class of unskilled blue-collar workers and the lower middle-class of skilled blue-collar workers.

early years of marriage, before children, couples tend to be syncretic—discussing and mutually deciding on major decisions, except perhaps about the husband's job and food and housekeeping matters.[47] Later in the family's life cycle, when children are being raised and the system is more complex, each spouse usually has clearly defined areas of power and decision making, although major decisions are still jointly made. Corrales confirms that when the dyad changes to a triad with the addition of a baby, some loss in the wife's power is seen.[48] Typically, mates discuss most areas less and less as time goes on, a sign that some estrangement from each other may also be occurring. In the later years of the family, the marital couple, returning to a dyadic relationship, again share decision making and power.

FAMILY POWER TYPOLOGIES

One of the hoped for, but sometimes unrealizable, aims of analyzing the assessment areas of bases for power, decision making, and the variables affecting power is to be able to classify a family as to its overall power structure. This involves being able to state whether a family is dominated by one member (usually one spouse), has an egalitarian power structure, or has no effective leadership (is chaotic). Some authors point out that most of the classifications used to describe families are too simplistic and do not adequately reflect the dynamic qualities of family power nor its complexity. Although we should retain an awareness that an overall labeling of family power may not be possible nor entirely accurate, we cannot overlook the value of classification: namely, that it permits a lot to be said in a few words. If a family displays an overall dysfunctional power structure, a statement of this conclusion may serve as a family nursing diagnosis.

Historically, the literature has described generalized, pure types of families, in particular, the patriarchal and the democratic families. In the patriarchal family, the father is an authoritarian figure, with family power vested in his hands, and his wife, his sons and their wives and children, and his unmarried daughters are subordinated to his rule. In contrast, the democratic family is based on the equality of husband and wife, with consensus in making decisions and an increasing participation by children as they grow older.[49]

The most frequently used typology today for classifying power in the marital subsystem or family was developed by Herbst. It divides marital power into autocratic, syncretic, and autonomic patterns.[50] Autocratic power patterns exist when the family is dominated by a single family member. In these families,

decisions on marital activities, and usually family activities also, are made solely by this individual. Syncretic power patterns exist when decisions involving the marriage, as well as the family, are made by both members of the marital dyad. In this case there is a greater mutual commitment and involvement in the marriage. An autonomic power structure is present when the two partners function independently of one another in both decision making and their activities. Other authors refer to this pattern at the family level as atomistic. Tinkham and Voorhies comment on this type of family:

> In the nuclear family today, with its emphasis on the individual and his achievements, the old stereotypes of the woman's role and the husband's leadership role do not have much relevance. Today's families are often more atomistic, with decisions being made by an individual on the basis of his own needs rather than on the basis of the family's needs.[51]

One of the problems with Herbst's original typology is that he assumed that the power always rested with one or the other parents (or was shared). This is a constricting approach, since the dominant individual may be a child, grandparent, or other family member if the family is other than a traditional two-parent nuclear family. Most research into family power has, in fact, dealt with conjugal power rather than family power, focusing on only husband–wife interactions to the exclusion of the child's role in the decision-making processes. The relative power of children in families has been found to be substantial, especially that of older children. For instance, Strodtbeck found that the power of an adolescent son in a family was almost as great as that of the mother.[52] Thus an adequate assessment of the power structure must include consideration of the children.[53]

In contrast with the analysis and classification of marital power relationships, the categorization of the parent–child subsystem has usually been quite simple: on a continuum from high to low parental control, for example.

In family process literature, which derives largely from family therapy, the categories most widely used are symmetrical (balanced), complementary (submissive–dominant), and metacomplementary (dominance through weakness) forms. These three types of marital role relationships are discussed in Chapter 11.

Lewis et al. developed a comprehensive model for summarizing a family's power structure which includes the chaotic or leaderless family not identified in the former models. Figure 10.1 modifies Lewis' model, incorporating the various types of power commonly observed in families. This continuum is suggested for use in assessing the overall family power dimensions.

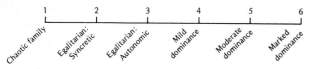

Explanation of the above terms:

Chaotic family: This refers to a leaderless family, where no member has adequate power to make decisions effectively.

Egalitarian syncretic and autonomic families: Here decisions and power are shared. In the syncretic form the decisions are made together; in the autonomic form the decisions are made independently.

Dominance (mild to marked): Dominance or power ranges from marked dominance, where there is practically absolute control and no negotiation to mild dominance, where there is a tendency for dominance and submissiveness, but most decisions are reached through respectful, mutual negotiation.

FIGURE 10.1
The family power continuum. The chaotic family (1) refers to a leaderless family, wherein no member has adequate power to make decisions effectively. In egalitarian syncretic and autonomic families (2–3), decisions and power are shared. In the syncretic form, the decisions are made together; in the autonomic form, they are made independently. Dominance or power (4–6) ranges from marked, where there is practically absolute control by an individual and no negotiation, to mild, where there is a tendency for dominance and submissiveness, but most decisions are reached through respectful, mutual negotiation.

Marital Satisfaction and Family Power Type

Research done in the 1950s and 1960s consistently demonstrated that the structure of decision-making power was significantly related to marital satisfaction. High levels of satisfaction were found most frequently among egalitarian couples, followed closely by couples where the husband was dominant. Wife-dominant couples showed the least marital satisfaction.[54]

More recently, Center et al. used a different typology of power and discussed some of the differences from earlier studies. They found that 75 percent of the mates in husband-dominated marriages perceived their marriages to be highly satisfying, while 70 percent of couples in syncretic marriages—where a preponderance of decisions were jointly made—reported being very satisfied. In autonomic marriages—where power was shared, but decisions were made independently—79 percent of the couples reported being very satisfied. Wife-dominated marriages were less satisfying, with only 20 percent of the couples perceiving their marriages to be highly satisfying.[55]

In discussing the findings of Center et al., Corrales notes two interesting trends:

First, is the high proportion of satisfied people who have an autonomic pattern. This is surprising since the equalitarian norm is syncretic by cultural definition. Perhaps the situation of equal but separate spheres is becoming a more viable arrangement. Second, is the very high proportion of satisfied persons in the husband-dominated category. There is no significant difference between these

and the equalitarian couples who report very satisfying marriages. This indicates, as do past studies, that the husband-dominated structure is apparently still quite viable.[56]

As mentioned, wife-dominated couples have generally been found to rate their marriages as less satisfying.[57] It is curious that these women classify themselves as the least maritally satisfied, far below their husbands' satisfaction. The tentative conclusion that may be drawn is that the wife is dominant by default, not choice, being forced to fill the vacuum created by a weak, passive, or incompetent husband. Wife-dominance also goes against the normative expectations, that is, the cultural prescriptions of either the traditional (husband-dominated) or the modern (egalitarian) marriage. Why are husbands in these marriages not also unhappy? Corrales[58] speculates that the reason might be because the wife not only makes most of the decisions, but probably also assumes most family roles.*

One of the family phenomena which Mead discusses is the position of the husband in many American families. She calls his position a "social accident" and points out that the woman's family involvement is generally quite extensive. In contrast, the man's socialization has been geared heavily toward his occupational role, which is basically outside of the family. His self-concept is to a large degree derived from his perception of how well he is carrying out this work role and the satisfactions to be derived from it. Because men have important alternatives to family satisfactions, they may reduce their involvement in family life. This lack of interest and involvement in the family may be one of the important reasons for the existence of wife-dominant families, at least among the middle-class. Thus, the wife may be saddled with most family responsibilities and decisions due to the husband's withdrawal from family life.[59]

CONTEMPORARY TRENDS IN FAMILY POWER

There has been a gradual shift from the traditional, patriarchal family structure toward a democratic equalitarian or egalitarian family structure. As egalitarianism in the family becomes more prominent, changes in women's base for power are occurring, albeit slowly. In 1974 Johnson demonstrated that men were more likely to use expert formal legitimacy or direct informational power as a base for influence in the family,

---

* Despite the wife's general feelings of dissatisfaction and the husband's relatively higher level of satisfaction in these marriages, it must be remembered that both of the spouses are intimately involved with establishing and maintaining the power structure within the relationship. Hence the end result is the responsibility of neither spouse exclusively.

while women used referent power, "helpless" power, and indirect informational power.[60] These bases for power were selected by women because of their greater acceptability to their mates. If women used the modes of expert power and direct informational power, they were seen as being masculine and aggressive. The common use of helpless power by women is more acceptable to their spouse, although at the expense of their self-esteem.

Raven sees these interactional and power strategies changing, however:

> There is good reason to suspect that the bases of power in conjugal relationships may be changing dramatically with the current changes in the sex roles. The problems in such changes would appear to be especially great for women, and we might well expect that changes in power choice in the family will be accompanied by increased personal threat for both parties and increasing tensions in the family.[61]

HEALTHY AND DYSFUNCTIONAL FAMILY POWER ATTRIBUTES

Lewis et al. conducted in-depth interviews with a group of middle-class families to determine their psychosocial health status and the family structural characteristics which correlated with it.[62] From these interviews and observational analysis, they grouped families into three categories of health, from the severely dysfunctional to optimally healthy. It was generally found that the most severely dysfunctional families presented chaotic family structures (see Fig. 10.1), and the most competent of families presented flexible structures. These researchers emphasized that, "The most direct measure of structure concerned the distribution of power or influence within the family."[63]

The power attributes of healthy families were seen to reflect the following:

> In healthy families the parental coalition played a crucial role in the determination of overall family competence.... Leadership was provided by the parental coalition as was a model of relating which appeared to be of great learning value to the children. Leadership was shared by the parents.... This trend toward an egalitar-

ian marriage was in striking contrast to both the more distant marriages of the adequate families and the marital pattern of dominance and submission that so often was seen in the dysfunctional families.[64]

In the healthy families the parents acting as a coalition did not exercise their power in an authoritarian or rigid way but, within their style of leadership, left room for options and negotiation. Nevertheless, power and boundaries were clear; there was no confusion as to the position and power of family members. Generally the father held the most power, the mother somewhat less, and the child distinctly least.[65] In contrast, the severely disturbed families studied all showed that the family had little power. The most inept families, they reported, had a powerless father, with strong coalitions between mother and child. In families labeled as midrange, a strong, healthy parental-marital coalition did not exist. These families characteristically maintained rigid, authoritarian structures via dominance by one mate.[66]

Concerning such findings on the healthy family's attributes, Minuchin expresses his belief that the most important aspect of power within a family is the presence of a clear and functioning hierarchy in which the parents and children have different levels of authority. For a family to function effectively, there must also be complementarity of functions, with the husband and wife accepting interdependency and working as a team.

Minuchin also mentions variations in power due to differing family forms. In large families, single-parent families, or families where both parents are employed, some allocation of parental power is usually given to an older child(ren). This arrangement may work well, for the younger children are cared for, and the parental child can develop responsibility, competence, and autonomy beyond his or her years. The family with a parental child structure may experience problems, however, when the delegation of authority is unclear or if the parents abdicate their authority, leaving the parental child to become the primary source of decision making, control, and guidance. In these situations, the child is given a task which exceeds his or her abilities and which interfere with the meeting of his or her childhood needs of support and dependency.[67]

ASSESSMENT QUESTIONS

In this chapter the various major areas germane to family power have been described. Family power is obviously not an easily inferred dimension to assess. In spite of these difficulties, the following summary of the primary facets of power, the areas to observe, and the questions to ask will hopefully make the assessment process more concrete and clear.

DECISION MAKING

Areas and Outcomes of Decisions: Who makes *what* decisions? And how important are these decisions or issues to the family? As some family workers have done, you may wish to ask more specific questions to elicit this information (and validate what you can with your own observations). General questions followed by more specific questions in these areas may be helpful:

    a. Financial: Who budgets, pays bills, decides on how money is spent?
    b. Social: Who decides on how to spend an evening or which friends or relatives to see?
    c. Major decisions: Who decides on changes in jobs or residence?
    d. Child rearing: Who disciplines and decides on children's activities?[68]

It must be remembered, though, when asking these questions, that *overall* power in the family often does not correlate well with specific task responsibilities.

Decision-Making Process: What specific techniques are utilized for making decisions in the family and to what extent are these utilized?

    a. Consensus.
    b. Accommodation.
      1. Bargaining
      2. Compromising
      3. Coercion
    c. De facto.

Specific questions eliciting decision-making techniques used would focus on *how* the family makes decisions.

BASES FOR POWER

This area deals with the source from which the power of individuals within a family is derived. To enumerate again these various sources:

    1. Authority (legitimate power) and helpless power.
    2. Referent power.
    3. Expert power or resources.
    4. Reward power.
    5. Coercive power.
    6. Informational power—direct and indirect

Questions asked to elicit information on the source of power might follow either specific questions about who makes certain decisions and how (sometimes how also reveals the source). For example, in speaking to the husband-father: "On what basis was it decided to send the children to summer camp?" Or you may suggest choices, such as, "Was your wife's suggestion agreed on because of her greater knowledge in that area, because of the children's positive feelings and respect for her, or for some other reason?"

VARIABLES AFFECTING FAMILY POWER

Several variables were discussed which affect family power. These are:

    1. The family communication network.
    2. Control for implementation of decisions.
    3. Interpersonal resources, including factors which explain why the family members will or will not use their interpersonal resources, e.g., lowered level of self-confidence, unimportance of issue under consideration, norms restricting use of interpersonal techniques, attitudes toward conflict, and the unequal nature of relationship.
    4. Formation of coalitions.
    5. Social class differences (cultural differences are discussed in Chap. 16).
    6. Family life cycle differences.

Recognizing the influence of other assessment areas will assist in more fully appraising and interpreting family power attributes.

OVERALL FAMILY POWER

From your assessment of all the above broad areas, are you able to deduce whether the family power can be characterized as dominated by wife, husband, child, or grandparent; as egalitarian-syncretic or autonomic; as leaderless or chaotic?

The family power continuum presented in this chapter can be used for a visual representation of the analysis.

If dominance is found, who is the dominant person? Power arrangements on this continuum in the 2 to 4 range have been found to be healthy and satisfying patterns (if mild dominance is by husband).

To determine the overall power pattern, asking a broad, open-ended question is often illuminating. For example, asking both spouse and children if feasible: "Who usually has the last say about important issues? Who is really in charge and why? Who runs the family? Who wins the important arguments or issues? Who usually wins out if there is a disagreement? Who gets his or her way when they disagree?"

Another significant follow-up question is, "Are you satisfied with how decisions are made and with who makes the decisions (i.e, the present power structure)?"

In concluding this discussion of the assessment of family power, it needs to be emphasized that the most accurate way to assess this area is to observe marital and parent–child interactions—and sibling interaction if indicated and feasible—and combine pertinent observations with the data gathered from the self-reporting by family members.[69]

REFERENCES

1. Cromwell RE, Olson DH (eds): Power in Families. New York, Sage Publications, 1975, p 3
2. Blood RO, Wolfe DM: Husbands and Wives: The Dynamics of Married Living. Glencoe, Ill, Free Press, 1960
3. Rogers MF: Instrumental and infraresources: The bases of power. Am J Sociol 79:1423, 1974
4. Satir V: Peoplemaking. Palo Alto, California, Science and Behavior, 1972, p 131
5. Blood, Wolfe, op. cit., p 11
6. Peters LR: Family team or myth. In Hall J, Weaver B (eds): Nursing of Families in Crisis. Philadelphia, Lippincott, 1974, p 226
7. Olson DH, Cromwell RE: Power in Families. In Cromwell, Olson, op. cit., p 5
8. McDonald GW: Family power, reflection and direction. Pacific Sociol Rev 20:612, 1977
9. Olson DH, Cromwell RE, Klein DM: Beyond family power. In Cromwell, Olson, op. cit., pp 236, 238
10. Blood, Wolfe, op. cit.
11. Reiss IL: Family Systems in America, 2nd ed. Hinsdale, Ill, Dryden Press, 1976, p 254
12. Johnson CL: Authority and power in Japanese-American marriage. In Cromwell, Olson, op. cit., pp 182–196
13. Sprey J: Family power structure: a critical comment. Marriage Family 34:235, 1972
14. Cromwell, Olson, op. cit., pp 7, 22, 144
15. Olson DH, Cromwell RE: Methodological issues in family power. In Cromwell, Olson, op. cit., pp 142–145
16. Raven BH, Centers R, Rodrigues A: The bases of conjugal power. In Cromwell, Olson, op. cit., pp 217–232
17. Turner RH: Family Interaction. New York, Wiley, 1970, p 133
18. Osmond MW: Reciprocity: A dynamic model and a method to study family power. J Marriage Family 40:51, 1978
19. McDonald, op. cit., pp 609, 610.
20. McDonald, op. cit., p 609
21. Raven, op. cit., p 219
22. Ibid., p 232
23. Blood, Wolfe, op. cit., p 2
24. Turner, op. cit., Chap. 5
25. Sprey, op. cit., pp 235–238
26. Komarovsky M: Blue-Collar Marriage. New York, Random House, 1964, p 221
27. Ibid.
28. Goode W: The Family. Englewood Cliffs, NJ, Prentice-Hall, 1964, p 75
29. Turner, op. cit., p 103
30. Ibid., p. 98
31. Ibid., pp 106–108
32. Ibid., pp 120–123
33. Ibid., pp 123–124
34. Ibid., p 125
35. Ibid., pp 126–127
36. Ibid., p. 127
37. Waller W: The Family: A Dynamic Interpretation. New York, Dryden Press, 1938
38. Gorman G: New families, new marriages. In Smoyak S: The Psychiatric Nurse as a Family Therapist. New York, Wiley, 1975, p 30
39. Satir, op. cit.
40. Minuchin S: Families and Family Therapy. Cambridge, Mass, Harvard, 1976
41. Lidz T: The Family and Human Adaptation. New York, International Universities, 1963
42. Turner, op. cit., pp 128–132
43. Jayaratne S: Behavioral intervention and family decision-making. Social Work 23:24, 1978
44. Besmer A: Economic deprivation and family patterns. In Irelan LM (ed): Low-Income Life Styles. Washington, DC, United States Department of Health, Education, and Welfare, 1967, p 19
45. Komarovsky, op. cit., pp 222–225
46. Kanter RM: Jobs and families: Impact of working roles on life. Children Today 7:13, 1978
47. Blood RO: Marriage, 2nd ed. Glencoe, Ill, Free Press, 1969, p 205
48. Corrales RG: Power and satisfaction in early marriage. In Cromwell, Olson, op. cit., p 214
49. Burgess EW, et al: The Family: From Institution to Companionship, 3rd ed. New York, American Book, 1963
50. Herbst PG: Conceptual framework for studying the family: Family living-regions and pathways, family living-patterns of interaction. In Oeser OA, Hammond SB (eds): Social Structure and Personality in a City. New York, Macmillan, 1954
51. Tinkham C, Voorhies E: Community Health Nursing, 2nd ed. New York, Appleton, 1977
52. Strodtbeck FL: Family interaction, values, and achievement. In McClelland DC et al. (eds): Talent and Society. Princeton, NJ, Van Nostrand, 1958, pp 135–194
53. McDonald, op. cit., pp 613–614
54. Corrales, op. cit., p 197
55. Corrales, op. cit., p 198
56. Corrales, ibid.
57. Ibid., p 211
58. Ibid., p 211
59. Ibid., pp 212–213
60. Johnson PB: Social Power and Sex-Role Stereotyping. PhD Dissertation, University of California, Los Angeles, 1974
61. Raven, Centers, Rodrigues, op. cit., p 232
62. Lewis JM, Beavers WR, Gossett JT, Phillips VA: No Single Thread. New York, Brunner/Mazel, 1976
63. Ibid., p 209
64. Ibid., p 210
65. Ibid., p 10
66. Ibid., pp 53–55
67. Minuchin, op. cit., p 52
68. Johnson, op. cit., p 185
69. Olson, Cromwell, op. cit., pp 142–145

STUDY QUESTIONS

1. Power is an important dimension in human relationships and groups because (select all appropriate answers):
   a. It is critical in understanding role relationships.

b. It greatly influences the establishment and the maintenance of communication channels.

c. It is the sole determinant on which an intimate relationship is formed and maintained.

2. Demonstrate your knowledge of several basic power concepts by matching the correct synonyms or definitions with the concepts on the left-hand column.

Concepts	Synonym/Definition
__a. Power.	1. Influence.
	2. Legitimate power.
	3. Primary authority.
	4. Dominance.
__b. Authority.	5. May involve individual.
	6. Family group dominance patterns.
	7. One facet is decision making.
__c. Family power.	8. Assessed within context of family interaction.

3. Identify three limitations cited relative to studies of family power.

4. Match up the appropriate definition with the specific bases for power.

Bases for Power	Definition
__a. Authority.	1. Dominant person's obligation to assist the needy.
__b. Referent power.	
__c. Reward power.	2. Dominant person's greater knowledge regarding issue.
__d. Coercive power.	3. Legitimate power.
__e. Helpless power.	4. Tradition-based power.
__f. Expert or resource power.	5. Based upon positive identification with influencing individual.
__g. Informational power (direct).	6. Belief in ability to inflict punishment.
__h. Informational power (indirect).	7. Based on belief in the ability to grant privileges.
	8. Based upon having greater competency in matter.
	9. Hinting or "putting suggestions into another's mouth."

Are the following statements True *or* False?

5. In cases where power is maintained by the husband because of his control over money, this type of power is called expert authority.

6. Among traditional patriarchal families, direct informational power is quite common.

7. Primary authority is based on tradition and acceptance of culturally based roles.

8. Identify and describe the three techniques used in making decisions.

9. Describe how each of the following variables affects family power.
   a. Family communication network.
   b. Control over implementation.
   c. Interpersonal resources.
   d. Coalition formation.
   e. Social class.
   f. Developmental or life cycle changes.

Choose the correct answers to the following questions.

10. The most commonly used and well-accepted typology of family power is:
    a. Democratic–patriarchal.
    b. Companionship–authoritarian.
    c. Husband-dominated, egalitarian, wife-dominated.
    d. Autocratic, syncretic, autonomic.
    e. Cohesive–atomistic.

11. Which type of overall power structure seems to be the least satisfying to both spouses?
    a. Husband-dominated.
    b. Wife-dominated.
    c. Syncretic.
    d. Autonomic.

12. What is the most outstanding contemporary trend relative to family power?
    a. The upsurge in tradition and conservatism.
    b. The trend toward egalitarianism.
    c. The atomistic trend in the family.
    d. The rise of the matrifocal, matriarchal family.

13. The healthy family, as described by Lewis et al. and Minuchin, is characterized by:
    a. A strong parent–child coalition.
    b. A clear power hierarchy.
    c. Husband having more power than wife.
    d. A strong parental coalition.

14. The following family roles and power relationships are frequently observed in poor families:
    a. Division of marital responsibilities is informal.
    b. Joint planning predominates.
    c. Father is bestowed titular authority.
    d. Father often plays a more passive, minimal role in the home.

15. Komarovsky found that the following factor played a significant role in the type of power structure present in working-class families:
    a. Occupational status.
    b. Residence (city or rural).
    c. Education.
    d. Ethnicity.

FAMILY CASE STUDY 1

From the following example, answer the two questions below.

Mr. G. walked in the door while Mrs. G. was discussing child rearing with the community health nurse. Mr. G. immediately "took over" the conversation, voicing his opinion about every parenting comment made by the nurse or Mrs. G. The children were heard to giggle about a couple of their father's assertions. Toward the end of the visit he shouted to the children to get up and clean the kitchen. The children did not respond, but looked at their mother. She paused and then said, "Children, please go clean the dishes." With this request the children left for the kitchen.

16. In this situation, which of the following most clearly describes the power and role relationships of the father and mother?
a. Male dominance.
b. Children actually manipulate parents, playing one against the other.
c. Insufficient data to clearly define roles.
d. Mother acts as final arbiter and dominant one.

17. Data substantiating above interpretation include:
a. Father asserting role in an exaggerated manner.
b. His assertions being responded to by giggles from children.
c. Need to show he is "leader."
d. Children looking toward mother and responding to her request.
e. No response to father's requests.

FAMILY CASE STUDY 2

Read the family history and then complete an assessment of family power from data presented in vignette by answering questions that follow.

The Simpsons are a middle-class WASP "reconstituted" or stepparent family living in a suburban area. John Simpson, age 37, recently (8 months ago) married Sylvia who had been divorced for 4 years. Sylvia (age 42) has three children, ages 13 (Joe), 10 (Mary), and 8 (Jimmie) from her former marriage. Mr. Simpson had no children from his former marriage. Mr. Simpson is a businessman; he owns and manages a hardware store. Mrs. Simpson is a registered nurse and works at a local hospital. Both have baccalaureate degrees from local colleges and their income level, due to their double income, is "quite comfortable." They live in a lovely, well-kept residential neighborhood. Their home is large and well-furnished, containing four bedrooms, a living and family room, and a large, spacious kitchen. They moved to this particular community from the nearby city when they married and formed their new family.

The Simpsons are bringing their 8-year-old child, Jimmie, to the family health center because of bedwetting (enuresis) and hyperactivity and inattention at school. He will be examined by a family practitioner but, because of the nature of his situation, is also being interviewed by a family nurse practitioner who is in the process of completing a family assessment and comprehensive history of Jimmie.

Sylvia, the mother, relates that things in the family have been difficult since John "moved in." "First we had to move and the children lost all their friends. And even though John used to come and take me out for the evening and visit with us—so that the children were able to get to know him—they now resent him terribly and I feel I'm in between the devil and the deep blue sea!"

When asked what seems to be the major area of family conflict and concerns, she mentions disciplining of the children. "John doesn't discipline them, which I wish he did, and when he does set some limits, due to my nagging, the children don't listen to him. Then, I have to come in and settle things myself. I married John because I felt the children needed a father to relate to. Their own natural father lives far away now and seldom keeps in contact with them. The children don't seem to respect John, and the only way he is able to manage them is by promising them something or threatening to punish them."

She says that she never fights or disagrees with her husband in front of the children (believing children should not hear such unpleasant things). But after the children go to bed, she finds herself berating John for not following through with his family obligations—paying bills, repairing house, yard work, etc. Sylvia sees herself as in charge of the children (primarily), housework, social affairs, cooking, and shopping, and feels that the rest is up to her husband. She does her work, in addition to a full-time job, and expects him to do his.

According to Mrs. Simpson, Joe, the 13-year-old, likes caring for his younger siblings, and Mary and Jimmie turn to him for help and advice if she is not home. She also comments that Joe is the child who really seems to resent John, and speaks to her husband only when necessary, with most messages pertaining to his father going through the mother.

When the nurse asks Sylvia how the family arrived at the major decisions they have made since she and John became involved with each other—such as marriage, moving, and buying the house—Sylvia says that she initiated all three of these conversations. "I'm a practical person. I could see that marriage would be good for all of us, and so suggested it to John!" The nurse then asks, "And what was his answer?" Sylvia replies, "I don't remember exactly. I think he kind of hemmed and hawed around, and then, anyway, agreed and I started making plans. He didn't want to move from the city or into such a big house, but I convinced him that it would be better economically and that the commuting time was reasonable for him. And I agreed to let him buy a more comfortable car to commute in, in return."

The assessor meets with the whole family twice more to discuss their "identified" problem (Jimmie) and the family dynamics and family problems. At these meetings she notices that when she speaks to the parents and the children became noisy or disruptive that twice the older son, Joe, takes over, scolding them. In their discussion she observes that this is a family in which there is a proliferation of "do's" and "don'ts" about everything—from the time they get up in the morning until the time they go to bed at night. Feelings are not openly expressed, and the two youngest children directly answered the nurse's questions in a short, incomplete manner, looking to the mother for approval. The mother appears quite committed to a particular home schedule. John mentions that it is hard to fit into someone else's schedule and way of doing things. Joe confirms this point with nurse in his statement, "We all know the rules better than he does, so why do we need him to tell us what to do." (Mr. Simpson just sits quietly, and neither parent responds to Joe's hostile statement.)

In discussing his own feelings and thoughts about the family, Mr. Simpson perceives that Jimmie may feel confused and insecure because of moving, their marriage, and the new school. He alludes to the difficulty he has faced in parenting his wife's children and to their negative reactions toward him. He also finds disciplining very hard because he never had children before and in growing up was treated very permissively ("anything at all seemed to be okay with my parents"). He comments that "he tries to stay out of child rearing as much as possible."

Mr. Simpson was married twice before and appears to be passive and easygoing with his wife. In contrast, Mrs. Simpson initiates topics, leads discussions, and is quite "definite" and opinionated in her statements.

18. Assess the family power pattern described in the above case.
    a. Who makes what decisions?
    b. What decision-making techniques are utilized?
    c. On what basis is family power derived?
    d. What variables affect family power?
    e. Using the family power continuum (see Fig. 10.1), where would you place this family?
    f. If dominance, indicate dominant family member:
       ———.

STUDY ANSWERS

1. a and b

2. a. 1, 4, 5, and 7
   b. 2 and 3
   c. 6 and 8

3. Limitations of family power studies (any three):
   a. Lack of good correlation between task allocation and decision making and overall dominance patterns in family.
   b. Focusing on outcome of decision making, which family members have difficulty reporting, rather than process, which gives much greater information regarding family interaction and dynamics.
   c. Methodologic: interviewing wife, rather than whole family.
   d. Methodologic: solely depending on the self-reporting of family member (interviews), rather than combining with actual observations.

4. a. 3 and 4   e. 1
   b. 5   f. 8
   c. 7   g. 2
   d. 6   h. 9

5. False

6. False

7. True

8. a. *Consensus.* Both parties discuss and mutually decide.
   b. *Accommodation.* One partner "convinces" other to adjust or they both make concessions.
   c. *De facto.* No conscious, overt decision made, "things just happen."

9. Description of how each of the following variables affects family power:
   a. *Family communication network.* The unequal intensity of family relationships influences power, especially the centrality of one or more member in the network of interactions (an intermediary or go-between). Persons holding these intermediary positions can screen information as they see

fit and can use more intimate knowledge of family members' attitudes and opinions to influence them and obtain more control over decisions.

b. *Control over implementation.* Generally, the person(s) having control over the implementation of a decision have some measure of power, since they can undermine or modify the decisions by virtue of the way the decision is implemented.

c. *Interpersonal resources.* Through masterful use of a range of interpersonal techniques, persons with much less objective resources can become dominant or enhance their power position. Conversely, some family members may not use their interpersonal skills effectively because of lowered self-confidence in a familial relationship, the unimportance of an issue, restrictive norms, such as avoidance of confrontation, or a relationship in which there is more involvement by one person than the other (thus the principle of less interest occurs).

d. *Coalition formation.* By forming coalitions, the members of the coalition increase their power vis-à-vis other family members.

e. *Social class.* Social class affects family power by setting up family life conditions which influence the resources which each spouse brings to their relationship, the role that tradition plays over new "scientific" or contemporary trends, and more generally, the basic conditions under which the family survives.

f. *Developmental or life cycle changes.* During the life cycle of the family, demands on the family unit vary, and in response to both internal and external demands, power patterns are altered. For example, couples when first married tend to share decisions more than after children arrive, since there is usually more emotional involvement at the start of their relationship.

10. d

11. b

12. b

13. b and d

14. c and d

15. c

16. d

17. All (a–e)

18. a. Who makes what decisions?
    Husband–father. Expected to pay bills, carry out home-maintenance work, garden (his degree of involvement and decision making here is in question).
    Wife–mother. She initiates and convinces husband of the "rightness" of her proposals in areas of major decisions. Also assumes responsibility and decision making in areas of child care, household management, and social activities. Both appear to be responsible for deciding their own work.
    Joe (oldest son). In charge of child-care activity in absence of mother.
    b. What decision-making techniques are utilized?
    No strong evidence of consensus used. (They may not have the communication ability to negotiate and discuss alternatives so that consensual decision making can take place).

Accommodation: Use of bargaining seen in moving to suburbs and in purchase of home and car.

No use of de facto technique noted (wife is probably too task oriented and too much of a planner for this to happen very often).

c. On what bases is family power derived?

Referent power. The children listen to mother, and although it is not clear if this is out of positive identification or authority, they seem to "mind" when she is not there to enforce the rules (which would indicate reward–coercive power).

Reward–coercive power. The stepfather appears forced to use this type of power base, although ineffectively, because he does not have children's respect, they do not recognize his authority, and he seems not to have expert or informational power to use.

Expert and informational power. It appears that Mrs. Simpson is perceived by Mr. Simpson as having some special competencies or resources which he needs, or greater information on which to base decisions, since he seems to concede to her wishes. Perhaps the "principle of less interest" is operating here.

d. What variables affect family power?

Family communciation network. Mrs. Simpson definitely is in a central position as go-between or intermediary between her husband and children. This increases her dominance.

Interpersonal skills. Mr. Simpson lacks confidence in his parenting skills, thus decreasing his effectiveness in this area. Mrs. Simpson undermines his parenting by taking over when the children do not listen to him. Also, he may need her more than she needs him. (Could he be seeking leadership, a mothering figure?)

Social class variables. Family is obviously middle-class, and even though the wife "takes over," she is dissatisfied in her husband's role performance. This may be an indication of the disparity between her expectations (the cultural norm of a husband being either a leader or sharing responsibility with wife) and her reality, or her feeling that he is incompetent.

Developmental variable. During this cycle of the family's life, there are many tasks to be fulfilled, and thus the strain is seen in Mrs. Simpson's feeling that she has to assume too much responsibility. Usually there is more division of role responsibilities and decision making.

e. Overall family power typology:

Family power continuum:

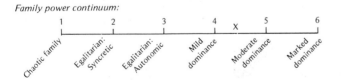

f. Mild to moderate dominance by Mrs. Simpson.

In all known societies almost everyone lives his or her life enmeshed in a network of family rights and obligations called role relations.[1] Family roles are critical, central roles an individual must learn and enact successfully. Adequate role functioning is critical, not only in terms of a person's successful functioning, but also for the satisfactory functioning of a family since it is through the performance of family roles that the functions of the family are fulfilled. In fact, family sociologists often define the family as an interacting, interdependent set of roles which are in a state of dynamic equilibrium.[2]

Because of the critical nature which family roles play in the organization of the family, it is imperative for the family-centered nurse to understand their relationships and, from this, be able to identify role problems, as well as role characteristics, that can direct the nurse to more effective interventions.

ROLE THEORY AND DEFINITIONS

Since role concepts and terms are fundamental to the discussion which follows, a number of basic definitions will be given. The reader is also directed to the works by Hardy and Conway[3] and Biddle and Thomas[4] for further understanding of these concepts.

Role

According to Nye, there are two basic perspectives on roles—the structuralist orientation, which stresses the normative (cultural) influence associated with particular statuses and their related roles,[5] and the interaction orientation of Turner,[6] which emphasizes the emergent quality of roles (generating from social interaction).

In this text, role will be defined in a more structural sense, since normative prescriptions are still relatively well defined within the family.[7] *Role is referred to as more or less homogeneous sets of behaviors which are normatively defined and expected of an occupant of a given social position,*[8] realizing, of course, that wide variations in role behavior exist today. The term role applies to a set of prescriptions (directions) and expectations which define what individuals in a particular situation should do in order to meet their own or another's expectations of them rather than the actual enactment or performance of a role.

Position or Status

Position or status is defined as a way of identifying categories of people for whom the basis of such differentiation is their common attributes, e.g., behaviors of persons in a certain occupation, or the common reaction of others toward them. Every individual occupies multiple positions, e.g., adult, male, husband, farmer, Elks member, and so on.[9] Associated with each of

11

Family Role Structure

LEARNING OBJECTIVES

1. Define and describe relative to the family:
   Role.
   Position or status (and paired positions).
   Role behavior (role performance or role enactment).
   Role conflict.
   Role strain.
   Normative dimensions of roles.
   Role sharing.
   Role taking and role making.
   Reciprocal or complementary roles (also principle of complementarity).
   Role patterning (role allocation).
   Family homeostasis.
   Role induction and role modification.
2. From the studies presented, summarize the findings of these with respect to the basic roles making up the wife-mother and husband-father positions and which roles are shared and not shared according to present trends.
3. Describe three types of marital relationships.
4. Describe the common role conflict experienced by the working wife–mother and her husband in dual-career families.
5. Define and give examples of covert roles which often exist in families (both healthy and detrimental roles). Describe why both covert and overt roles are assessed in the family, as well as the purpose that covert roles serve.
6. Explain the process and effects of labeling on individuals in the family.
7. With the use of a family case example, complete an assessment of the family role structure.
8. Describe the frequently observed role characteristics in:
   Lower- and middle-class families.
   The single-parent family.
   The reconstituted family.
   The family during health and illness.

these positions are a number of roles. In the case of the mother position, some of the associated roles are housekeeper, child caretaker, family health leader, cook, and companion or playmate. Merton explains:

> A particular social status involves, not a single associated role, but an array of associated roles. This is a basic characteristic of social structure. This fact of structure can be registered by a distinctive term, *role-set*, by which I mean that complement of role relationships which persons have by virtue of occupying a particular social status.[10]

Thus for each position there exist a number of roles, each of which is composed of a more or less related homogeneous set of behaviors culturally defined as expected of those in that position or status. They might, however, be shared with other members of a group; in the family, for example, the child-care role is now a shared responsibility of both the mother and father.[11]

Role Behavior, Role Performance, or Role Enactment

Role behavior is a term applied to what a person actually does in response to role expectations. What does the process of learning and performing a role actually involve? Expectations and/or prescriptions for the sets of behavior appropriate for the basic social positions and their associated roles (family roles, occupational roles, etc.) evolve and are developed by society. This process may involve the wider society alone or the wider society and a particular reference group for some families. These expectations are modified or refined as a result of an individual's exposure to role models and the person's individual personality, that is, his or her capacities, temperament, attitudes, and interests. An individual accepts a particular role based on societal expectation and as modified by his or her identification with role models and individual personality characteristics. The outcome is his or her actual role behavior or performance. Figure 11.1 illustrates the process by which role behavior actually develops.

Role Conflict

Role conflict occurs when the occupant of a position perceives that he or she is confronted with incompatible expectations.[12] The source of the incompatibility may be due to changes in expectations within self, others, or environment. Thus the conflict can be conceptualized, as is usually the case, as interrole conflict, in which the norms or behavior patterns of one role are incongruent with those of another role which the same individual plays. There may also be intrarole strain, in which two or more categories of people, including the

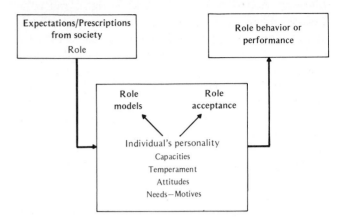

FIGURE 11.1
Development of Role Behavior.

person involved, hold conflicting expectations concerning the behavior appropriate for a role. Interrole conflict occurs when an individual's role complex—that is, the group of roles he or she enacts—involves several roles which are incompatible due to the excessive amount of energy these roles demand, such as the familiar case of performing the student, housekeeper, cook, marital, and child caretaker roles concomitantly. An illustration of the second type of role conflict—intrarole conflict—is the presence of conflicting expectations on how one's occupation role should be performed. For example, the head nurse may expect efficiency of actions; the patient may expect patient-centeredness, based on his or her perceived needs; and the nurse expects to be able to give individualized care as defined by him- or herself, rather than by the patient. In the family one can easily see how intrarole conflict often occurs in parent-teenager conflicts.

Role Strain

Role strain is indicative of problems of role enactment[13] or role conflict. Nye defines role strain in terms of such mental states as worry, anxiety, or guilt (interrelated mental states) and feels that since strain is a "cost," the presence of role strain among family members could be used as one predictor of marital dissatisfaction or emotional illness.[14]

Normative Dimensions of Roles

As outlined under the description of role, roles are normatively or culturally defined, i.e., the culture in which one participates and/or with which one identifies prescribes and proscribes the behavior of the occupants of various positions. However, "not all the family roles are equally normative."[15] Jackson notes that some family roles are more "crystallized"—clearly spelled out as expected behavior—than others.[16] For instance, in the past the affective (Nye calls it therapeutic) role of the spouses was not crystallized; that is, it was not *expected* of mates to listen to each other's problems. Today, however, spouses see therapeutic assistance not as permissive behavior, but as an obligation, since it is a duty to help one's spouse.[17] Thus the therapeutic role for spouses has been "crystallized."

One can infer the strength of a role (whether it is a strong norm or not) in a specific position by assessing the sanction(s) applied when the role is not performed. Certainly social ostracism as a sanction against lack of role fulfillment, as in the case where the wife-mother is not carrying out her housekeeper role, is less strong or intense than imprisonment, as might result from failure to carry out the child-care role when it reaches the point of child neglect. Sanctions provide evidence that the society or parts of the society perceive a particular role to be sufficiently important that conformity to the norm be enforced.[18]

Role Sharing

Role sharing refers to participation of two or more persons in the same roles even though they hold different positions. Differentiated, technologically sophisticated societies such as the United States are characterized by their extensive role sharing. Sharply segregated role structures are unusual within families today. As noted previously, an example of this normative role sharing in the family is the case of the child-socialization role where both mother and father jointly participate, in addition to the school teacher, youth leaders, minister, and so on.[19] In the older family, the housekeeper and shopping roles are often shared by the retired couple.

Role Taking

Another essential concept within role theory is that of role taking. In order for family members to play roles, they must be able to imagine themselves in the role of a counterpart, or role partner; in this way they are able to assign a role to the other and also better understand how they should behave in their own roles.[20] Through socialization family members acquire a repertoire of roles through which they can act and interact with others. "Roles are never learned singly, but always as pairs or sets of interacting roles. Because the individual learns the role of alter [his role partner] while playing his own role, he is able to play the role of the alter when others in the situation are playing his usual role."[21] Over a period of time, however, the self-conception incorporates certain roles and denies others, so that the individual no longer plays past roles.

Reciprocal or Complementary Roles

A basic concept in role theory is that of the complementarity of roles. A role is interdependent with and patterned to mesh with that of a role partner. In other words, a role is always paired with a reciprocal role of another person. One can never look at a role in isolation. To use a teacher as an example, one must look at the teacher's role vis-à-vis the student's role, since both are necessary for either to function. Society specifies behaviors for each person in these reciprocal arrangements so that each will know what is expected of both role partners. Both role partners are constantly influencing each others' role behavior through their many interactions with one another. For instance, if students become more verbal and assertive with teachers, the teacher responds by modifying his or her expectations and behaviors toward the students. Likewise, as society changes and family systems evolve, changes in social and family roles become necessary. Thus if a wife begins working, she may become more instrumental in financial decisions and the husband may become more involved with household tasks and child-rearing.

Parsons coined the concept of "the principle of complementarity," referring to the functional adequacy of roles in social situations which are based on the match between the performances and the expectations of the partners in the relationship.[22] The principle of complementarity is of great significance because it is chiefly responsible for that degree of harmony and stability which occurs in interpersonal relations.[23]

Whenever there is dissimilarity in expectations and performances of family roles—due to cultural, social class, or individual differences—the potential lack of role complementarity exists. "The presence of conflict produces dynamic shifts in the equilibrating mechanisms of the family, which function to reduce the conflict and restore some measure of complementarity in the role patterning."[24]

Role Patterning or Role Allocation

The patterning or allocation of roles provides for definitions of what is to be done in the family, who is to do it, and who is to decide on the allocation of tasks (leadership). Role patterning makes provision for carrying out tasks on the basis of age, sex, personality characteristics; it also provides sanctions for dealing with the neglect or poor performance of agreed-on tasks.

In the family role allocation is largely defined by culture and social class, albeit more latitude and flexibility exist today. Furthermore, family roles are also the result of each member's searching for a viable position for him- or herself (a group of roles which give a person some feelings of satisfaction, competency, and dominance in a "sphere of influence") and the functional requirements of the family.[25]

Family Homeostasis

Family homeostasis refers to the family's use of regulatory mechanisms to maintain the equilibrium of the family. The family achieves this homeostasis through adaptation, i.e., by altering family structure or bringing in assistive outside resources, and integration (mobilization of inner resources such as cohesiveness). This concept did not directly evolve from role theory but is closely related and critical to an understanding of family role relationships. Family roles can be both dynamic and/or inflexible. Turner remarks that once a system of roles is established within the family, family processes proceed laboriously unless the members play their expected role.[26] Families become dependent on the existence of certain informal roles to be enacted so as to maintain family homeostasis. For example, if the family is used to having the middle daughter act as the mediator in disputes, this encourages other family members to be less restrained in their sentiments. When the mediating daughter is not present, conflicts are handled in a much less effective manner due to the absence of the go-between.

Role Induction and Role Modification

The techniques families use to "persuade" family members to change their role behavior during times of intrarole conflict, and thus restore family equilibrium, involve the use of either role induction or role modification. In the case of role induction, a family member changes role behavior as a result of coercion, coaxing, or other manipulative techniques. Because role induction is primarily defensive and the basic value conflict is only temporarily avoided, the same conflict will reappear. On the other hand, role modification involves a change in both parties to a conflict. Complementarity is achieved once more, but it is mutually agreed upon. Role modification, which leads toward insight, begins with (1) joking; (2) referral to a third party; (3) exploring, a testing phase that may involve the work of the helping person who assists the family to find solutions to conflicts; (4) compromising, the phase in which parties to the conflict perceive the need for a change of goals; and (5) consolidating, or learning how to make the compromises work.[27]

Criteria for Adequate Family Functioning

In respect to role relationships in the family, what does the adequate family look like? If we have an understanding of satisfactory family functioning, we may better be able to understand families who are marginally or inadequately coping. Glasser and Glasser summarized their findings of working with a number of families in which one member of the primary group was undergoing psychotherapy. From their observations and analysis they identified five general criteria necessary for adequate family functioning.[28] They underscored the importance of role complementarity; compatibility of family roles and norms with societal norms; the presence of roles in families which meet the psychological needs of family members; and the ability of the family to respond to change via role flexibility.[29, 30]

FORMAL FAMILY ROLES

Family Positions

There are a limited number of positions defined as normative within the most common type of family form, the traditional nuclear family. These positions are referred to as *formal* and *paired* and consist of father-husband; wife-mother; son-brother; and daughter-sister. Although a variety of other family positions may be seen today, they can be viewed simply as variations of the traditional two-parent nuclear family structure.

Although the variant family is increasingly common and more acceptable today, the traditional nuclear family is still the predominant pattern of family life. Thus it is perceived as "out of the ordinary" for married couples to live with either set of parents. If an aging parent is a member of a given family, he or she is usually viewed as an "extra" person. And other persons who may form part of a particular household are similarly viewed as being outside the normal situation, and frequently the family will go to great lengths to explain the presence of unexpected "members." Furthermore, each of the normative positions of the family group is associated with its related roles. Husband-fathers are expected to be wage earners, among the other roles which they may possess. Wife-mothers are viewed as homemakers. When a wife-mother is employed outside the home, as often occurs in American society, this role is not viewed as her primary responsibility, whereas the wage-earner role of the husband-father is certainly viewed as his primary role.

Formal Roles

Associated with each formal family position are related roles, i.e., clusters of more or less homogeneous behaviors. The family apportions roles to its family members in a manner similar to the way society apportions its roles: according to how critical the role performance is to the system's functioning. Some roles require special skills and abilities; others are less complex and can be assigned to less skilled and/or to those with the least amount of power. Standard formal roles exist in the family, e.g., breadwinner, homemaker, house repairman, chauffeur, child rearer, financial manager, cook, and so forth. When there are fewer persons in a family the number of persons to fulfill these roles is limited; thus there will be more demands and opportunities for family members to play several roles at different times. If a member leaves home or becomes unable to fulfill a role, someone else fills this vacuum by taking up his or her role to keep the family functioning.[31]

Marital and Parental Roles

Nye has identified eight basic roles making up the husband-father and the wife-mother social positions:

> Provider role.
> Housekeeper role.
> Child-care role.
> Child-socialization role.
> Recreational role.
> Kinship role (maintaining relationships with paternal and maternal families).
> Therapeutic role (meeting the affective needs of spouse).
> Sexual role.[32]

In this scheme the companionship role has been subsumed under the recreational and therapeutic roles.

Many persons fail to separate parental roles from marital roles, but in reality the two roles are quite distinct, and marital roles should not be short-changed due to overinvolvement in the other.* The marital roles are focused on the husband–wife interactions, while the parental roles are focused upon the parent–child interactions and the parental responsibilities. Nevertheless, performance of marital roles will certainly have impact on parental roles and vice versa.

Minuchin stresses the importance of the spouse role relationships: the need for mates to maintain a strong marital relationship. Children especially can interfere with the marital relationship, creating a situation where the husband and wife have a relationship based not on their own personal relationship with each other, but on their parenting role.[33] Maintaining a satisfying marital relationship is identified as one of the vital family developmental tasks of the family as it progresses through its life cycle. In the previous discussion of family development, the stress which children put on the marital relationship is quite evident.

What are marriages supposed to be like? In the past, behavioral scientists put together a composite picture of the well-functioning marriage that we now think of as biased, simplistic, and rarely found in reality. Moreover, two fairly well-conducted studies have shown the variety of relationships present in marriages generally[34] and also in stable, longstanding marriages.[35] In both of these studies the researchers found that no one pattern of marital adjustment existed. A wide range of behaviors and marital roles were found among persons who felt content with, or at least remained in, their marriages.

One of these studies was conducted by Cuber and Harroff. They interviewed about 400 upper-middle-class couples who had been married at least 10 years and had a stable marriage. From this data they devised a typology of marital relationships illustrating the diverse types of stable marriages. These ranged from conflict-habituated relationships through devitalized relationships and passive, congenial relationships to vital and total relationships. Cuber and Harroff estimate that roughly 80 percent of the marriages they studied were utilitarian oriented, while only 20 percent were vital or total relationships.[36] Thus the American ideal of a marriage where most of one's intimate and social needs are met by a spouse is a widespread myth.

Bott attempted to explain some of the differences apparent in the extent of involvement and intimacy in marital relationships, and she theorized that when marriages were superimposed on a social network of friends, neighbors, and relatives among whom there was frequent and meaningful interaction that met many of the needs of the husband and wife, the impetus for the mates to become deeply involved with each other and share roles was decreased. Thus a sharper demarcation of roles would be seen, in addition to a lower value being placed on the marital relationship itself. It may well be that the social environment in which the family is embedded is of vital importance in determining the nature of the marital relationship.[37]

Types of Marital Relationships

In addition to studies demonstrating the wide diversity of marriages, efforts have also been made to classify the types of dyadic (two-person) relationships. For assistance in assessing the marital relationship in families, one of these typologies will be explained briefly.

Basically three types of relationships are found in dyadic relationships. These are termed complementary, symmetrical, and parallel relationships.[38]

---

* The reader is referred back to Chapter 6, to the section exploring the vital nature of family subsystems and how these need to be kept intact and strong.

Complementary Relationships. Mates in this type of dyad exhibit contrasting behavior. One spouse is the leading, dominant personality and decision maker, whereas the other partner is the subservient follower. They accept and enjoy these differences and there exists a strong element of dependency between them.

The positive element in this type of relationship is that it allows one to give and the other to receive. The inherent danger lies in its tendency to become increasingly rigid, thus stifling the growth of both persons.

It is necessary that both partners of a complementary relationship play their "proper" role. If either mate does not continue to perform his or her respective functions, the relationship will come to an end, with each feeling disconfirmed by the other.

Symmetrical Relationships. This type of relationship is based on the equality of the partners. The partners demand equality through the character of their mutually exchanged messages and behavior, and each mate has the right to initiate action, to criticize the other's behavior, and to have a voice in family decisions.

The positive aspect of this type of relationship is that it allows for mutual respect, trust, and spontaneity, with the optimal effect being that each partner is free to be him- or herself, knowing that each will be accepted and respected by the other. The danger inherent in this type of relationship is that the competitive aspect of the relationship may become over-emphasized. When this happens there is increasing frustration and a decrease in cooperative behaviors (mutual assistance and support). Egocentricity by one or both partners may preclude the mutual accommodation and giving needed to enhance and nurture the intimate, affectional part of a marital relationship.

Parallel Relationships. This type of relationship is viewed as a healthy, stable type of relationship, in which both the complementary and symmetrical patterns are seen. Depending on the situation and the partner's areas of competence, there is an interchange and flexibility in relationship patterns. This switching from one pattern to the other restores the stabilizing properties when either pattern threatens to break down.

Because of the greater flexibility and individual growth-enhancing properties, since each partner is able to contribute according to his or her competencies and the situational needs, this type of relationship is seen as the most mature form of the three types of relationships according to Watzlawick et al. Developmentally, if maturation is allowed to occur, a relationship should evolve from a complementary form to a symmetrical form to a parallel form. If one visualizes this in terms of the dependency factor, the relationship undergoes a change from dependency (complementary) to independence (symmetry) to interdependence (parallelism). The value judgment placed on these types of relationships and their perceived degree of maturity, however, does not take into account the cultural background of the individuals involved—an obvious limitation.

Contemporary Family Role Changes

The roles of family members have become more variable, flexible, and complex. In the past, there was "women's work" and "men's work," and very little role sharing existed. The family lived according to relatively rigid, traditionally established rules that were maintained by the social and moral pressures of the entire society. Today, great variation in the roles of both sexes is feasible. The expectations and practices differ tremendously. In one family, both adult members may be expected to work and jointly share in all family affairs and responsibilities; in another family, traditional roles are expected and performed; and in yet another situation, the single-parent family, the adult assumes the roles of both parents.

Since the normative limits of family roles are now so broad, a wide range of behaviors are acceptable as appropriate to a particular position. Turner pointed out that the requirements of the situation and the individuals in it determine specific behaviors found in a role. Thus the individual tentatively makes his or her role in response to the cues given by other(s) in the situation, i.e., his or her role partner(s).[39]

For Aldous, this role taking and social interaction generates much *role making* in present-day marriages and families. She states that "there is a great deal of role-making in families today since changing conditions have rendered suspect or inappropriate age and gender norms." And she points to changing marital roles as a prime example of role making in process.

> When gender norms dictated that men were the bread-winners and women were responsible for the family, a segregated conjugal role organization, in which women saw to the day-to-day operation of the family and men provided the economic resources, made a certain kind of sense. With 65.7 percent of married women presently engaged in gainful employment, including 20.6 percent of women with children under six years of age, people no longer are willing to accept the norms legitimating and prescribing a segregated conjugal role organization. The questioning particularly comes from women who according to gender norms are the most responsible for household affairs even though they are holding full-time jobs. They experience "role overload" with all the attendant problems of mental and physical strain.[40]

Whereas most family studies have surveyed middle-class populations, Cronkite investigated approximately 700 low-income families of different ethnic groups in the Denver area, querying husbands and wives about their beliefs concerning appropriate patterns of spousal behavior.[41] Her findings showed that the earnings of the employed wife significantly altered the role preferences of both spouses. Nevertheless, husbands with working wives still believed that housework and child care was the wife's role. In contrast, working women in Cronkite's sample expected and wished that husbands would assist them in household and child-care tasks.[42] An obvious discrepancy in expectations exists. Recent studies show that the role behavior of husbands has not much changed; it is the wives who have had to adapt to the increased load by spending less time working in the house through such measures as using preprocessed, ready-prepared foods, dining out more frequently, employing part-time house cleaners, and utilizing child-care facilities.[43, 43a]

Cronkite discusses the common dilemmas of the dual-career family and the stresses generated by role changes. She describes how couples see the benefit of the additional income outweighing their objections and reluctance to the wife's working. But at the same time, the husband is anxious about his diminished power in the role of breadwinner, and the wife—though enjoying the challenge of work and adult social interaction—often feels guilty about hurting her husband's pride in being the sole provider or about not spending enough time with her children.[44]

More nontraditional role and task allocations were preferred in these low-income families when one or both spouses were more highly educated (had some college education). If the wife had more education, she valued working jointly and a cohesive, affective (therapeutic) role in marriage; if the husband had more education, he believed that it was acceptable for married women to be employed.

Findings from multiple studies report that attitudes about family roles are moving in a direction of favoring egalitarianism. For example, Gecas found that the majority of parents in his sample viewed the responsibilities associated with socializing children as belonging to both partners.[45] Other researchers found that the sex of the child influenced which parent assumed more socialization responsibility—fathers being more involved with their sons and mothers with their daughters.[46]

Although attitudes about family roles may be moving to favor egalitarianism, Araji asserts that there is a lag in concomitant role behavior. Women, by far, were found to be experiencing greater discrepancy between their role attitudes and their actual role behavior. Araji supports Aldous' findings that there is little evidence to suggest that husbands are assuming a larger share of household-related activities even when the wife works.

Her findings do suggest, however, that "more husbands are helping with the child care role—possibly in response to their wives being committed to working outside the home."[47]

Nonetheless, as masculine and feminine adult roles are changing in families, especially among the middle class, so are the socialization experiences of children. Because motherhood has come to occupy a less significant aspect of a woman's adult life and because there are so many married women working, socialization practices are changing, there being less sex-based differences in socialization patterns.[48]

Thus Nye,[49] Gecas,[50] Araji,[51] and others have discovered that the child-care and socialization roles are becoming the shared responsibilities of both spouses. Bronfenbrenner points out that among middle-class families there has been a continual shift over the years in the model-parent role. The relative position of the father vis-à-vis the mother is shifting, with the former becoming increasingly more affectionate, nurturant, and less authoritarian and the latter becoming relatively more important as the agent of discipline, that is, having greater parental authority, especially for boys.[52]

Another apparent change in roles within the spouse positions involves the sexual role. In the past men had the right to regular sexual activity with their wives, but felt under no obligation to be concerned about the wives' feelings of satisfaction. Today the wife's right to sexual enjoyment and equality is growing in importance, changing the nature of the sexual role for both mates.[53] Lastly, in regard to the kinship role—maintaining relationships with both sides of the family—the wife-mother still generally assumes this role.

Role Change Problems

It should also be acknowledged that the advent of role changes in families does not come without a cost to the individuals involved. It is well recognized that when individuals deviate from normative role expectations and/or take on new roles, they may lack the role preparation or previous socialization needed to perform these new roles comfortably and adequately. In addition to lacking the necessary training, the family member may not feel the new roles meet his or her interests or needs. In some families, role changes such as brought by having a new baby, wife's employment, or husband's unemployment may create confusion, generate anxiety and unhappiness, and heighten familial conflict.[54] Meleis and Swendsen have written a series of articles promulgating the use of role supplementation to assist individuals who are trying to cope with role transitions and role change. They have used role models, groups of persons experiencing the same role changes, and counseling as ways in which to provide role supplementation.[55-57] Certainly assistance to families undergoing role change and experiencing role problems should be considered a vital nursing function.

The status and associated roles of individuals in a family will change in many ways throughout a person's life cycle and that of his or her two families (family of orientation and family of parenthood). The change in role relationships, expectations, and abilities is referred to as *role transition*.[58] Role transitions occur at clear demarcations of the family life such as marriage, divorce, or the death of spouse, as well as more subtly as an ongoing response to life experience. A role change experienced by one family member necessitates role changes in other family members, that is, complementary adjustments of the role partner(s).*

INFORMAL FAMILY ROLES

As stated previously, there are specific explicit *formal* family roles operating in families: husband-father, wife-mother, and child-sibling. Within each of these positions are associated roles and clusters of expected, homogeneous behaviors. Family roles can be classified into two categories: formal or overt roles and informal or covert ones. Whereas formal roles are explicit roles which each family role structure contains (father-husband, etc.), informal roles are implicit, often not apparent on the surface, and are played to meet the emotional needs of individuals[59] and/or to maintain the family's equilibrium.

Feldman and Scherz underscore the salience of looking at both types of roles within a family:

> The family operates through roles that shift and alter during the course of the family's life. Roles can be explicit or instrumental; they can be implicit or emotional. . . . The healthy family carries out explicit and implicit roles appropriately according to age, competence and needs during all the different stages of family life.[60]

A family member will play many roles in a family, both covert and overt, with some of these roles being shared. The existence of informal roles is necessary to fulfill the integrative and adaptive requirements of the family group. Kievit explains that

> Informal roles have different requirements, less likely based on age or sex and more likely based upon the personality attributes of individual members. Thus, one member may be the mediator, seeking possible compromises when the other family members are engaged in conflict. Another may be the family jester, who provides

gaiety and mirth on happy occasions, and a much needed sense of humor in times of crisis and distress. Other informal roles may exist and emerge, as the needs of the family unit shift and change. In working with families, awareness of the informal roles may facilitate insight into the specific nature of problems faced and in turn possible solutions. Effective performance of informal roles can facilitate the adequate performance of the formal roles.[61]

The following are some examples of other informal or covert roles described by Benne and Sheats and Satir which are commonly seen in families and may or may not contribute to the stability of the group—some of them being adaptive and others apparently detrimental to the ultimate well-being of the family.

Encourager. The encourager praises, agrees with, and accepts the contribution of others. In effect he is able to draw out other people and make them feel that their ideas are important and worth listening to.

Harmonizer. The harmonizer mediates the differences that exist between other members by jesting or smoothing over disagreements.

Initiator-Contributor. The initiator-contributor suggests or proposes to the group new ideas or changed ways of regarding group problems or goals.

Compromiser. The compromiser is one of the parties to the conflict or disagreement. The compromiser yields his or her position, admits error, or offers to come "halfway."

Blocker. The blocker tends to be negative to all ideas, rejecting without and beyond reason.

Follower. The follower goes along with the movement of the group, more or less passively accepting the ideas of others, serving as an audience in group discussion and decision.

Dominator. The dominator tries to assert authority or superiority by manipulating the group or certain members, flaunting his or her power and acting as if he or she knows everything and is the paragon of virtue.

Recognition Seeker. The recognition seeker attempts in whatever way possible to call attention to self and his or her deeds, accomplishments, and/or problems.[62]

Martyr. The martyr wants nothing for self but sacrifices everything for the sake of other family members.

The Great Stone Face. The person playing this role lectures incessantly and impassively on all the "right" things to do, just like a computer.

Pal. The pal is a family playmate who indulges self and excuses family members' behavior or his or her own regardless of the consequences. He or she usually seems irrelevant.[63]

---

* The changes in family roles throughout the family life cycle are explored in Chapter 5.

How do family members come to play these various informal roles within the family? Most learning of these roles occurs through role modeling, as well as through the emotional responses received to behaviors a child exhibits in the family when he or she imitates adult members. The child experiments with various roles in play, receives selective reinforcement for certain roles, and eventually finds informal roles that are comfortable. Moreover, family members, as do the members of other small groups, "fill in vacuums" where they exist. If there is no leader or decision maker playing the instrumental role, a member of the group will naturally emerge to fill this role.

Two additional covert roles will be described since both are common and important to identify and comprehend. The first of these is the scapegoat role, a role adopted by a member to preserve the family and maintain homeostasis. The family member who is constantly scapegoated usually serves to divert attention from a disturbance between the spouses. As described by Ackerman,[64] when the marital pair is in conflict, the attention is focused on the scapegoat and the system is preserved.*

Another role which is adopted in families is that of the go-between.[65] The go-between or intermediary role is usually taken by the mother. In this role the person acts as a "switchboard" between family members, relaying communication from one member to another. In so doing, the direct communication between other family members is blocked. As the switchboard through which all communication must go, the go-between assumes a covert position of power, and by passing along only those messages considered suitable, the go-between acts as a censor. She or he thus becomes a central figure in the family, acting as a confidant to its members. And as the center of the family communication network the go-between is typically in charge of settling all disputes and insuring fairness to all sides. However, when disputes or conflicts do not become resolved, the go-between often gets blamed. Consistently having one person act as an intermediary is dysfunctional in that it is an emotional distancing mechanism and promotes estrangement between the other members of the family, since they are discouraged from communicating directly with each other. Satir discusses the consequences of communicating via a third person:

> If the family habitually transacts business without all the members present, and also has little spare time, then family members get to know each other through a third person. I call it *acquaintance by rumor*. The problem is that most people forget about the rumor part and treat whatever it is as fact.[66]

The presence of a go-between role is revealed in the family's communication patterns. In interviews, it will be observed that the go-between answers for the children or other spouse when not directly questioned. In addition to talking for other family members, she or he usually gets in the way of all messages which are elicited from or received by family members.

Hence through selective reinforcement of certain behaviors by parents and significant others, children are molded to play specific informal, covert roles. This selective parental reinforcement may occur because of early *labeling* of the child; this labeling leads to a self-fulfilling prophesy. Parents label children for a variety of reasons: projection, comparison with siblings, past unresolved personal needs, and so on. A study of large families found that there were a number of specialized roles and labels given to the children. Eight informal roles, which resullt in or from labels, existed: (1) the responsible one, (2) the popular one, (3) the socially ambitious one, (4) the studious one, (5) the family isolate, (6) the irresponsible one, (7) the sickly one, and (8) the spoiled one.[67] Additionally, these labels are likely to exist in complementary pairs. Thus if a "sickly" child is identified in a family, the family usually labels another as the "healthy one"; if a "dumb one" is deemed to be present, there is usually a "smart one." Thus children are compared and contrasted with each other.

Labeling is often not positive because it suggests limits to the way the child may act or develop. True negative labeling—where adverse adjectives are used—occurs when parents and/or significant others label a child according to an attribute or behavior which indicates the child is inferior or unlovable. Because the parents see these labels as bad, the child sees him- or herself in the same light. Initially parents condemn the child; later the child, through identification with them, internalizes the parental label and condemns him- or herself. Negative labeling has been identified as an antecedent to both depression and lowered self-esteem.[68]

As a result of early negative labeling and the internalization of these labels, individuals often develop certain limited ways of perceiving themselves and of reacting to others called "life games" or "scripts"; these restrict and limit a person's adaptability and repertoire of interpersonal skills.[69] In other words, a script is formed in early childhood based on messages and labels (both verbal and nonverbal) that a child receives from his parents, such as parental perceptions of the child related to his worth, lovableness, sexual status, work, responsibility, and dependency. "Life patterns," which include suicide, obesity, and recurrent physical illness—especially when treatable and preventable—are all examples of tragic scripts.[70]

---

* Chapter 16 discusses this problem in greater detail.

ASSESSMENT QUESTIONS AND TECHNIQUES

There are three broad areas for the assessment of the family role structure:

1. The formal role structure.
2. The informal role structure and types of relationships.
3. The analysis of role models.

FORMAL ROLE STRUCTURE

Each family member's positions and roles would be described by asking and answering the following questions:

1. What formal positions and roles do each of the family members fufill?
2. Are these roles acceptable and consistent with the individual's and family's expectations? In other words, is there any role strain or role conflict?
3. How competently do members perform their respective roles?
4. Is there flexibility in roles when needed?

INFORMAL ROLE STRUCTURE

Questions pertinent to this area include:

1. What informal or covert roles exist in family, who plays them, and how frequently or consistently are they enacted? Are members of the family covertly playing roles different from those which their position in the family demands that they play?
2. What purpose does the presence of the identified covert or informal roles serve?

In analyzing the informal role structure, an important area to describe relates to the types of role relationships within the subsystems of the family. Role relationships can be observed and assessed within each of the usual three family subsystems, thus adding further information on both the adequacy of those sets of relationships and also the covert roles played within them. In assessing marital, parent–child, and sibling relationships, it is suggested that reference be made to the types of dyad relationships discussed previously (complementary, symmetrical, and parallel), which will assist in describing the nature of the subsystem role relationships and covert role structure.

In identifying the formal and informal roles which family members play, Satir questions patients about their roles by asking:

> "You wear three hats . . . individual, marital partner, and parent. I can see the parent, but where are the other two?"
> "Before marriage you were Miss So and So. What happened to her?"

Satir also explicitly teaches family members about their roles by listing the three basic roles—individual, marital partner, and parent—on a blackboard and explores their responses to interactions in these different roles and what other response options are available.[71]

THE ANALYSIS OF ROLE MODELS

In addition to an assessment of the overt and covert roles, role-model analysis is also helpful *when role problems exist.* This analysis is aimed at finding how the early life of the family members has affected their present behavior. It is not uncommon to find people tending to treat their children as their parents treated them in the past. These questions are suggested:

1. Who were (or are) the models that influenced family members in early life, who gave feelings and values about, for example, growth, new experiences, roles, and communication techniques?
2. Who specifically acted as role model for the mates in their roles as parents, and as marital partners, and what were they like? From this information a family member can be helped to see how past models influence his or her expectations and behavior.[72]

SOCIAL CLASS AND FAMILY ROLES

Lower-Class Families

The functions of family life in terms of family roles is, of course, greatly influenced by the demands and necessities put upon the family by the larger social structure. Thus, in response to our society's "benign neglect" of the poor, lower-class families, of all ethnic groups, have evolved a variety of subcultures as one means of solving the recurrent problems and issues arising from their class position.

Marital Roles

The marital stability of the lower-class families is far more precarious than for other groups, with divorces being two to six times greater among the unskilled labor group than among the professional middle class. The high rate of unemployment among the very poor is a major stressor in the marital relationship and significant cause of its dissolution. Twenty-five to forty percent of all poor families are headed by a woman, with serial monogamy—one mate after another—being a more common characteristic than with families of higher socioeconomic status.[73]

Several studies have found that lower-class marriages tend to provide less companionship than middle-class marriages. Furthermore, the marital therapeutic role is usually attenuated, or hardly present, in that emotional isolation from each other is expected. Personal and marital happiness are positively correlated with companionship and sociability with the spouse. In studying marriages among the lower-class, Bradburn found that a strong relationship existed between personal happiness and marital satisfaction and that the marital relationship was much less satisfying to mates among the lower social class.[74]

The lower-class family is a relatively loose-knit structure, although the roles of the marital partners and their division of responsibilities are formal. In many poor families there is a sharp demarcation of family roles based on whether the jobs are located inside or outside the home. These firm lines of authority serve to reinforce the emotional distance of the mates. The husband generally plays a minimal role in the low-income family, often conceiving of his role as being simply the provision of money to meet material needs. The lower-class wife's role, in turn, is expanded, and she often performs the majority of functions in the home, in addition to child rearing.[75]

Parental Roles

Since typically the affective and social needs of women are not met by their husbands, they develop greater emotional attachment to children as compensation for the emotional distance and lack of communication with their husbands. A peer relationship often develops between mother and her children of either sex. A son may be expected to contribute economically at an early age and become the man of the family.[76]

In the poor family, the parenting role is of central importance to the mother. There is a tendency to be more traditional in her outlook of child rearing, e.g., a greater emphasis on respectability, obedience, cleanliness, and discipline of young children, when compared with the middle-class parent, who centers more on developing self-reliance and independence in children and takes more cognizance of developmental and psychological principles in their parent–child relationship. To elaborate further, the focus of parenting in the poor family is on fulfillment of maintenance functions—providing food for the children, making sure they eat, have adequate rest, bathe, get to school on time—and on the maintenance of order and discipline in the home.[77]

Sibling Roles

When the children are older, the sibling roles acquire significance as a socializing agent far beyond that seen in the middle class. When there is a breakdown in communication between parents and children, the sibling subsystem tends to encourage expression of opposition to parental control.[78] Peer groups are also very important, especially for boys who seek masculine models, given the central role of the mother and the more passive role of the father in child rearing.

Working- and Middle-Class Families

Komarovsky found in her study of unskilled and skilled blue-collar workers and their families that the more educated the husband, the greater the degree of emotional closeness and companionship in marriage.[79] This was confirmed by later studies. In middle-class marriages companionship is a strong reason for the initiation and continuance of a marriage, an aspect that is stressed by a large number of families as being the chief end of marriage. In Blood and Wolfe's large study of the marital relationships of working-class and middle-class families from both urban and agrarian settings, about one-half of the wives from both environments identified "companionship in doing things together with the husband" as the most valuable aspect of marriage.[80] Additionally, middle-class couples report more sexual satisfaction in their marriages than do partners of the lower-class.

Working-class families generally tend to have more traditionally based family roles than middle-class families—the husband being more authoritarian in his role as head of the household. There is less joint planning and less of an egalitarian role relationship than in the middle-class family, but again there is wide variation, with the educational level of the spouses a prime factor (see Chap. 10).

Child rearing is now generally a shared role of middle-class parents, and their role behavior toward their children differs qualitatively from the lower-class family. It has been pointed out that one major reason for this may be the unconscious molding of a child to survive in the world as experienced by the parents. For instance, if a family is poor and parents expect that their boys will probably have to work in a menial position where obedience and comformity are stressed, training which promotes creativity, questioning, and independence would be counterproductive to what that child needs when he matures and has to relate and survive in society. In contrast, middle-class parents are more concerned with psychological growth, individual differences, independence, and self-reliance in their children. These traits encouraged by middle-class parents are functional to success in the middle-class occupational life, whereas those encouraged in lower-class parents—obedience, politeness, and respect for authority—are functional to low-status occupations.[81]

ROLES IN THE SINGLE-PARENT FAMILY

In Chapter 1, Introduction to the Family, the single-parent family was specifically discussed because of the large numbers of such families in our society today.* Most of these families are headed by mothers, although fathers are increasingly also heading single-parent families.

Two prominent role features of these families are (1) role overload and role conflicts and (2) role changes. In these families, the parent must fulfill both mother and father roles, in addition to lacking the support of the marital relationship. Single parents tend to be either overloaded with roles or in conflict over their various role commitments, since they have double tasks to assume. With a spouse to depend on, there is some role flexibility (if the child-care and housekeeping roles are shared). And even though the single parent is freed from the responsibilities of marital roles, other adult relationships often enter in and create demands on the single parent's precious time. Eighty to ninety percent of the mothers who are single parents will eventually remarry, necessitating another role change—relinquishing the father's role and forming new marital and parental roles.[83]

Significant research has been generated by behavioral scientists who have studied the single-parent family with a view to determining whether the single-parent family is detrimental to children. Herzog and Sudia, in summarizing research findings in this area, point out that there is little convincing evidence that the *mere absence* of a father in a family has a detrimental effect on a child's psychosexual or intellectual development. Factors such as how competently the mother handles her child-care roles are more crucial.[84]

ROLES IN THE RECONSTITUTED FAMILY

With the tremendous increase in the number of divorces (over a million recorded in the United States in 1975) and remarriages (80 percent of the divorced re-

marry), we have another type of family emerging, referred to as the reconstituted family or the stepparent family. In 75 percent of these cases, this type of family form denotes the entry of a new husband and surrogate father (stepfather), rather than stepmother, into a previously established single-parent family.

Reconstituted families pose greater problems than families of "first marrieds" or "second marrieds" with no children: 59 percent of all second marriages end in divorce as compared to 37 percent of all first marriages.[85] One of the primary reasons for this is the greater complexity involved integrating the stepfather into an already established family, especially owing to the mixed allegiance of the wife-mother to her new husband, on the one hand, and her children, on the other.

There has been a paucity of research on the reconstituted family and the adjustments and the roles of its members. Of the limited studies done in this area, Fast and Cain identified role confusion as a major familial problem. The stepfather and mother were both uncertain about whether the stepfather should assume the role of parent or nonparent. These authors noted the following problem areas:[86] (1) denial that any interpersonal problems were present; (2) hypersensitivity of stepparent to any suggestions or criticism; and (3) the newly formed couples' scapegoating of the children, perceiving them to be the source of all their conflicts and marital problems.*

Perhaps the underlying issues creating role confusion for the stepfather and the resultant family disequilibrium are the issues of child rearing and disciplining of children. As discussed in Chapter 14, the diversity in child-rearing practices and values is great. Each parent draws on his or her own family background when defining child-rearing beliefs, practices, and discipline. And it is difficult to compromise on these values and beliefs, since many of them are not objectively based. When parents enter into a relationship in which the stepfather heads the household but is not really the parent, synthesis of these values and rules is further complicated. Furthermore, the children, through exposure to their natural parents' child-rearing practices, have developed their own behaviors and expectations of what is acceptable or unacceptable behavior, for both themselves and their parents. In the reconstituted family the stepfather has no biological rights over the children, and whatever parental rights he may have must be granted him by his wife. This places the stepfather into a rather untenable position. When conflict arises over the disciplining of a child, the mother feels a natural right to decide the issue. If

---

*At least 17 percent of households in the United States in 1978.[82]

---

*It is clear that if conflict exists between stepfather and child (due to lack of clarity as to whether he should be a parent or not), the entire family is negatively affected, including the marital relationship.

the stepfather goes ahead and disciplines the child, she will often either directly become angry or, more often, indirectly strike back by undermining him. This latter course is particularly devastating to the entire family and often exacerbates the conflict, with the mother being torn between the loyalty to her children and to her husband.

FAMILY ROLES DURING HEALTH AND ILLNESS

Chapter 15 elaborates on the entire area of the family's involvement in health care and health practices. One aspect of this broad area is the issue of who is the decision maker, especially in the health–illness area, what happens when family members are sick or disabled, and what factors influence the family role structure during illness. These are all broad, significant questions and will be covered only in summary form in this section.

Role of Mother in Health and Illness

It has become increasingly clear that in most families an important role subsumed under the mother-wife position is that of health leader. Whatever criteria have been used in studies to measure health decision-making and roles, including such measures as illnesses incurred and treated, medical and health services used, and primary source of family assistance, the pervasive and central role of the mother as prime health decision-maker, educator, counselor, and "nurse" within the family matrix has remained a constant finding.[87] In this role, the mother defines symptoms and decides the "proper" disposition of resources. She also exerts substantial control over whether the children will receive preventive and curative services,[88-90] as well as acting as the main source of comfort and assistance in times of illness.[91]

One of the ways one can surmise the importance of the mother's health leader role is by observing what happens to her and the family when she is ill and unable to carry on her wife-mother roles. First of all, the mother-wife has been observed to assume the sick role only when it is absolutely mandatory, and then only reluctantly. Because her role performance is considered essential to family functioning, her illness tends to be quite disruptive and disorganizing.[92] Usually, severe illness or prolonged incapacitation of the mother-wife is seen as a more serious blow to the family's functioning than is the incapacitation of the husband-father (although if his illness is prolonged, adverse economic reverberations are felt).[93]

Role Changes during Illness and Hospitalization

In a period of crisis, such as that caused by the serious illness of a family member, the family structure is modified, the extent of modification depending on (1) whether the sick member is able to carry out his or her usual family roles and to what degree and (2) the centrality of the family roles or tasks which are vacated. The roles taken on by the mother are, as discussed previously, a good example of the centrality of a member's roles as compared to those of a young child in the family. When illness results in the vacancy of critical roles the family often enters a state of disequilibrium in which role and power relationships are altered until new homeostasis is achieved.[94]

The role changes which occur due to the loss or incapacitation of a family member may be of two basic types. Either the remaining family members have enough inner and outer resources that they are able to fulfill roles by shifting the basic and necessary role obligations and tasks which the sick family member is unable to assume—this is the functional way to handle the situation—or they do not have the capacity for role flexibility and adaptability, with the result that certain basic and necessary roles in the family are not performed or performed unsatisfactorily. In other words, the adequately functioning family can flexibly modify family roles to meet the demands of the situation or may call in resources and assistance from the outside to fill the vacuum, whereas dysfunctional families cannot.

Because of the role changes necessitated due to the loss of a family member, role conflicts and role strain are often present, especially during the stage of family disequilibrium immediately following the loss, when family structure is in the transitional process. Either interrole or intrarole conflict may exist, since the family members are "forced" to accept new roles and have had little opportunity to learn these roles and rearrange all their other role responsibilities. Role strain is often the outcome. The family members burdened with the acquisition of new roles may feel worried, anxious, and guilty because of feelings that they are not doing a competent job in their new roles or that with these added responsibilities, their role complex is excessively demanding and unmanageable.

Once a family has achieved a new equilibrium in response to a sick member's inability to perform his or her roles adequately, a similar reintegration must take place when that member resumes his or her place in the family unit. Understandably, having once gone through the process of adapting, the other members may well be reluctant to again "reshuffle" family roles and tasks, despite the recovery or reentry of the "lost" member. One sees this reluctance even in the most well functioning families, since the process of reintegration must entail the difficulties and problems that are part of any disorganization before a new (in this case, renewed) balance is achieved.

NURSING PRACTICE IMPLICATIONS

Assessment of family roles enables one to determine whether role changes or problems exist. Both role transitions and other types of role problems can create substantial disequilibrium and tension within the whole family and compromise the family's level of wellness. Hence for the benefit of the family members and the family as a whole, attention should be directed toward assisting the individuals and families by providing (1) information and demonstration on the role(s) being learned or support persons or groups who can help; (2) supportive help and counseling; and (3) direct physical assistance to family members in carrying out new roles or roles creating strain.

A second benefit in assessing family roles is that a knowledge of the formal and informal role structure helps our understanding of family strengths and resources. This supplies us with important data for planning interventions to resolve other health problems.

In conclusion, the provision of nursing assessment and intervention services in the area of family role adjustments and problems is a vital, rich area for family-centered nursing care.

REFERENCES

1. Goode W: The Family. Englewood Clifs, NJ, Prentice-Hall, 1964, p 1
2. Turner RH: Family Interaction. New York, Wiley, 1970
3. Hardy ME, Conway ME: Role Theory: Perspectives for Health Professionals. New York, Appleton, 1978
4. Biddle BJ, Thomas EJ: Role Theory: Concepts and Research. New York, Wiley, 1966
5. Linton R: The Cultural Background of Personality. New York, Appleton, 1945, p 77
6. Turner, op. cit.
7. Nye FI (ed): Role Structure and Analysis of the Family, Vol 24. Beverly Hills, Calif, Sage, 1976, p 7
8. Nye, op. cit.
9. Biddle, Thomas, op. cit., p 29
10. Merton RK: Social Theory and Social Structure. New York, Free Press, 1957, p 3
11. Nye, op. cit., p 10
12. Love L: Process of role change. In Carlson C (ed): Behavioral Concepts and Nursing Intervention. Philadelphia, Lippincott, 1970, p 305
13. Nye FI: Role constructs: Measurement. In Nye, op. cit., p 23
14. Ibid., p 23
15. Ibid., p 15
16. Jackson J: A conceptual and measurement model for norms and roles. Pacific Sociolog Rev 9:35–47, 1966
17. Nye FI: Emerging and declining roles. J Marriage Family 36:238, 1974
18. Nye, op. cit., p 17
19. Ibid., p 19
20. Turner, op. cit., p 186
21. Ibid., p 215
22. Parsons T, Bales RF, Shills EA: Working Papers on the Theory of Action. Glencoe, Ill, Free Press, 1953
23. Spiegel J: The resolution of role conflict within the family. Psychiatry 25:1, 1957
24. Peters L: Family team or myth. In Hall J, Weaver B (eds): Nursing of Families in Crisis. Philadelphia, Lippincott, 1974, p 35
25. Turner, op. cit., p 187
26. Ibid., pp 185–186
27. Spiegel J: Cultural strain, family role patterns and intrapsychic conflict. In Howells J (ed): Theory and Practice of Family Psychiatry. New York, Brunner/Mazel, 1971
28. Glasser P, Glasser L: Families in Crisis. New York, Harper & Row, 1970, pp 290–301
29. Ibid.
30. Messer A: The Individual in His Family: An Adaptational Study. Springfield, Ill, Thomas, 1970
31. Murray R, Zentner J: Nursing Concepts for Health Promotion. Englewood Cliffs, NJ, Prentice-Hall, 1975, p 350
32. Nye FI, Gecas, V: The role concept: Review and delineation. In Nye, op. cit., p 13
33. Minuchin S: Families and Family Therapy. Cambridge, Mass, Harvard University Press, 1974, pp 60–66
34. Cline CL: Five variations in the marriage theme: Types of marriage formation. Bull Family Dev 3:10, Spring 1966
35. Cuber JF, Harroff PB: The more total view: Relationships among men and women of the upper middle class. Marriage Family Living 25:140, May 1963
36. Cuber, Harroff, op. cit.
37. Bott E: Family and Social Networks. London, Tavistock, 1957
38. Watzlawick P, Beavin JH, Jackson DD: Pragmatics of Human Communication. New York, Norton, 1967
39. Turner RH: Role taking: process vs. conformity. In Rose AM (ed): Human Behavior and Social Processes. Boston, Houghton-Mifflin, 1962, pp 20–40
40. Aldous J: The making of family roles and family change. Family Coordinator 23:232, 1974
41. Cronkite RC: The determinants of spouses' normative preferences for family roles. J Marriage Family 39:575, 1977
42. Ibid.
43. Block F: Allocation of time to market and non-market work within a family unit. Unpublished doctoral dissertation, Stanford University, 1974
43a. Meissner MW et al: No exit for wives: Sexual division of labor and the cumulation of the household demands. Can Rev Sociol Anthropol 12:424, 1975
44. Cronkite, op. cit., pp 580–585
45. Gecas V: The socialization and child care roles. In Nye, op. cit.
46. Araji SK: Husbands and wives attitude—behavior con-

gruence on family roles. J Marriage Family 39:311, 1977

47. *Ibid.,* pp 318–319
48. Hoffman LW: Changes in family roles, socialization, and sex differences. Am Psychologist 32:644, August 1977
49. Nye, *op. cit.*
50. Gecas, *op. cit.*
51. Araji, *op. cit.*
52. Bronfenbrenner U: The changing American child—a speculative analysis. In Coser RL (ed): Life Cycle and Achievement in America. New York, Harper & Row, 1969, p 6
53. Reiss IL: Family Systems in America, 2nd ed. Hinsdale, Ill, Dryden Press, 1976, p 278
54. Aldous, *op. cit.,* p 234
55. Meleis AI: Role insufficiency and role supplementation. Nurs Res 24:264, 1975.
56. Meleis AI, Swendsen LA: Role supplementation—an empirical test of a nursing intervention. Nurs Res 27:11, 1978
57. Swendsen LA, Meleis AI: Role supplementation for new parents—a role mastery plan. Am J Maternal-Child Nurs X:84, March-April 1978
58. Meleis, *op. cit.,* p 265
59. Satir V: Conjoint Family Therapy, rev ed. Palo Alto, Calif, Science and Behavior Books, 1967
60. Feldman F, Scherz F: Family Social Welfare. New York, Atherton, 1967, p 67
61. Kievit MB: Family roles. In Parent-Child Relationships—Role of the Nurse. Newark, NJ, Rutgers University, School of Nursing, 1968, p 7
62. Benne KD, Sheats P: Functional roles of group members. J Soc Issues 4:41, Spring, 1948
63. Satir V: Peoplemaking. Palo Alto, Calif, Science and Behavior, 1972, pp 208–209
64. Ackerman N: The Psychodynamics of Family Life. New York, Basic, 1966
65. Zuk GH: The go-between process in family therapy. Family Process 5:162, 1966
66. Satir, *op. cit.,* p 266
67. Bossard JH, Boll ES: The Large Family System: An Original Study in the Sociology of Family Behavior. Philadelphia, University of Pennsylvania Press, 1956
68. Mishel MH: Patient Problems in Self-Esteem and Nursing Intervention. Los Angeles, California State University at Los Angeles, Trident Shops, 1974, p 43
69. Lange S: Transactional analysis and nursing. In Carlson, *op. cit.,* pp 247–248
70. *Ibid.,* p 147
71. Satir, *op. cit.,* pp 174–175
72. Satir, *op. cit.,* pp 105, 173–174
73. Chilman C: Growing Up Poor. Washington, DC, Department of Health, Education, and Welfare, Welfare Administration Publication No. 13 (U.S. Government Printing Office), 1966, p 67
74. Bradburn NM: The Structure of Psychological Well-Being. Chicago, Aldine, 1970, p 163
75. Besmer A: Economic deprivation and family patterns. In Irelan LM (ed): Low-Income Life Styles. Washington, DC, Department of Health, Education, and Welfare, Social and Rehabilitation Service, 1967, pp 17–18
76. *Ibid.,* p 17
77. Besmer, *op. cit.,* p 24
78. *Ibid.,* pp 193–194, 219
79. Komarovsky M: Blue Collar Marriage. New York, Random House, 1964
80. Blood RO, Wolfe DM: Husbands and Wives. Glencoe, Ill, Free Press, 1960, p 150
81. Besmer, *op. cit.,* p 25
82. Woodward KL et al: Saving the Family. Newsweek, May 15, 1978, p 64
83. LeMasters EE: Parents without partners. In Skolnick A, Skolnick JH (eds): Intimacy, Family and Society. Boston, Little, Brown, 1974, p 524
84. Herzog E, Sudia CE: Children in fatherless families. In Caldwell BM, Riccuti HN (eds): Review of Child Development Research, Vol 3. Chicago, University of Chicago Press, 1973
85. Kiester E: Marriage the Second Time Around. New York, Family Circle, February, 1976, p 82
86. Fast I, Cain AC: The step-parent role: Potential for disturbances in family functioning. Am J Orthopsychiatry 36:485, 1966
87. Litman TL: The family as a basic unit in health and medical care: A social behavioral overview. Soc Sci Med 8:505, 1974
88. Aday LA, Eichhorn R: The Utilization of Health Services: Indices and Correlates—A Research Bibliography, 1972. Washington, DC, Department of Health, Education, and Welfare, Publication No. (HSM) 73-3003, National Center for Health Services Research and Development, 1973, pp 29–30
89. Diosy LL: Socioeconomic status and participation in the poliomyelitis vaccine trial. Am Sociol Rev 21:185, 1956
90. Rayner JF: Socioeconomic status and factors influencing the dental health practices of mothers. Am J Public Health 60:1250, 1970
91. Litman TJ: Health Care and the Family: A Three Generational Study. An Exploratory Study Conducted under the Division of Community Health Services and Medical Care Administration, US Public Health Service, 1974
92. Mechanic D: Influences of mothers on their children's health attitudes and behavior. Pediatrics 33:445, 1964
93. Litman, *op. cit.*
94. Hill RR: Social stresses on the family. Social Casework 39:142, 1958

STUDY QUESTIONS

1. Match the correct definition or description with the appropriate term.

Terms
a. Role.
b. Role taking.
c. Position.
d. Role making.

Definitions
1. Status.
2. Described as being empathetic.
3. Incompatibility of the role(s) (intrarole or interrole).

Terms		Definitions	
e.	Role enactment.	4.	Normative behavioral expectations of person occupying a particular position.
f.	Socialization.		
g.	Role conflict.	5.	The process of learning family and adult roles in preparation for societal responsibilities.
h.	Reciprocal roles.		
i.	Role strain.		
j.	Role patterning.	6.	Balancing in family structure to maintain stability.
k.	Family homeostasis.		
l.	Role sharing.	7.	Joint participation in fulfilling same role.
		8.	Complementary role.
		9.	The worry or guilt felt as a result of lack of role enactment or presence of role conflict.
		10.	The actual behavior exhibited in a role.
		11.	Allocation of roles and their associated tasks.
		12.	The generation of new prescriptions and expectations of appropriate behavior for a certain position.

Are the following statements True *or* False?

2. The most functional way of maintaining equilibrium in a family in the face of change is by use of role induction.

3. The principle of complementarity states that there must be a match in expectations and performance of roles by mates in order for stability and harmony to be present in the relationship.

4. Paired relationships in the family refer to father–son and mother–daughter relationships.

5. For each of the roles making up the wife–mother and husband–father positions listed in the following table, indicate whether these roles are normatively shared or the primary responsibility of one or the other partner. If the trend is toward sharing or being more or less a single partner's role, indicate this with an arrow pointing up (increasing emphasis) or down (decreasing emphasis).

Role	Shared Role	Role of Wife-Mother	Role of Husband-Father
Provider			
Housekeeper			
Child Care			
Recreational			
Kinship			
Therapeutic			
Sexual			
Companion			
Health Leader			

6. From the two studies presented on the observed types of marriages (by Cline, and Cuber and Harroff), which conclusion would be the most accurate and practically significant?
    a. Well-functioning or longstanding marriages are distinguished from poorly functioning marriages.
    b. It was discovered that diverse patterns of marital relationships existed.
    c. A wide range of behaviors and roles existed in the marriages studied.
    d. Because there is no one type of marriage which fits the needs of most couples, acceptance and understanding of this diversity among couples is indicated.

7. When a wife is employed in a two-parent nuclear family with children, what are the common role changes and conflicts experienced by the husband and the wife?

8. Identify three commonly seen differences in role structure between the lower- and middle-class families.

9. List five examples of covert or informal roles seen in the family, indicating which of them could be functional.

10. The maintenance of informal or covert roles is vital to the family because (select *the* best answer):
    a. It relieves the role overload of some members.
    b. Without covert roles the family could not exist.
    c. Each formal role has an associated informal role.
    d. Through the assumption of informal roles, family homeostasis is maintained and individual socioemotional needs are met.

11. Why are both overt (formal) and covert (informal) roles important to assess?

12. Give reasons why labeling is restrictive to individual's growth and development.

13. Identify two role characteristics of single-parent families which act as stressors to the family and its members.

14. What are two prominent role problems within the reconstituted family?

Are the following statements True *or* False?

15. When a family member is ill, the functional way of handling the situation is to leave the roles unfulfilled until he or she returns.

16. Role flexibility suggests that family members have the motivation and capacity to shift and reenact new roles when needed.

17. Middle-class parents are generally more concerned with promoting self-reliance and independence in their child-rearing practices, while lower-class parents stress respect and obedience.

FAMILY CASE STUDY*

After reading the following case study, answer questions 18 through 23.

Mr. and Mrs. G. are a young couple, married for three years, with a 2-year-old son. The 23-year-old husband is a garbage collector, earning $12,000 a year. He completed two years of high school; his 22-year-old wife is a high school graduate. (But the family nurse commented: "It is hard to believe in view of her poor vocabulary and illiterate handwriting that she had completed high school." The husband said: "She was sort of a dumbbell at school, but people liked her and she got through.")

Mr. G. is a slim tall man, slow moving and soft spoken. When asked what he liked about himself, he replied, "People tell me I'm easygoing but not a chump." The assessor observed his deceptively lazy attitude as the manner of a man who thinks that most people, particularly women, become too excited about things and foolishly so. He reports that he quit school at 14 because he did not like it. Since then he has held a number of unskilled jobs. Concerning his present occupation as garbage collector, he stated: "People laugh at you for being in this line of work. I don't know what's so funny about it. It's got to be done. There is no future in it, though, and the pay is terrible. I'm going to make a break for it as soon as I can. Everybody's looking out for me now, and something is bound to turn up pretty soon."

Both Mr. G. and his wife express satisfaction with their sexual relations and with the marriage in general. Mr. G. is in charge of the outside of house and repairs to their home, and Mrs. G. is in charge of the interior of the home and child.

A good deal of the communication between them is nonverbal. This type of communication pattern began during their courtship. When asked whether her husband had said he loved her when he proposed, Mrs. G. answered, "He just got softer and softer on me and I could tell that he did and we got to necking more and more and he wanted to go all the way and I didn't want to unless we were going to get married." The nurse asked whether he had ever said out and out that he could go for her or wanted her or anything like that. Mrs. G. said, "No, we don't go in for that kind of stuff." When she told him that she was pregnant, "He looked a little funny when I told him, but he didn't say much. You know that's what's going to happen. After a while, when I began to show a lot, he asked me sometimes how I felt."

Mrs. G. was asked to describe their quarrels. She said they quarrel little, but when they do, it is about such things as his failure to help move the furniture or her failure to do something he demands. "We just get over it." He might "crab around and then he would know that he had been mean to me and makes it up." There is no conversation about such quarrels, but Mr. G. helps to dry the dishes or asks her if she likes a television program or wants something else. Mrs. G. felt that talking does no good, since it might worsen things.

When asked whether they like to talk about what makes people tick or to discuss the rights and wrongs of things, each said in separate interviews, "No, we don't hash things over." Mr G. added, "It's either right or wrong—what is there to discuss?"

This "conversation of gestures" between Mrs. G. and her husband contrasts sharply with the communication characterizing her relationships with female relatives and friends. On many counts Mrs. G. reveals her emotional life to the latter. And this extends to spheres of experience beyond the "feminine world" of babies, housework, or gossip.

Mrs. G. sees her sister and her mother daily. "Oh yes," she said about her sister, we tell each other everything, anything we have on our minds. We don't hold nothing back. We discuss the children, the house, cooking, and 'female

---

*Adapted by permission of Random House, Inc., from Blue-Collar Marriage, by Mirra Komarovsky with the collaboration of Jane H. Phillips. Copyright 1962, 1964, 1967 by Random House, Inc.

things.'" But when asked whether she can talk to her husband, she answered, "Sure, I can talk to him about anything that has to be said." Her view is that "men and women do different things; he don't want to be bothered with my job of cleaning and children and I don't want to be bothered with his. He makes the big decisions and I don't have to bother with it. Sometimes we got to do the same things, something around the house and we have to tell each other."

When asked what helped her when she was in the "dumps," Mrs. G. replied, "Talking to my sister or my mother helps sometimes." When asked directly whether conversations with her husband ever have a similar effect, she replied, "No."

Mr. G. enjoys an active social life with his male friends and relatives. Mr. G. revealed to his father and his brother he fears that Mrs. G. was making a "sissy" out of their son, and he regularly consults with them about his occupational plans. He does not discuss the latter topics with his wife because "there is no need of exciting her for nothing. Wait until it's sure. Women get all excited and talk too much."

Mr. G. thinks the world of the fellows in his own clique whom he sees after supper several times a week and on Saturday afternoons. Mrs. G. does not always know where he meets his "friends" when he leaves in the evenings. Mr. and Mrs. G. testified independently that having a beer with the fellows is the best cure for his depressions.

Select the one best answer referring to the family case study.

18. This marriage was characterized as "happy" by both marital partners. This was because:
    a. Both come from same social class.
    b. Both shared same marital role expectations.
    c. Both were denying how really alienated they were from each other and how unsatisfactory their marriage was.
    d. Their sex life was adequate.

19. This marriage illustrates:
    a. A lack of psychological intimacy.
    b. Meager verbal communication in meaningful areas of family life.
    c. That companionship is not essential to make a satisfactory marriage.
    d. That both mates did not communicate openly with anyone.

20. This type of marriage is frequently seen in:
    a. Lower-class families.
    b. White, skilled working-class families.
    c. Disorganized families.
    d. Middle-class WASP families.

21. Through the couple's communication we can gather that:
    a. Both mates carry out traditional male–female roles.
    b. Mrs. G. would rather move out and be with her sister and friends.
    c. Mr. G.'s occupational role is of central concern to him.
    d. Mr. G. desires to raise his son to be "a man."

22. Which type of relationship does this marriage most closely fit?
    a. Symmetrical.
    b. Parallel.
    c. Complementary.

23. Complete a brief description of the couple's formal roles from what can be inferred from the narrative.

STUDY ANSWERS

1. a. 4   g. 3
    b. 2   h. 8
    c. 1   i. 9
    d. 12   j. 11
    e. 10   k. 6
    f. 5   l. 7

2. False

3. True

4. False

5.

Role	Shared Role	Role of Wife-Mother	Role of Husband-Father
Provider	—	—	√↓
Housekeeper	—	√↓	—
Child Care	√↑	—	—
Recreational	√↑	—	—
Kinship	—	√	—
Therapeutic	√↑	—	—
Sexual	√↑	—	—
Companion	√↑	—	—
Health Leader	—	√	—

6. d

7. *Husband:*
    Feels partial role loss having to share the enacting of provider (breadwinner) role.
    Necessitates role transitions when he assumes greater (shared) responsibility for child care and perhaps other areas.
    Usually experiences role changes rather than role conflicts.
    Wife:
    Feels role conflict and strain.
    Most often still retains the housekeeper role and child-care role (although this is often shared) into addition working.
    Her other shared and assumed roles remain, also producing role overload.
    Commonly feels role strain as a result of role conflict, feeling worried and guilty that she is not spending enough time with children or is hurting husband's pride in being sole provider. (This is true in more affluent, especially upper-middle class, families.)

8. *Lower-Class Family:*
    Marital Roles
    Sexual role less satisfying and diminished in importance.
    Companionship role attenuated.
    Therapeutic role attenuated.

Parenting Roles
Child-care role is the mother's exclusively (and the central role in her life).
Middle-Class Family:
Marital Roles
Sexual role is shared and more satisfying.
Companionship and therapeutic roles are strong basis for marriage.
Parenting Roles
Child-care role shared.

9. a. Integrator (functional).
    b. Mediator (functional).
    c. Scapegoat.
    d. Jester (functional).
    e. Child (when formal role is parent).
    f. Blocker.

10. d

11. They describe how family members have allocated tasks to fulfill family functions; they disclose the socioemotional needs of family member(s) and the family and whether and how these needs are being met.

12. Individual cannot fully develop; he or she is rewarded only for certain behaviors and thus matures only in these rewarded areas.

13. a. Role overload.
    b. Role changes or shifts, which occur if there is remarriage.

14. a. Whether the father (in the case of a stepfather family) is a parent or not (role confusion).
    b. The incompatibility of her wife role vis-à-vis her husband versus her mother role vis-à-vis her children (role conflict). Often plays a go-between informal role which also has its hazards.

15. False

16. True

17. True

18. b

19. c

20. a

21. a

22. c

23. *Formal Role Structure of Hypothetical Family:*
    The family was characterized by a sharp demarcation of roles (traditional pattern).
    Husband-Father:
    Sole provider—breadwinner role.
    Home repairman and gardener role.
    Wife-Mother:
    Child-care role.
    Housekeeper role (inside the house).
    No roles are shared, nor do they wish to share any roles.
    The companionship and therapeutic roles are not present in their marriage.
    Sexual roles are not clear.

No family health assessment is complete without an analysis of a family's central values, since the value system is one of the four highly interdependent structural dimensions of a family. Understanding what is important to a particular family is vital in terms of assessment, diagnosis and health care intervention, for we know that what a family believes and values broadly affects both the family's and its members' behavior. Hence when family values and beliefs are identified, we may be better able to understand the reasons for family dynamics, thereby enhancing our interpretation of family behavior.

In addition, we must realize the tendency of health professionals to diagnose or label a family as pathological when they demonstrate deviation from the dominant cultural values and norms. Most research on families is based on the majority culture (described below), and we must be particularly cautious about extrapolating these findings to all social classes and cultural groups, whose life conditions and traditions differ greatly from those of the dominant culture.

An accurate assessment of a family's value system should help us tailor our nursing interventions to a particular family or groups of similar families. We need to work within the family's value system and relate our services to goals that are important to the family being assisted. For instance, it is well accepted that "ideas and methods which least affect the patient's habits, beliefs, and values meet less resistance than those that attempt to alter existing behavior patterns and values."[1]

In assessing a family's value system it is also imperative for us, as health providers, to recognize our own priorities and values and to examine carefully how our values and attitudes subtly—and sometimes not so subtly—affect our family-centered care. One ultimate goal in assessing family values is to demonstrate to families an appreciation of the inherent worth of different value systems.[2]

BASIC DEFINITIONS

Values are defined as a system of ideas, attitudes, and beliefs about the worth of an entity or concept and which consciously and unconsciously bind together the members of a family in a common culture.[3] The family group is a prime source of the belief systems, value systems, and norms that determine an individual's understanding of the nature and meaning of the world, his or her place in it, and how to reach his or her goals and aspirations. Thus values serve as general guides to behavior. For instance, if a person values health and feels it is a desirable state, he or she is much more likely to engage in preventive health care and salubrious health habits. These positive values are learned from the family of origin, which is the basic transmitter of values from one generation to the next.

12

Family Values

LEARNING OBJECTIVES

1. Define the terms *value* and *norms* and their significance relative to family assessment.
2. Describe the common outcome of a disparity in value systems between health worker and client.
3. Identify and briefly explain four important changes which have taken place in society and family values in recent years.
4. Discuss the major value orientations of American society in terms of their significance today and their interrelationships with each other.
5. Identify four of the variables which influence the family's value system and create value conflicts.
6. Describe some of the differences in values and norms among the social classes.
7. Given a case situation and utilizing the values assessment process, identify the salient values operating within the hypothetical family.

It should be understood, however, that values are not static. The potency, or primacy, of a family's values change over time, as the family and its members are exposed to different subcultures, as societal values undergo change, and as particular situations demand a shift of priorities by the family.

Families and individuals rarely behave according to consistent value patterns. Also certain values are amenable to conscious identification, whereas others are less susceptible to conscious expression. Hence values can be distinguished as to whether they are consciously held (overt or manifest values) or unconsciously held (latent or covert).

There is a hierarchical nature to values. Some values are more central, molding or influencing most aspects of our lives, while other values are more peripheral and have less influence or involve only certain aspects of our life style and daily functioning. In other words, certain values have a greater priority or potency than other values, particularly when looking at a family at a given point in time.

An individual's or family's configuration of values ascribes meaning to certain critical events and at the same time suggests ways to respond to these situations. This configuration of values provides definitions of the time dimension; contains concepts concerning the responsibility and worth of the individual members of the family; ranks certain commonly held life goals; imposes a framework within which the pursuit of risks connected with the pleasure impulse takes place; defines what messages, thoughts, and feelings should and should not be shared and with whom; and lastly, involves a system of sanctions.

An individual's or family's values are very much a reflection of the community in which the individual or family resides and the subculture(s) with whom they identify. Most persons belong to a number of subcultures based on social class, ethnic background, occupational groups, peer groups, religious affiliation, and so forth. Since subcultures exist within the larger, dominant culture, aspects of that value system also pervade the subculture. Thus members of a particular subculture respond to both subcultural and dominant value systems, although at different moments the values of one or the other may be more relevant to the individual or family. Obviously the greater the degree of congruence between a family's subcultural values and the community's values, the easier the individual's and family's adjustment, and the greater degree of success the family will meet in relating to the community.

Norms are patterns of behavior considered to be right in a given society and, as such, are based on the family's value system. They are also modal behaviors. In other words, norms prescribe the appropriate role behavior for each of the positions in the family and society and specify how reciprocal relations are to be maintained, as well as how role behavior may change with the changing ages of occupants of these positions.

DISPARITY IN VALUE SYSTEMS

One of the primary stressors in relationships between health workers and clients (family) is the social distancing created because of social class and/or cultural differences. When the health professional and client do not possess the same basic beliefs and values, the results are often divergent goals, unclear communication, and interactional problems.

In order to effectively explore the area of values and norms, it is first necessary to look at the values of the health care system and of nursing. As health professionals working within the health care system, we generally uphold the values of the white, Anglo-Saxon Protestant (WASP) dominant culture. Brink describes this situation:

> The American nurse, educated in the United States, falls within the "Old Yankee" classification of value systems. American nurses are future-oriented, belong to a doing-oriented profession, are individualistic in decision-making, but lineally-oriented in the health institution, believe that disease is controllable, and view the human being as neither good nor evil, but ill.[4]

If the health care system is to be successfully integrated into American society, its values and practices must be consonant with society's value orientation. This does not negate the reality that many nurses and nursing students come from diverse cultural and social class backgrounds and possess their own configuration of values and goals, although also conforming to the dominant cultural values.

Two serious reservations regarding the studies and literature of societal/family values need to be pointed out. The numerous investigations of different value orientations among the various social classes betray a repeated tendency toward ethnocentricity and overgeneralization. Sweeping conclusions have been made from limited or biased observations. Individual variations, and even variations in the same individual or family in different contexts, are not sufficiently emphasized.[5] We need to have some basic information on social class and cultural differences, but must at the same time realize the limitations inherent in characterizing groups of people. As health professionals, our assessments must be individualized, recognizing the unique attitudes and qualities of the client involved. Yet to have any practical significance, of course, one must generalize and synthesize from relevant studies.

Murillo, in writing about the Mexican-American family, speaks to the problem of generalizing and perhaps "stereotyping." In pondering on how to describe a traditional Mexican-American family, he writes:

> In an effort to solve this problem (there being no uniform pattern of family life), I have tried to temper my description of the "traditional" Mexican-American by describing it also in the context of a comparative cultural value system. . . . I will go further, however, and make explicit that the values discussed must be viewed from a probabilistic approach. That is, every value I attribute to a Mexican-American person or family should be understood basically in terms of there being a greater chance or probability that the Mexican-American, as compared with the Anglo, will think and behave in accordance with that value. . . . In the final analysis, one must come to know and accept the uniqueness of the individual or specific family. Many Mexican-Americans are not only bilingual, but bicultural, and it is very worthwhile to ascertain the special blending of cultures one may encounter in a person or family in order to acquire a realistic understanding.[6]

CHANGES IN AMERICAN SOCIETY AND ITS VALUES

The central, unifying theme of the dominant American culture has always been that cluster of values Weber called the Protestant ethic, in which a person's virtue has primarily been measured in terms of occupational success for men and being a good wife and mother for women. The most valued role model in the past, and to a large extent today, is the rational, hard-working, self-denying, risk-taking entrepreneur.[7]

In recent years, a number of authors[8-12] have suggested, however, that the vitality of the Protestant ethic has declined; some, like Reich, who predicted that the values of the 1960s "counterculture" would remake America, see a greater alteration in values than others. Although his thesis was overstated, those counterculture values are indeed becoming more widespread and have led to articles such as Flacks' "Growing Up Confused: Cultural Crisis and Individual Character" and Slater's "Cultures in Collision," which describe the value differences and conflicts between the old traditional values and the new cultural values.

Flacks illustrates the enormous influence economic changes in American society during the twentieth century have had in weakening many of its central values:

> The American economic system in the past was organized around problems of capital accumulation and the need for saving, entrepreneurship, and self-reliance . . . a system of free market and individual competition . . . has been replaced by an economic system organized around problems of distribution and the need for spending, interdependence, bureaucratic management, planning, and large-scale organization. . . . This situation requires that men consume; and obviates the need to save, postpone gratification, and be self-denying.[13]

Not only have there been vast changes in our economic system, but profound physical and social changes have also taken place. For example, in the last 200 years, the United States quadrupled in physical size and its population grew 52 times greater. We have gone from an overwhelmingly rural society to become a highly urbanized nation. Whereas only 1 percent of Americans were high school graduates in 1800, 76 percent of Americans now graduate from high school. And more recently, the country changed from an overwhelmingly white, Anglo-Saxon Protestant country to one with increasingly significant Catholic, Jewish, Asian, black, and Hispanic populations.

Despite these major changes and the resultant modification of values and priorities, a substantial amount of continuity in the American value system has prevailed. Nevertheless, five broad changes are well recognized and will be briefly discussed here. These are a decrease in the salience of the work ethic; an increasing tolerance of diversity; an increasing egalitarianism or equalitarianism; consumerism; and an increasing value placed on health and the quality of one's life.

The Work Ethic

According to Inkeles, the ethic of hard work is fast eroding. "Between 1958 and 1971, increasing numbers of Americans considered the most important attributes of a job to be high pay and short hours, not the intrinsic importance and a promise of advancement."[14]

Few persons in our society obtain sufficient rewards over and above the paycheck. The blue-collar worker especially bemoans this fact. Nevertheless, society attempts to inculcate the value of work, no matter how demeaning or repugnant the job. The youth of today particularly question this ethic. Moreover, widespread discontent with work is present throughout society as evidenced by symptoms such as alcoholism, absenteeism, the weekend flight from cities, movement from job to job, early retirement, increased filing for disability benefits, and a rise in filing for workmen's compensation and unemployment insurance benefits.[15]

But even if work is not the central overriding value today that it was in the past, it would be premature to prepare for a demise of the Protestant ethic of work and the desire to "get ahead." Several noted authors have written that when jobs were easily found and available, as in the 1960s, they were less valued. Now that jobs have become scarcer, work will correspondingly become more valued again.[16]

Tolerance of Diversity

Perhaps due to the civil rights and antiwar movements of the 1960s and/or because of the increasing number of minorities in the United States, a greater tolerance of diversity has been noted. This diversity includes greater acceptance of ethnic peoples, women, and variant life-styles. Weaver states that the major and most significant result of these two movements was the growth of popular questioning of cultural assumptions held by Americans for generations. "Rather than having values of a subcultural group dissipated and absorbed by the dominant culture, these two groups have undermined the values and assumptions of the dominant culture."[17]

Foremost among the numerous assumptions made in America has been the myth of the "melting pot." The pot never really melted out the differences, but the myth has tended to downgrade these differences and elevate and validate the standardized WASP values and norms. This cultural imperialism (as opposed to cultural pluralism) is a result of racism, technological advances, urbanization, and a progressiveness that holds everything scientific and new good and roots and traditions obsolete.[18]

Increasing tolerance of diverse life styles and family forms has also occurred.* Boulding predicts that "family living in the twenty-first century will probably provide more options than are open to today's individuals seeking familistic groups."[19] As mentioned in Chapter 7, the new diverse experimental families have certain common features, one central one being a strong rejection of the privatistic family values of "middle America." These new forms are concerned with a more equitable distribution of goods, services, and role responsibilities, and greater opportunities for personal growth among family members.[20]

Equality

The growing importance of equality is closely linked with an increasing tolerance of diversity and the growing tendency to pursue individualistic personal goals, where freedom, independence, and autonomy, as well as greater expression of feelings, are paramount. The rise of egalitarianism is a major change in family life. According to Arnold Toynbee, the noted historian, the most vital revolution of our time is the emancipation of women, because ultimately their emancipation will affect everyone's life. "Above all, it is going to demand an immense and disturbing psychological adjustment on the part of men, because it implies a revolutionary change in the traditional relations between the sexes."[21] In addition to the women's movement and the affirmative action programs, there has been considerable progress in protecting the rights of the mentally

ill and of children. These legislative trends also demonstrate the rising potency of equality as a value.

Quality of Life and Health

Middle-class persons today are becoming increasingly interested in making qualitative changes in their lives, including such life style improvements as curtailing smoking, making dietary changes, partaking in self-help stress reduction and other mental health programs;* environmental alterations such as moving from city and suburban areas to small towns and sometimes rural environments; reducing the amount of work and changing type of work; and participating in creative and leisure endeavors. All these signify a basic modification of values away from the achievement orientation in which materialism, competition, possession of goods and power reigns, to a more introspective orientation where personal and familial happiness and personal independence in decision making have greater priority. While it is difficult to measure how highly health is valued and how widespread this shift is, available evidence suggests that maintaining health is not generally at the top of American hierarchy of values, although it is gaining in significance. The importance of this value is probably influenced, not only by social class, but also by age and ethnicity. A national survey of high school students' values found that being healthful ranked fifth in a list of twelve personal values.[23]

The Consumption Ethic

The consumption ethic has now replaced the thrift ethic according to Inkeles, who sees that the "put-away" society has become the "throw-away" society.[24] Credit policies in America have so greatly encouraged material indulgence on a pay-later basis that we now refer to our "plastic money."

MAJOR VALUE ORIENTATIONS OF AMERICAN SOCIETY

In spite of the declining state of the Protestant ethic and the existence of other, strongly conflicting values, this cluster of core values still molds and shapes American society, and thus family life, as well as the behavior of health professionals. Yankelovitch, Skelley, and White, in a study based on a national probability sample of 1,247 families and 2,194 interviews, confirmed the continuity of the Protestant ethic. In an-

---

* There appears to be some backlash or reaction to this growing tolerance of differing life styles, as seen in the antihomosexual legislation proposed and/or enacted recently in Florida, Oregon, and California, as well as in areas of women's rights, and especially abortion.

* Since 1975 U.S. mortality figures have shown significant decreases in cardiovascular deaths. This has been largely attributed to a decrease in smoking among those persons at risk for heart disease.[22]

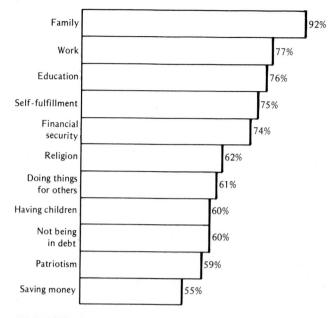

FIGURE 12.1
Most important personal values. (*From: Yankelovitch, Skelley, and White, Inc.: The General Mills American Family Report, 1974–1975. General Mills, Inc., Minneapolis, Minn, p 55.*)

alyzing their results they reported that the Protestant ethic "continues to dominate the value structure of the American family. Fifty-six percent of all Americans are strongly committed to such traditional beliefs as 'duty before pleasure,' 'hard work pays off,' religion, and 'saving even if it means sacrifice.' "[25] Figure 12.1 illustrates the salience of the traditional values of family, work, and education.

According to these authors, families which highly subscribe to the dominant American value orientation tend to be secure and confident. More specifically, they tend to be "savers" (financially), optimistic about the future, more likely to enjoy life, more satisfied with their degree of success, and more confident that they have the ability to handle emergencies.[26] The fact that the families who subscribe to the Protestant ethic, or dominant culture, tend to be well adjusted and confident provides further evidence that society's central values are still grounded in the Protestant ethic, since family conformity with the values of its society is one of the essentials for family health and adjustment.

Productivity

The most ubiquitous and significant value of our whole culture or society is that of productivity. In *Social Class and Family Life*, McKinley compiles impressive evidence of how family life and behavior respond to and are structured by the extrafamilial aspects of the society. His thesis is that we need to understand so-

ciety's norms and the standards by which it evaluates—ranks and rewards—people to comprehend family behavior. And in our society, the one dominant and unifying standard or set of values used to evaluate individuals in their groups is the secularized Protestant ethic, which focuses on solving adaptive problems, the postponement of gratification, and the pursuit of an assured sense of personal worth.[27] The major component within the value cluster of the secularized Protestant ethic is the value of productivity. By stressing productivity, the ultimate goal of American society, that of providing energy, products, and services, is obtainable.

Success and achievement, the reputed outcomes of being productive, are also identified as predominant social values. Extensive stress is placed on personal achievement, especially secular occupational achievement. Each person, particularly the adult male, must prove himself basically worthy of approval by acting in a productive manner toward some higher goal—namely, in his occupation—which will indirectly benefit society. No one in our society is exempt from finding his "calling," for no one is "good" until he proves himself productive. Thus personal worth is paired with occupational excellence and how much individuals have contributed to society.

The value placed on achievement strongly affects family and individual behavior. For example, in today's families much more emphasis is placed on individual interests and fulfillment—rather than family interests and activities—since it is the individual who is expected to make it on his or her merits. The individual is socialized to believe that he or she need not always respond to the needs and feelings of family members or friends, since he or she is a private individual, responding to a higher and more general value system.

Because so much apprehension surrounds choice of occupational goals, there is an anxious postponement in selecting one's career ("the professional student syndrome"). Many Americans also have not learned how to relax and enjoy life, as seen by their anxious preoccupation with activity and productiveness and the enormous numbers of persons suffering from stress-related illnesses. Another behavioral consequence of our achievement value is its effects on individuals who do not have the required position and role adequacy for productiveness. For those persons, the emphasis on achievement often leads to a lack of goals and norms and to alienation.

In order for a value to continue to mold a person's goals and behavior, a powerful system of social sanctions and rewards must be present. According to McKinley, there are four major rewards available to the "successful," which are referred to as the "American Dream": material possessions, interpersonal approval and status, control over others, and control over self (autonomy).[28]

Interpersonal approval and status is seen when individuals and society's institutions—such as the workplace, family, and school—convey positive feelings toward a person's accomplishments. Coupled with the positive reinforcement individuals receive is the expectation that they will maintain acceptable goals and accomplishments. Those persons who withdraw from their ambitions or do not reach their potential are admonished "not to give up." The American manifesto is clear: one must not quit, must not cease striving, must not lessen his goals, for not failure, but low aim, is a crime.[29]

Various types of interpersonal sanctions are employed against those individuals who are "unproductive," including the unemployed, those on welfare, or those who choose values markedly different from society's values. These responses range from gossip, laughter, and ridicule to social ostracism, isolation, or rejection. Members of society will vary their reactions depending on the society's evaluations of where the responsibility for unproductiveness lies and how important the deviation is. As a result of society's disapproval, many times the individual adopts those same attitudes toward him- or herself generally (i.e., low self-esteem, lack of self-worth), a phenomenon referred to as "self-fulfilling prophesy."

Two other rewards of being productive involve having power and authority over others and having control over self. These rewards involve autonomy and personal freedom—important values in themselves. McKinley sees the latter reward, control over one's own life, as probably the most important reward a society can offer its compliant members. This reward is often felt to be more satisfying and meaningful to an individual than the actual salary or remuneration received on a job.[30]

Work Ethic

The rule of "He who does not work should not eat" expressed the deadly struggle of the early settlement and frontier days and explains the primacy of this ethic as due to the objective conditions of want that existed historically. As part of Puritanism and the Protestant ethic, however, work literally became an end in itself—not the means to an end. Americans were obsessive about work, and even today we meet individuals who are "work-aholics." However, the importance of this value, along with several others, is considerably attenuated, as previously mentioned. Although the work ethic has lost much of its potency, it is still part of our dominant culture and upheld by our societal institutions, and the success of modern industrial states remains dependent on work-oriented indi-

viduals. In surveying youth from 1968 through 1973, Yankelovitch reports a slow resurgence in the value of work among college-aged students. "In 1973 most college students go to college for very pragmatic, work-oriented reasons."[31] And in spite of the lack of sufficient meaning associated with work for so many persons, the work ethic is sufficiently established so as to stifle many individuals in their enjoyment of leisure-time activities and relaxation. "Working at play becomes the norm."[32, 33]

Schools have been very aware of the declining interest in work, self-discipline, and learning the prerequisite skills. To counteract this trend, the Department of Health, Education, and Welfare recently advocated the inclusion of work-ethic content into educational curricula. Community and government concern about this area is seen in the recent local and Federal funding to plan and implement "Push for Excellence Programs," the purpose being to encourage restoration of work ethic and achievement in students. This program involves parents, schools, and community leaders as resources to motivate students. The approach of Reverend Jesse Jackson, the project's director, includes asking students to pledge to do two hours of homework a night with no distractions and asking parents to make sure they do it. Teachers are asked to assign sufficient homework and notify parents when a student misses two or more days of class.

Materialism

The possession of money and goods is not only an essential reward for being productive, but is also a central value of society in and of itself. This value is referred to as materialism. Money and wealth are both the foundation for power and prestige and the primary symbol of success and achievement. Money has been consecrated as a value over and above its use in procuring goods and services or for the enhancement of power. Merton underscores the centrality of this value:

> To say that the goal of monetary success is entrenched in American culture is only to say that the Americans are bombarded on every side by precepts which affirm . . . the duty of retaining the goal even in the face of repeated frustration.[34]

Society, through its major institutions, reinforces this cultural emphasis except perhaps among the lower class. These institutions join to provide the disciplining and training required for an individual to retain this illusive goal and at the same time be properly motivated by the promise of gratification.

Along with materialism has come a relaxation of prohibitions against expressiveness and hedonism. In a society in which the consumption of goods has become a fundamental issue, people are required to cease being ascetic and self-denying and to abandon guilt about spending and expressing their pleasure impulses.

Individualism

Individualism, intricately related to productivity and materialism as another prerequisite to success, is derived from Puritanism and Protestantism. It is a reversal of the traditional Catholic doctrine or ethic of reciprocity in which "you are your brother's keeper." Individualism suggests that an individual is not his "brother's keeper," but rather that every person has to make it on his or her own merits. Whereas in the traditional Catholic culture, the extended family is expected to assist a needy cousin or adult brother, the WASP family today would meet such a situation with questions, only responding under "justifiable" circumstances.

Individualism also involves the associated values of self-reliance and self-responsibility. Starr points out that today young people still tend to interpret failure in personal terms. The prevalent belief remains that a "strong" person can control his or her own life and that lack of such control is evidence of their own weakness.[35]

In summary, productivity, achievement, success, work, individualism, and materialism are all interrelated values—reinforcing and strengthening each other. Together they form the central cluster of the dominant culture's value orientation.

Education

Education is seen by the middle class as the means by which to achieve productivity, and the value placed on education is therefore closely aligned with the work ethic, materialism, individualism, and progress. Although education is much more emphasized among the middle and upper classes, its value has also become much more prominent within the working class.[36]

Consumption Ethic

The moral values of thriftiness and saving were parts of the Protestant ethic. As with other traditional values, their importance arose partly from the short supply of material goods and money that existed in the past. In fact, often the ability to save and conserve was critical to survival. In other words, there was a much narrower "margin of safety" between "making it" and "going under," and every saved resource might make the difference.

In more recent times Americans seem to have entirely disregarded these values (except perhaps by members of the older generation) as evidenced by our wasteful habits of acquiring vast goods and constantly replacing material items. Toffler calls this "planned obsolescence."[37] We have acted as if there were a limitless supply of goods and resources. This consumption ethic has now largely replaced the thrift ethic, and the "put-away" society has become the "throw-away" society.[38]

We may now be seeing a slight swing back to "conservation" goals, however. There is a noticeable attitudinal change, among some Americans at least, that our habits of waste and enormous consumption of the world's resources must be altered. More concern is voiced about ecology, dwindling resources, and environmental impact. In 1974 Yankelovitch reported that financial security was one of the priority values of Americans, and since saving is inherent in financial security, the value of thrift has not been entirely lost (see Fig. 12.1). In spite of these encouraging signs, Americans continue to consume goods and resources at increasingly high levels.

PROGRESS AND MASTERY OVER ONE'S ENVIRONMENT

Kluckholm refers to this area of concern as the "man–nature relationship," i.e., whether man is viewed as subjugated to nature, as part of nature, or as lord over nature. Traditional Spanish-American culture in the American Southwest illustrates the first relationship. To the average rancher in the Southwest, there is little or nothing which can be done if a storm damages his range lands or disease destroys his flocks. He simply accepts these events as inevitable. This fatalistic attitude may also be found in dealing with illness and death in a statement such as, "If it is the Lord's will that I die, I shall die."[39] The second relationship, in which man and nature are viewed as aspects of a harmonious whole, is found in many of the North American Indian tribes and traditional Chinese cultures. The dominant American culture, however, views this relationship in the third way—that of man against, or over, nature. Natural forces are seen as things to be overcome, mastered, and utilized by man. We build bridges, blast through mountains, create lakes and massive dams, and exploit all of nature's resources—all to serve mankind.[40]

It is this general attitude of being able to problem solve and overcome seemingly impossible obstacles which here is referred to as progressiveness. Change is seen as progress or going forward, even though it sometimes seems the pendulum swings backward. The opposite of "progress" is "tradition" to many Americans. Inkeles reports that in recent surveys, innovativeness and openness to new experiences is still very marked, coupled with an optimism or the confidence that striving and change are positive.[41]

Future Time Orientation

Obviously all societies must deal with three time dimensions—past, present, and future. All cultures have some conception of the past, all have a present, and all give attention to the future time dimension. They vary, however, in the emphasis they place on each dimension. For example, Kluckholm[42] and Murillo[43] report that in contrast to Americans, Mexican-Americans are more present oriented. Historically, China and Japan, on the other hand, were societies which put their main emphasis on the past. Ancestor worship and strong family traditions were both expressions of this time orientation. Many modern European countries, such as England, have also tended to stress the past much more than America.

Americans place their emphasis on the future—which we anticipate optimistically will be "bigger and better." Past ways are considered "old fashioned," and we are seldom content with the present. With the trend toward hedonism there is also a greater emphasis on the present and meeting of short-term gratification. The value put on the future correlates closely with the value on change and progress. A Frenchman, Servan-Schreiber, wrote, "We Europeans continue to suffer progress while Americans pursue it, welcome it and adapt to it."[44]

Efficiency, Orderliness, and Practicality

In frontier society, being practical—learning to improvise and make the best out of one's resources—was tied up with survival. Individuals and families concentrated on obtainable goals in the immediate situation—"If it works, it must be good." Today, this same kind of pragmatism views technical advances with great appreciation, especially those resulting in savings of time and manpower—after all, "time is money." Science is highly valued as an endeavor through which efficiency, practicality, and progress can be achieved.

Rationality

In order to be efficient, orderly, progressive, productive, and practical, one must be rational and able to react by problem-solving and logically thinking through one's situation and goals. Foresight, deliberate planning, allocation of resources in the most efficient way, and long-term gratification are involved. Rationality became a prime value during the Enlightenment in the late 1700s and early 1800s, and science was a natural outgrowth of its rational philosophy, since it depends on the same logical cognitive approach to the

world and its problems. Applied science is highly esteemed in the dominant culture as a tool for controlling nature and the environment.

This value has led to the "rational scientific man" becoming the exemplar of our society. Women, in contrast, have historically been stereotyped with the opposite of these desirable attributes, i.e., women have been deemed irrational, illogical, and emotional, albeit this stereotyping is losing its potency as women move into cognitively challenging fields and succeed admirably.

Cleanliness

Another highly prized value among the Puritans was cleanliness, which remains something of a fetish with many Americans and especially those involved with health care. Culturally this value has great moral implications, hence the saying, "Cleanliness is next to Godliness." It is important for nurses to understand this value, since we often devalue both hospitalized patients and clients/families in clinics and homes for their "unkempt," dirty appearance or that of their homes. The distinction needs to be clearly made between characteristics that are deleterious to health and those that are offensive due to our biases.

One can judge the strength of a value by the interpersonal and legal sanctions a society imposes for those who "break the unwritten rules." Note the abhorrence and revulsion the middle-class displayed for the "hippies," and youth generally, during the 1960s because of their unacceptable appearance and personal hygiene, or the negative reactions and often compromised services health workers provide to clients who do not display a clean, neat appearance.

Democracy, Equality, and Freedom

These three values describe America's ideal, but only partially real values. What one says and what one does are sometimes very much in opposition with each other! Thus our aspirations bespeak these values—and to an extent our society has fashioned itself on these ideals—at least for the middle-class WASP male.

The United States has been known as "the land of opportunity," and in comparison to the countries of the Third World and the communist bloc, it may still be. This is important to understand since we care for many immigrants who see America very much from this perspective, despite the fact that few other value complexes are more subject to strain in modern times.

The dominant culture does value equality in personal relationships much more than many other societies, and antiauthoritarianism is still a very important characteristic of the present-day American.[45] Flacks found that children in today's society are dissatisfied about the use of arbitrary or coercive power, feelings that are derived from the family values favoring a power structure based on egalitarianism, as well as expectations resulting from parental fostering of participation, independence, and autonomy.[46] On the other hand, there exists a strong hierarchal and authoritarian emphasis in large-scale organizations. And running through the whole of our society is the thread of nonequalitarian beliefs and practices concerning interpersonal relations with persons of different ethnic groupings and women, which is to say, prejudice and bigotry.

Americans emphasize freedom of speech, a multiparty representative political system, "private enterprise," and freedom to change employment and residence. These values stem from a basic conception of the person as a relatively autonomous and morally responsible individual. Individualism is equated with the right of persons to use their property as they see fit within very broad limits and to compete freely with others. Competitiveness is exalted above cooperation.

Voluntarism

The value of participating in voluntary community activities is a singularly American one that has persisted for two centuries. Middle-class Americans are joiners.[47] A case in point is this country's huge number of voluntary health and welfare organizations, many of which have existed for over a hundred years and have had a major impact for the betterment of our country. Because of the value of voluntarism, many diverse, important community health resources are available to families, resources such as the American Heart Association, the American Cancer Society, and the multitude of self-help groups.

The "Doing" Orientation

Kluckholm refers to the normative interpersonal behavior valued in American society, or its national character, as being exemplified in the "doing orientation." Its most distinctive feature is its demand for action in terms of accomplishment and in accord with external (societal) standards. Again, the person who "gets things done" is productive or finds ways to do something, and the rational problem solver is much esteemed.[48]

MAJOR VARIABLES AFFECTING FAMILY'S VALUE SYSTEM

There are several important variables or factors which greatly influence whether a family assimilates the "major value orientation" of American society, or

whether differences in priorities and values or divergent norms continue to operate. The most important variable is social class, which will be elaborated on below. In addition, a family's ethnicity or cultural heritage, including religious background; degree of acculturation to the dominant culture; whether a family resides (or has resided for a long period of time) in a rural, urban, or suburban community; the life cycle phase and age of the family members; and the family and personal idiosyncrasies are other important variables. The chapter on ethnic differences explores the effects of ethnicity and acculturation.

Religious value differences, some effects of which have been mentioned previously, are certainly important. Geographic factors also play a significant role. In terms of country versus city residence, rural dwellers tend to be more traditional and conservative than their urban or suburban counterparts. Suburban communities are primarily residential and middle-class, and usually espouse WASP cultural values. In contrast, urban, inner-city populations are diverse, generally containing families from the whole social class spectrum, as well as families from various ethnic/racial groups; thus urban families usually show a greater diversity of values, although generally tending to hold more liberal social and political views.

Another variable influencing the values and norms of a family is the life cycle of the family and age of its members. As we know, certain values were predominant when persons were in their early adulthood years in, say, the 1930s. These individuals are now most likely in the phase of retirement/death or the contracting family phase, and they retain many of their traditional work-oriented Protestant ethic values (values which have more potency in their lives than for younger adults). Slater illustrates the drastic differences in values when he compares the values of the "youth generation" with the old values of the dominant culture.[49]

Value Conflicts

Because there are so many factors which serve to alter an individual's or a family's values and norms, conflicts inevitably exist. Issues or unresolved conflicts are present because the traditional and emerging sets of norms exist simultaneously, both within and outside of the family. Within communities certain groups and individuals resist the emerging norms and cling vehemently to the more traditional patterns, whereas other individuals and groups find the traditional patterns unacceptable and adhere to the new set of norms and values. The result of this social change is that areas of major conflict arise. Although our society values its pluralism, where both traditional and emerging family value systems and patterns can exist side by side, this social diversity also results in conflict and confusion in the family system. A very common family value issue is that concerning the meaning of marriage. Whereas traditionally marriage was viewed as sacred and binding, today it is increasingly viewed as a contract to be voided when either or both parties have legitimate grievances.[50]

Another common source of value conflict is a clash between the values of the dominant culture and a family's cultural reference group. Larrabee, a Cheyenne Indian, describes this clash of values and one of its effects:

> The value systems of any group lie in the cultural differences; the assessments of what is and what ought to be determine the actions of the group. In trying to teach our young about themselves, we must tell them about the Indian values of compassion, respect for elders, sharing, and wisdom. We want our children to have these values and to know about them. When our children go to school and are told by the teacher that they must learn to be saving instead of sharing, the child becomes confused. This terrible conflict of values contributes to the high suicide rate among our youth.[51]

When we consider the family as the mediating agent between the culture (or the wider society) and the individual, it follows that a basic incompatibility in values between the family and wider society generates certain value conflicts which increase stress within the family as a system and also negatively affect family members. Cleveland and Longaker examined the impact of cultural factors on the mental health of family members by analyzing the transmission and mediation of values in a family setting. Based on extensive data collected from interviews, home visits, testing, and therapeutic sessions, they concluded that the emotional problems in family members studied were a function of two processes: (1) a value conflict between the society the family resided in and the family and (2) a culturally recurrent mode of self-disparagement linked to the failure of individuals to adjust to incompatible value orientations. These are the findings of only one study, but they aptly demonstrate the potentially disruptive effect that value conflicts may have on families and their members.[52]

A third source of value conflict within families lies in generational differences in values, as mentioned previously. A family may be composed of several generations of individuals, each bringing to the family group his or her generationally based values.

Social Class Value Differences

A family's social class is probably the prime molder of its value system. Social class refers not only to educational level, occupation, and income, but also to the intricate interplay of these variables. Persons with different basic conditions of life and different levels of social order, by virtue of their varied experience and exposure, come to see the world differently, to develop different conceptions of social reality, as well as different aspirations, fears, and values.

Social classes will be defined as aggregates of individuals who occupy broadly similar positions on the scale of prestige.[53] Occupational position, weighted somewhat by education and income, is used as a serviceable index of social class in American society. It has been frequently assumed that the husband's occupational status is the best single index of family ranking. Currently, however, it is being acknowledged that the wife's occupational level and income also have a major impact on the life style and social class of a family.

Six discrete classes have been described by Warner: the upper-upper, lower-upper, upper-middle, lower-middle, upper-lower, and lower-lower.[54] In the American class structure it is the family, not merely the individual, that is ranked. Goode, along with other sociologists, states that the family is the keystone of the stratification system, the social mechanism by which it is maintained.[55]

Presently there is much blurring between the social classes; moreover, within each of the groupings relative to their values and status there is certainly not homogeneity.[56] Other factors are also significant in creating diversity within a social class grouping—religion and ethnicity being two prime examples. But even when all such considerations are accounted for, the evidence clearly shows that being in one group or another has profound effects on life style, values, and behavior.

Earlier in this chapter the extensive discussion of the core values of the dominant culture made the point that the configuration or clustering of values was representative of WASP culture and the middle-class in general. One of the important corollaries to this premise is that when a family and its reference group subscribes to the central core values of a society, adjustment to society is relatively easy. In contrast, the greater the distance from this core value system, the more difficult family adjustment to community life becomes and the greater social stigma it experiences.

Using Warner's schematization of social class in America, the subsequent section of this chapter will briefly describe some characteristics of each of the six social classes, with an emphasis on value differences. Again, these classes are not precise explanations of reality, but are constructs designed to show the patterned relationships and life style differences.

Upper-Class Families

Upper-class families, according to Warner, are divided into two groupings: the established upper-class family (upper-upper) and the "nouveau riche" (lower-upper). Families who have possessed wealth for more than two generations are classified in the established group, while families of more recent affluence are placed in the second group.[57]

The family and its members are closely protected and guarded from social exposures involving other social classes. The upper-upper class is very firmly entrenched in its culture, as well as in an extended family and a patriarchal kinship system. Protestant ethic values are subscribed to, to some extent, but these values do not have to be strictly upheld behaviorally, since professional and occupational security and monetary resources are provided by the family.

The New Lower-Upper Class Family.
The "nouveau riche" lack the financial security provided by the kinship group in the upper-upper class family. Its members are able to engage in a life style resembling that of the established upper class, but they lack the long history of prestige and family lineage.

In contrast with the upper-upper class, the newly affluent families are less likely to inherit their wealth, have a greater cultural diversity, income which is earned rather than inherited, and some differences in values, e.g., spending patterns (being symptomatic of priorities in values) vary between the two upper-class groups. Whereas upper-upper class members spend more in the areas of culture and philanthropy, the lower-upper class spends more on conspicuous goods and products—automobiles, clothes, expensive recreation, and large houses. Since these families are upwardly mobile, they tend to pursue friendships with socially prominent individuals, rather than maintain close ties with their extended family. Thus the predominant family structure is nuclear and husband dominated, and its members act independently of kin.

Middle-Class Families

The middle class is considered *dominant* numerically and in the sense that middle-class people are most able to disseminate their views on what is right, proper, and expected behavior—whether in the family, school, or health agency. This dominance is due primarily to the key positions of the upper middle class in government, education, and mass communications.

The Upper-Middle Class Family.
This class is comprised of a group of substantial businessmen and professionals, who often also serve as leaders in civic affairs.[58] Being the career-oriented bearers of "American success syndrome," most of this class are college graduates and comprise the "solid, highly respectable" people in the community. Individualism and personal achievement and the other secular Protestant ethic values (mastery, future-orientation, work, etc.) are stressed.[59]

The nuclear family of the upper-middle class tends to be one in which the husband has more power than in the lower-middle class family, although he is easily influenced by the other members' opinions and reactions. The roles of husband and wife are differentiated but strongly interlock. It is expected that the husband will be the major producer of a stable and significant income. The home, the children, and social activities of the family rest primarily in the hands of the wife and mother, although there is increasing involvement of the husband in these areas.[60]

The Lower-Middle Class Family.
The lower-middle class is made up of small businessmen, clerical workers, other low-level white-collar workers, and some skilled tradesmen. This class represents a wide variety of national and ethnic backgrounds. Like those in the class above them, the families are relatively stable in spite of problems connected with their economic security and the education of their children. Frequently students report the conflicts that exist between themselves and their parents. The parents work, to provide an education for their children, which in turn introduces the children to a set of values that is often in conflict with those of the parents.

In the lower-middle class family today, the power structure is usually egalitarian or mildly husband dominated. Socially the kinship group is close, and major social activities often take place with relatives from the husband's or wife's family.[61]

Lower-Class Families

The Blue-Collar (Upper-Lower) Family.
The lower class is frequently divided into two groups: the upper-lower class, referred to as the working-class or blue-collar workers, and the lower-lower class. The job of a blue-collar worker generally requires some sort of manual skill. The difference between the two lower-class groups is greater than the difference between lower-middle and upper-lower classes, since the "working class" is often difficult to distinguish from the lower-middle class today. The upper-lower or working class is made up of skilled workers, semiskilled workers in factories, service workers, and a few small tradesmen who usually have steady jobs, even though they often do not pay well. In 1971 these workers constituted 45 percent of employed white persons and 67 percent of employed black workers.[62] The elite of the working class—electricians, plumbers, and other highly skilled operators—frequently earn more than members of the middle classes and are sometimes viewed as part of the lower-middle class group. For members of this class who are in trades dependent on

the swings of the business cycle, economic stability is lacking.

A considerable proportion of wives are employed outside of the home. Unlike a sizable proportion of female workers from the middle and upper classes, the upper-lower class wife takes a job more out of economic necessity than from the desire for a career. Family strains are associated with the uncertainties of many economic facets of life.

It is within the blue-collar family more than any other class that one still sees many husbands and wives conforming to the traditional husband and wife roles. Komarovsky found that the majority of men and women in blue-collar families believe that the woman's place is in the home. Both of the sexes tended to think that friendship and companionship were more likely to exist between members of the same sex, and they saw the principal marital ties as involving the sexual union, complementary tasks, and mutual devotion.

When there is need of assistance, relatives are likely to be called on before turning to a public agency.[63] The extended family, the neighborhood peer group, and the informal work group provide much social interaction for blue-collar families, as well as actual assistance.

The Lower-Lower Class Family. Lower-lower class families are at the impoverished level of existence, although their degree of impoverishment varies. Wide variations also exist in life style, as seen in rural versus urban areas, regional differences, and in ethnic/social lower-class communities. Generally, however, the common social characteristics of the lower-lower class include the following:

1. A formal education of eight years or less.
2. The male's occupation is almost always semi-skilled or unskilled, and his work pattern is often sporadic, with long periods of unemployment. There is also a strong probability that the woman works in unskilled or service occupations.
3. Because of unemployment or underemployment and low wages, lower-lower class families make up a large number of those on the public assistance rolls.
4. Their place of residence is typically in the slum areas of the city, often in old, dilapidated homes and buildings converted into small apartments. The ratio of persons per room is often three or four to one, and frequently as many as 20 people share the use of a single toilet.[64]

About 25.6 million persons, or one-eighth of the population in the United States, were below the low-income or poverty level in 1971, according to the re-

sults of a survey conducted by the Bureau of Census. One-tenth of all white persons were in the low-income category in 1971 as compared to about one-third of blacks.

It is difficult for most students and teachers to describe the life style of the lower-lower class without imposing middle-class evaluations on them. Even the use of the term lower class probably imposes a negative connotation and interpretation to persons who occupy this class level. As stated by Rodman, "It is little wonder that if we describe the lower-class family in terms of promiscuous sexual relationships, illegitimate children, deserting men, and unmarried mothers, we are going to see the situation as disorganized and chock-full of problems."[65] In observing social conditions of lower-class life from a middle-class perspective, we should not become so engrossed in looking at the victims that we fail to understand the reasons for the problems. Perhaps it is more realistic to think of these conditions as consequences of, or in some instances solutions to, other issues faced by lower-class persons as they experience all the social, economic, political, and legal realities of life.[66] Oscar Lewis has termed this class "the culture of poverty," in the belief that the lower-lower social class life style is the direct result of poverty and that this "culture" is not just an American phenomenon, but represents values and patterns that can be found cross-culturally.[67]

In contrast with the upper-lower class, the lower-lower class does not have the respect of the larger community. Its members are likely to be stigmatized and characterized as being lazy, shiftless, and dependent. The source of the stigma is usually the inability or lack of fulfillment of our number one cardinal value—productivity.

The lower-lower class, although having a stable population, is also disproportionately composed of internal migrant groups such as those from the rural South; of certain personally disorganized persons such as the emotionally ill, alcoholics, and drug addicts; of unskilled laborers and unemployable persons on relief; and of low-income single-parent families.

Directly related to the poverty of the lower-lower class is the irregularity of employment, and thus income. Because income is irregular, a considerable amount of insecurity exists in regard to food, clothing, shelter, transportation, and other essentials. Children may be forced or encouraged to contribute to the financial needs of the family, and few remain in school beyond the minimum legal age.

Both stable marriages and legal divorces tend to be luxuries in this class. Toughness is a desirable interpersonal trait. Children are frequently taught to defend themselves physically rather than with mental or psychological tactics. The poor cannot "afford" such values of the middle class as productivity, achievement, work, long-range planning, and so forth. It is interesting to note, however, that the aspirations of parents for their children are very "middle class," despite their inability to provide the ways and means of achieving such goals.

A large portion of the poor are now termed "the American underclass."[68] These are the people who remain more or less permanently at the bottom of the social ladder, completely removed from "the American Dream." Although its members come from all races and live throughout the United States, the underclass is made up primarily of (1) impoverished urban blacks, who still suffer from the heritage of slavery and discrimination; (2) the Hispanics, primarily Chicanos and Puerto Ricans, who have recently immigrated into cities and rural areas (as migrant workers); and (3) Appalachian migrants who live in dilapidated neighborhoods of some cities. This group now amounts to about 3 to 5 percent of America's population.[69]

Their bleak environment nurtures values that are often at radical odds with those of the majority—even the majority of the poor. Thus the underclass minority is disproportionately represented in the nation's juvenile delinquents, social dropouts, drug addicts, and single-parents on welfare, and are "responsible," therefore, for a considerable amount of the adult crime, family disruption, urban decay, and need for social expenditures. The underclass remains a nucleus of psychological and material destitution despite some two decades of civil rights gains and antipoverty programs. Even though this fact is disheartening, the proportion of the nation officially listed as living in poverty has dropped from 22 percent in 1959 to 12 percent in 1977.[70]

Unemployment has also decreased, but the underclass is made up of people who lack the necessary education, skills, discipline, and self-esteem to succeed. Long-term unemployment is certainly a large factor here, coupled with the large numbers of single-parents on welfare. A substantial proportion of the 4.4 million disabled on Aid to the Totally Disabled who receive welfare should also be included.

More jobs and a better education are clearly two pressing needs. In our achievement-oriented society, work is more than a source of income. It is also a source of being productive, which brings self-esteem, status, a point of identification with the system, and a satisfying social environment. Stanford University black Historian Clay Carson comments: "Permanency of jobs, stability in an economic situation, is important. Even if someone is only a janitor, his job still means stability. Those who can get established with a job in an urban environment can pass this stability on to their kids."[71]

People from the underclass subculture within our communities, especially our cities, are in the greatest need of our health and social services. In official health agencies, much of the nurse's effort is necessarily concentrated on the very poor. And, of course, it is only through our understanding and appreciation of some of the major problems and daily realities of the poor that we can even begin to assist these families with the resolution of their health needs.

ASSESSMENT QUESTIONS

An understanding of the prevailing value system of American society and hence the health care system, as well as an appreciation of social class and concomitant life style differences, provides the foundation for the specific observations and areas to consider in completing an assessment of family norms and values.

Values and norms cannot be seen directly, but must be inferred from observations and assessment of family roles, power structure, and communication patterns, since these dimensions are strongly influenced by the underlying values held by family members.

It is suggested that one way of simplifying the assessment of norms and values is for nursing students to make use of a "contrast and compare" method. This involves comparing and contrasting a specific family's values with those of the dominant culture. This enables the assessor to identify various areas which need assessment and to appraise how much conformity to or disparity with the dominant culture exists in the value set of the family under consideration. If an assessor is familiar with the values and norms of a specific ethnic group, then this same comparison process could be applied, using the family's cultural reference group as a basis for comparison. In either case, this process should assist the nurse to accomplish the following:

1. Estimate the extent of compliance and the rewards a family is receiving from their reference group and society in general. (The lack of compliance and rewards will be present if there is moderate or marked value disparity, as well as stigmatization of the family by the community.)
2. Degree of acculturation.
3. Social class identification.
4. Identification of possible health problems, i.e., value conflicts, low value in areas leading or contributing to a lowered level of family wellness.

5. Identification of appropriate community resources.
6. Mutual formulation of goals and approaches to resolve health concerns.

To illustrate this process more concretely, it is suggested that a list of the central values be utilized as a guide for this assessment. Using a list of central values of the dominant culture on one side of the assessment form, the assessor can then discuss a family's particular values in each of these areas.

American Core Values	Family's Values
1. Productivity.	
2. Work ethic.	
3. Materialism.	
4. Individualism.	
5. Education.	
6. Consumption ethic.	
7. Progress and mastery over environment.	

8. Future time orientation.
9. Efficiency, orderliness, and practicality.
10. Rationality.
11. Cleanliness.
12. Democracy, equality, and freedom.
13. Voluntarism.
14. "Doing orientation."
15. Health.

Following this listing, the following questions can be posed:

How important are these identified values to the family?
Are these values consciously or unconsciously held?
Are there any value conflicts evident within the family?
How do these family values affect the health status of the family?

REFERENCES

1. Dougherty MC: A cultural approach to the nurse's role in health planning. In Spradley BE (ed): Contemporary Community Nursing. Boston, Little, Brown, 1975, p 441
2. Clemen S, Will M: Family and Community Health Nursing: A Workbook. Ann Arbor, Mich, University of Michigan, 1977, p 189
3. Parad H, Caplan G: A framework for studying families in crisis. In Parad H (ed): Crisis Intervention. New York, Family Service Association of America, 1965, p 58
4. Brink P (ed): Transcultural Nursing. Englewood Cliffs, NJ, Prentice-Hall, 1976, pp 63–64
5. Kluckholm F: Dominant and variant value orientations. In Brink, op. cit., pp 66–67
6. Murillo N: The Mexican-American family. In Hernandez M et al: The Chicanos. St. Louis, Mosby, 1976, p 17
7. Flacks R: Youth and Social Change. Chicago, Markham, 1971, pp 20–34
8. Ibid.
9. Reich C: The Greening of America. New York, Bantam, 1970
10. Slater P: Culture in collision. Psychology Today, July 1970, pp 31–33, 66–68
11. Inkeles A: Paper presented to American Sociological Association, Washington, DC, September 1977. Los Angeles Times, September 20, 1977, Part 1, pp 1, 10
12. Starr SF: Color the generation very light green. In Eldridge E, Meredith N (eds): Environmental Issues: Family Impact. Minneapolis, Minn, Burgess, 1976, pp 148–151
13. Flacks, op. cit., pp 21–22
14. Inkeles, op. cit., p 10
15. Terkel S: Why should Sammy run anymore? In Eldridge, Meredith, op. cit., pp 132–133
16. Starr, op. cit., p 149
17. Weaver GR: American identity movements: A cross-cultural confrontation. In Eldridge, Meredith, op. cit., p 123
18. Ibid., pp 123–129
19. Boulding E: Familism and the creation of futures. In Eldridge, Meredith, op. cit., p 82
20. Ibid., pp 81–82
21. Toynbee AJ: We must pay for freedom. Women's Home Companion, pp 52–53, 133–136, March 1955. Reported in Duvall EM: Marriage and Family Development. New York, Lippincott, 1976, p 67
22. National Center for Health Statistics: Death rate for United States reaches new low. The Nation's Health, June 1978, p 5
23. Remmers HH: Report of Poll 74: The Purdue Opinion Panel. Lafayette, In, Purdue University, Purdue Research Foundation, 1965
24. Inkeles, op. cit., p 10
25. Yankelovitch, Skelley, and White, Inc: The American Family Report: A Study of the American Family and Money. Minneapolis, Minn, General Mills, Inc., 1975, p 100
26. Ibid.
27. McKinley D: Social Class and Family Life. Glencoe, Ill, Free Press, 1964, Chap 1
28. Ibid.
29. Merton RK: Social Theory and Social Structure. Glencoe, Ill, Free Press, 1957
30. McKinley, op. cit.
31. Yankelovitch D: The New Morality: A Profile of American Youth in the 70s. New York, McGraw-Hill, 1974, pp 60, 87
32. Terkel, op. cit., p 134
33. Orthner DK: Familia ludens: Reinforcing the leisure component in family life. In Eldridge, Meredith, op. cit., p 153
34. McKinley, op. cit., Chap 1
35. Starr, op. cit., pp 148–151
36. Inkeles, op. cit., p 10

37. Toffler A: Future Shock. New York, Random, 1970
38. Inkeles, *op. cit.*, p 10
39. Kluckholm, *op. cit.*, p 69
40. *Ibid.*
41. Inkeles, *op. cit.*, p 10
42. Kluckholm, *op. cit.*, pp 70–71
43. Murillo, *op. cit.*, p 18
44. Inkeles, *op. cit.*, p 10
45. *Ibid.*
46. Flacks, *op. cit.*, pp 20–34
47. Inkeles, *op. cit.*, p 10
48. Kluckholm, *op. cit.*, pp 72–73
49. Slater, *op. cit.*
50. Eshleman JR: The Family: An Introduction. Boston, Allyn & Bacon, 1974, pp 33–34
51. Larrabee E: Comments stimulated by Dr. Ford's research: An ethnic perspective. Community Nursing Research: Collaboration and Completion, Denver, WICHE, 1973
52. Cleveland EJ, Longaker WD: Neurotic patterns in the family. In Handel G (ed): The Psychosocial Interior of the Family, 2nd ed. Chicago, Aldine-Atherton, 1972, pp 159–185
53. Williams RM: American Society: A Sociological Interpretation, 3rd ed. New York, Knopf, 1960, Chap 4
54. Warner WL; American Life. Chicago, University of Chicago, 1953
55. Goode WJ: The Family. Englewood Cliffs, NJ, Prentice-Hall, 1964, p 80
56. Kohn ML: Social class and parent-child relationships: An interpretation. In Coser RL (ed): Life Cycle and Achievement in America. New York, Harper Torchbooks, 1969, p 25
57. Hollingshead AB: Class differences in family stability. Ann Am Academy of Political and Social Science 272, 1950
58. Warner, *op. cit.*, pp 55–56
59. Schulz DA: The Changing Family. Englewood Cliffs, NJ, Prentice-Hall, 1972, pp 120–121
60. Eshleman, *op. cit.*, pp 250–251
61. Schulz, *op. cit.*, p 121
62. U.S. Bureau of Census. Statistical Abstract of the U.S., 93rd ed. Washington, DC, US Government Printing Office, 1972, No. 367, p 231
63. Komarovsky M: Blue-Collar Marriage. New York, Random House, 1962
64. Bell R: Marriage and Family Interaction. Homewood, Ill, Dorsey Press, 1971, p 45
65. Rodman H: Marriage, Family and Society. New York, Random House, 1965, p 223
66. Eshleman, *op. cit.*, p 258
67. Lewis O: Children of Sanchez. New York, Random House, 1961
68. Russell G: The American underclass. Time, August 29, 1977, pp 16–19
69. *Ibid.*, p 18
70. *Ibid.*, pp 16–19
71. *Ibid.*, p 18

STUDY QUESTIONS

Choose the correct answers to the following questions.

1. It is true that:
   a. Values are defined as a system of beliefs and attitudes which bind families together.
   b. Values serve as general guides to behavior.
   c. The family is the basic transmitter of values.
   d. Values are relatively fixed and change very little over time.
   e. All values have the same or similar weight as far as their influence and centrality in a person's life are concerned.

2. The *best* definition of *norms* is:
   a. Patterns of personal behaviors.
   b. Modal behaviors.
   c. Role behaviors or expectations.
   d. Clustering of attitudes and beliefs.

3. When a social class difference exists between a middle-class health worker and a lower-class client, the usual outcome(s) is(are):
   a. An increase in information and communication occurs to clarify messages.
   b. The health worker negatively evaluates or judges client's behavior.
   c. A social distancing in the relationship.
   d. Divergent goals and unclear communication.
   e. Family tries harder to communicate their concerns to health worker.

4. List and briefly explain four major, recent value changes which have occurred in society and within families.

Choose the correct answers to the following questions.

5. In American society, the one dominant and unifying standard or set of values is (select the *best* answer):
   a. Puritan ethic.
   b. Catholic ethic.
   c. Protestant ethic.
   d. WASP culture.
   e. Secularized Protestant ethic.

6. The major component within the value cluster of the dominant culture is:
   a. Religion.
   b. Scarcity and thrift value.
   c. Productivity.
   d. Work ethic.
   e. Consumerism.

7. In today's family there is greater emphasis on family interests and goals, rather than individual interests and activities (answer *True* or *False*).

8. Several values cluster together, comprising the central configuration of values in the dominant culture. List six values.

9. There are four variables which influence the family's value system. List these. Which is most important generally?

Choose the correct answers to the following questions.

10. Which of the following are sources of value conflicts?
    a. Past versus present mores.
    b. Social class differences.
    c. Acculturation differences.
    d. Idiosyncratic (personal) differences.

11. Social class is based generally on three criteria: income, education, and occupational status. Identify which of these is the most important determinant.
    a. Income.
    b. Occupational status.
    c. Educational level.

12. One of the concepts germane to social class is that when a family and its reference group do not subscribe to the central core values of a society:
    a. The adjustment to wider society is relatively easy.
    b. The family is able to gain compliance from society.
    c. The more difficult the family adjustment to community life becomes.
    d. The family experiences social stigma.

13. The primary difference between the "nouveau riche" and the upper-upper class families is:
    a. Wealth.
    b. Spending patterns.

c. Ethnicity.
d. Family background.

14. The upper-middle class highly values (choose the applicable values):
    a. Education.
    b. Productivity.
    c. Materialism.
    d. Community involvement (voluntarism).
    e. Individualism.

15. Lower-middle-class families, in contrast with upper-middle-class families, tend to (choose all correct answers)
    a. Value education highly.
    b. Be more racially and ethnically mixed.
    c. Have closer kinship relations.
    d. Put more emphasis on individualism and productivity values.

16. The blue-collar or working class is often difficult to distinguish from the lower-middle class, especially because there may be little income difference. Nevertheless, the most obvious differences between the two groups are (choose all correct answers):
    a. Wife's employment.
    b. Emphasis on family background.
    c. Spending patterns.
    d. Husband's type of employment—manual to nonmanual labor.
    e. Education.

17. The lower-lower class consists of the poor. In this social class the following characteristics are prevalent (choose all correct answers):
    a. Most often families live in rural or suburban areas.
    b. Men have unskilled jobs (sporadic and underemployed) or are unemployed.
    c. The family may receive welfare.
    d. A larger percentage of whites are poor in comparison with ethnic minorities.

18. The poor's value system is substantially different from the dominant culture values. Identify three examples of these contrasting values.

FAMILY CASE STUDY—THE GARDINERS*

After reading the family case study, answer the questions which follow.

The Gardiner family members are Harry, age 37; May, 28; Len, 11; Joanie, 7; and Ann, 3. The family, black Americans, came to the attention of the public health nurse working in a pediatric outpatient clinic when appointments arranged for Len at the diabetes and urology clinics were repeatedly not kept. Although appointments to the diabetes clinic were kept occasionally, no urology visit was

---

* Family case study adapted from: Sobol EG, Robischon P: Family Nursing: A Study Guide, 2nd ed. St. Louis, Mosby, 1975, pp. 97–100. This compilation of family case studies is designed to cover the range of families and common health problems family-centered nurses face. These case studies are excellent teaching tools.

made, and the chart showed that the mother at one time had reported continual bedwetting.

Len was originally diagnosed as having juvenile diabetes when he was hospitalized at age 6. After the child was diagnosed and stabilized, the family was counseled as to treatment regimen. Subsequent to this time, four hospitalizations occurred because of diabetic crises.

During the nurse's first visit, Mrs. G. appeared very anxious, explaining that she always anticipates "bad news" about Len. In response to inquiries about Len's missed clinic appointments, Mrs. G. seemed indifferent, stating that they have been too busy and that arranging child care for Ann was a problem. On a later visit other factors, more covert, which contribute to the family's reluctance to keep Len's appointments were noted. The mother's statements clarify these factors: "When they told me what was wrong with Len I worried day and night and wouldn't let anyone play with him or take him any place. I was constantly with him. Then I decided I couldn't worry like that anymore. I know he really isn't sick. No one could play as hard as he does and still be sick!" Mrs. G. seemed unwilling to discuss Len's fainting episodes except to say they were Len's way of getting attention. She also refused to discuss his four diabetic crisis hospitalizations.

Data concerning the health status of other family members was also noted. Mrs. G. was of average weight and neatly dressed. She was quite gregarious as long as she could control the conversation. Her knowledge about nutrition and other aspects of family welfare important to her—shelter, cleanliness, adequate child care arrangements, regular school attendance—were satisfactory. Mrs. G. claims good health, although she has not received any preventive care from a physician, with the exception of prenatal care in the past, and even this was obtained late in the pregnancy.

Mr. G. had been in the Army many years ago and since this time has been under the care of a Veterans Administration Hospital. Here he regularly receives tranquilizers and occasional counseling. His wife reported that his physical health is average, stating: "He doesn't get sick or go to the doctor, but he sure is tired all of the time."

Joanie, the seven-year-old, was reported to be in good health, attended school regularly, and was doing all right there. Her mother termed her "a good girl." Ann, the preschooler, was active, friendly, and healthy appearing. Mrs. G. complained of her "overactivity." She explained that Ann was constantly into things and interfered with her efforts to keep the house clean and picked up. Ann's health supervision was irregular and her immunizations incomplete. After well-baby care was completed at one year, health care has been sought only for acute illnesses.

The family's economic situation has been unstable. Mr. G. works irregularly in a factory, while Mrs. G. works off and on at a car washing business. To supplement their insufficient earnings, they receive welfare.

Mrs. G.'s primary expressed concerns had to do with her husband's lack of responsibility for helping with the household and child-care tasks, as well as his overall neglectfulness and his irregular employment. She openly berated her husband in front of him, the nurse, and their children, complaining that he did not bring home enough money for the family to live on and lacks interest in the home, the children, and money matters. Mr. G. sat silently as his wife verbally assaulted him.

There was an impression of little communication or companionship among family members, except in those areas related to the daily activities of living and taking care of the apartment. The children's play was kept at a minimum due to the noise they created. Most communication was in the form of commands, emanating from the mother to the husband and children. The home was viewed as a place to be kept clean and organized, so that everything was put away; the children were expected to be "seen but not heard"; they were to be home exactly on time; attend school regularly; keep themselves and their surroundings clean; and obey and respect their mother. There were no toys or reading materials visible. The only discernible source of recreation for the entire family was the television set, which was on constantly. Family recreational pursuits were practically unheard of. Life was virtually task oriented, and no enjoyable and fun activities were included.

The family lived in a low-income housing project, for which they were charged a minimum rent. Kitchen equipment, food, and clothing storage facilities were adequate as was their furnishings. Although the outside appearance of the housing project was dirty and visually in a state of disrepair, the inside of their apartment was orderly and well maintained.

Both Mr. and Mrs. G. dropped out of high school in the ninth and tenth grades, respectively, in order to start working to help out their parents. No further education or skill training had been received since that time. Relatives did not reside near them, nor were they affiliated with any religious or other community groups.

The community in which the family lived was part of a large inner-city area which was deteriorating rapidly. Transportation and social, health, and welfare facilities were easily accessible. Shopping for food and other necessities was limited to small neighborhood shops in the area, since they did not own a car. The schools and churches were nearby. The mother felt the neighborhood was crime-ridden (which the nurse confirmed), and hence she kept the children indoors most of the time.

19. From the limited information contained in the family case study, what are the salient values operating in this family?
    (Use the assessment process that was suggested in this chapter.)

20. How important are these identified values to the family?

21. Are these values consciously or unconsciously held?

22. Are there any value conflicts evident within the family itself?

STUDY ANSWERS

1. a, b, and c

2. b

3. b, c, and d

4. Four major, recent value changes (any four):
   a. *Work ethic.* A change from seeing work as an end in itself to a means for obtaining other important aspirations. Decline in belief that hard work will pay off and a decline in the intrinsic meaning of work to many individuals.

    b. *Tolerance of diversity.* Studies show that Americans are becoming increasingly tolerant of variation in life styles and also of ethnic differences. Weakening of the myth of the "melting pot."

    c. *Equality.* Egalitarianism in families and in society is increasing. Women's liberation is probably the strongest force in bringing about this change, but other oppressed groups have also sought and are receiving a fairer share of the resources and more consideration of their rights. These groups include children, the mentally ill, and other stigmatized groups.

    d. *Consumerism.* There has been an increased exploitation of resources and a rise in material indulgence involving the discarding and replacement of goods rather than saving.

    e. *Health and quality of life.* The increasing numbers of middle-class Americans engaging in life-style improvements are evidence of this value change.

5. e

6. c

7. False

8. a. Productivity   d. Work ethic.
    b. Materialism.   e. Progress.
    c. Individualism.   f. Education.

9. a. Ethnicity, including religious background.
    b. Social class.
    c. Rural versus urban or suburban (geographical location).
    d. Degree of acculturation to dominant cultural values.
    Most important generally: Social class (b).

10. All (a–d)

11. b (usually of husband)

12. c and d

13. d

14. All (a–e)

15. b and c

16. c, d, and e

17. b and c

18. Any three:
    a. Productivity versus "getting by."
    b. Education versus less value on education.
    c. Mastery over environment versus fatalism, powerlessness against environment.
    d. Future-oriented, long-range planning versus present-oriented, immediate gratification.

19. *American Core Values*
     1. Productivity.

   Gardiner Family Values
     1. Probably aspired to being successful—at least get by and be self-sufficient—but were not able to succeed. (Note wife's frustration and hostility toward husband because of employment problem.)

American Core Values	*Gardiner Family Values*
2. Work ethic.	2. Wife appears to be committed to work ethic at home. Husband is not in conformity with this value.
3. Materialism.	3. Not present (not realistic for family).
4. Individualism.	4. Not evident.
5. Education.	5. Not one of the central values for this family. Note lack of educational pursuits by parents and total lack of books at home.
6. Consumption ethic.	6. Not present (economically unrealistic).
7. Progress and mastery over environment.	7. Progress. Not implied. Mastery over environment not present. (Again powerless position makes this value unrealistic.)
8. Future orientation.	8. Future-time orientation not seen; no planning observed during the time reported.
9. Efficiency, orderliness and practicality.	9. Mrs. G. seemed to place a high value on all these areas.
10. Rationality.	10. Value not seen.
11. Cleanliness.	11. An important value. The home environment, especially, bespoke of the high value that Mrs. G. placed on neatness and cleanliness.
12. Democracy, equality, and freedom.	12. Democratic functioning not observed in home (authoritarian, wife-dominated power structure).
13. Voluntarism.	13. Absent; this type of activity is real luxury for the poor.
14. Doing orientation (national character).	14. Wife appeared to be a very active person at home, but her doing was limited to her mother and housekeeper roles.
15. Health.	15. Health was not seen as an important (prime) value. Preventive care not sought. Child-care services utilized due to the obvious necessity of receiving treatment for acute problems.

20. Practicality, orderliness, cleanliness appear highly valued.

21. Not known.

22. Wife—work oriented; husband—unable to succeed in this area.

It is generally recognized that the family exists so as to fulfill certain basic functions that are necessary for the survival of the species (societal needs), namely, procreation and child rearing. Additionally, it acts as the necessary mediator between the society and the individual and forms the matrix in which personal needs are met. As mentioned previously, the family is more specialized today, and activities that traditionally took place within the home and/or involved the whole family now take place elsewhere and engage only segments or individual family members. For example, the economic activity in which the whole family was traditionally engaged is now the purview of the father, and perhaps also of the mother, and takes place outside of the family. In addition, extrafamilial social organizations and institutions now share in, if they have not actually taken over, many of the traditional functions of the family. However, a number of extremely vital functions remain and of these socialization and affective functions are perhaps the most important. Two other significant functions also remain family responsibilities: the health care function, covered in Chapter 15, and the family coping function, Chapter 16.

IMPORTANCE OF AFFECTIVE FUNCTION

The individual's self-image, his or her sense of belonging, of the meaningfulness of existence, and of sources of love, approval, reward, and support are most frequently derived through primary group (familial) interactions.[1] Fulfillment of the affective function is critical to the healthy development and growth of all family members,[2] and the central basis for both the formation and continuation of the family unit. The family accomplishes this task largely through the meeting of the socioemotional needs of its members, starting with the early years of an individual's life and continuing throughout his or her lifetime. Adams, a family sociologist, describes the family function in this way: "The family has become a specialist in gratifying people's psychological needs—the needs for understanding, affection and happiness."[3]

In attempting to fulfill the role of meeting its members' socioemotional needs, the family assumes a heavy responsibility, especially in view of the fact that families move frequently and often do not have the social support systems needed. Moreover, today's families are generally smaller in number, and thus there are fewer members to share the tasks of meeting each other's needs for companionship, love, and support.

In view then of the increased emphasis on the importance of family relationships, it is not surprising to find a parallel rise in divorce rates. Permissive laws and a concomitant lessening of social stigma, along with other factors such gains made by the women's movement have also facilitated this national trend by making this option more accessible to all sectors of society.

13

The Affective Function

LEARNING OBJECTIVES

1. State three reasons why the affective function is a vital family function.
2. Explain briefly the three components of need-response patterns.
3. Explicate how mutual support and emotional warmth originate and continue in a family as an inherent part of the "spiral phenomenon."
4. Describe the aims of a family in achieving a mutual respect balance.
5. Define concepts of bonding or attachment, response bonds, identification and crescive bonds, and their significance to the family's fulfillment of the affective function.
6. Discuss the prime task of parents in assisting their children to form a stable, sound identity in the area of separateness and connectedness.
7. Compare and contrast the marital therapeutic role with the affective function of the family.
8. Name two underlying values and/or priorities present in energized families related to the affective function area.
9. Utilizing assessment questions pertaining to the family affective function, describe assessment data culled from a family case situation.

It may then be said that those families that do remain together do so more and more because the members want to as a result of enduring affection than because of necessity or coercive social pressures.[4]

The importance of assessing a family's affective function is self-evident. Since the affective function is so vital for both the survival and functioning of the family as a whole and its individual members, assessment and intervention in this area are crucial. Thus if families are having difficulties fulfilling the demands of this function, the problems should be identified and discussed with them. Both health counseling and education are critical strategies to employ in helping families shore up their relationships and better meet each other's needs. This is particularly vital in working with young families with newborns and infants, where parent–infant relationships are so significant in terms of the individuals' and family's future.

COMPONENTS OF THE AFFECTIVE FUNCTION

The affective function involves the family's perception of, respect accorded to, and care of the socioemotional or psychological needs of its members. Through fulfillment of this function, the family serves the major psychosocial purposes of building within its members the qualities of humanness, stabilization of personality and behavior, relatability (ability to relate intimately), and self-esteem.

In meeting this tremendous mental health responsibility, the family provides the following:

1. A social milieu for the generation and maintenance of affectional bonds within family relationships, where one is first loved and given to, and in turn, learns to love and give in return.
2. An opportunity to develop a personal and social identity tied to family identity.
3. An opportunity for individuals to be themselves. The family provides a home base where its members are permitted to express their true feelings and thoughts, e.g., hostility with less fear of consequences, and experience security and love without fear of rejection.

Mutual Nurturance

Fulfilling the affective function first and foremost involves creating and maintaining within the family a system for mutual nurturance. A prerequisite to achieving this is the basic commitment of a couple to each other and a nurturing, emotionally satisfying marital relationship. This becomes the emotional foundation on which the parents can build their supportive structure. The nurturing attitudes and behavior flowing from parents and siblings to younger children will result in a return flow from children to parents as well. Brown views this flow as a spiral phenomenon. As each member receives affection and care from others in the family, his or her capacity to give to other members increases, with the result being mutual support and emotional warmth. The key concepts here are *mutuality* and *reciprocity*. Parents give emotionally to children; this, in turn, is received and fed back to parents and siblings.[5] (The opposite also occurs: rejecting and angry parents breed angry and rejecting responses in their children.) By maintaining this kind of environment in which its members' needs are adequately responded to, the family provides the opportunity for individuals to form and maintain meaningful relationships not only with family members, but with other individuals also.

Hence through the family's fulfilling of the affective function, individuals develop the ability to relate intimately with others. Intimacy is vital in human relationships, since it fulfills the psychological need for emotional closeness with another human being and allows individuals in the relationship to know the full range of each other's uniqueness.[6] A person usually first experiences an intimate relationship with his or her parents, beginning with early mother–infant bonding and continuing to grow and develop during the years which follow in the family of origin. When achieved, this sense of closeness and trusting gives the person the confidence to reach outside the family confines and establish close and emotionally satisfying relationships. As he or she then starts a family, this sense of intimacy and closeness is passed on to the next generation. Conversely, if this early bonding and sense of trust and intimacy does not occur in the family of origin, the individual will not have the confidence and ability to relate intimately with others. Unfortunately this inability is usually passed on to the next generation also, unless some intervening factor such as personal experiences and growth at a later stage in life occurs.[7]

We are reminded by Satir that it is impossible for a family to meet the emotional needs of its members without the presence of functional, clear family communication patterns.[8] Hence such communication becomes the vehicle through which the psychological needs of family members are recognized and responded to.*

Maintaining a nurturing familial environment is often a formidable task, as many stressors tend to dis-

---

* This statement provides a cogent basis for health or welfare professionals working with families to direct their efforts toward helping families shore up and improve their interactional patterns.

rupt family homeostasis and make family members less sensitive and loving toward each other. Brown further explains that when these stressors occur, "the system for mutual nurturance is subject to disruption; once such disruption occurs, there is a strong tendency for interpersonal tension to reverberate throughout the family system and for the disruption to escalate."[9]

When the psychological needs of family members are not being adequately perceived and addressed, the usual consequence is the overt appearance of symptoms in the form of distress signals from one or more family members. These symptoms of family dysfunction include various emotional responses such as anger, anxiety, and depressions; delinquent or acting-out behaviors; and somatic complaints and illness. This dysfunction, in turn, further inhibits clear, functional communication within family relationships, resulting in a downward spiraling process until some positive step is taken to curtail further disorganization and reverse the tailspin.

Parad and Caplan do not believe that the temporary periods of low response to members' needs are necessarily harmful to their mental health. However, persistent, longstanding need frustration is deleterious, and even a temporary inattentiveness to a family member's needs may be harmful if the loss occurs when that individual is particularly vulnerable, such as during a critical phase of his or her development.[10]

Mutual Respect Balance

The literature of parent–child guidance presents a well-respected approach to parenting termed the mutual respect balance.[11] When operationalized it helps family members to fulfill the affective function. The primary thrust in this approach is for families to maintain an atmosphere in which positive self-regard and the rights of parents and child *both* are highly valued. Thus it is acknowledged that each person in the family has his or her own rights as individuals, as well as developmental needs specific to his or her age group. A mutual respect balance can be achieved when each family member respects the rights, needs, and responsibilities of other members.[12]

Maintaining a balance between the rights of individuals in the family means creating an atmosphere in which neither parents nor children are expected to cater to the whims of the other. Parents need to provide sufficient structure and consistent guidelines so that limits are set and understood. Yet enough flexibility must also be built into the family system to allow for the freedom and room to grow and individuate.[13] Mutual nurturance is also made possible when a mutual respect balance exists.

Bonding and Identification

The sustaining force behind the perception and satisfaction of the needs of individuals in the family is *bonding* or *attachment.* Bonding is first initiated in marital relations when a couple discovers their common interests, goals, and values and finds that the relationship validates each of them, carries with it certain tangible benefits (prestige among friends, community privileges, etc.), makes possible the meeting of certain goals which could not be accomplished alone (having children and a home),[14] and provides a mutual enjoyment and comfortableness due to their sustained contact with each other. This kind of attachment develops later between parents and children and between siblings as they continually and positively relate to each other through the process called identification.

Identification is the critical element in bonding, as well as being at the heart of family relationships. Turner explains that in its most uncomplicated definition, identification refers to "an attitude in which a person experiences what happens to another person as if it had happened to himself."[15] In other words, when a family member identifies with another member, he or she experiences the joys and the sorrows of the other as if these experiences were his or her own.

In order for bonding or attachment to occur in family relationships, positive identification must first be present. As the most pervasive aspect of attachment, it may be based on sympathy or libidinal mechanisms or be solely derived from the internalization of the attitudes of the other whom he or she cares for and depends on. Once established, the long-term consequence of identification and bonding is a change in the individual's self-image toward the characteristics of the other person with whom he or she has identified. Through identification, children attempt to imitate the behavior of their parents (the parents with whom they identify become their role models). As the child's identity is thus enhanced by the learning behaviors, attitudes, and values of parents, a bond is formed.[16] Through identification and bonding, parents obtain referent power over their children.

The identification or identity bond depends on positive, giving responses from persons in the relationships. Even an infant gives or rewards mother in its earliest beginnings of their relationship by feeding, snuggling up, letting the mother comfort him or her, and so forth. Thus, for bonding to be effective there must be "support and enhancement of ego's identity through his/her association with alter, . . . Whenever a child shows admiration towards his parent or spontaneously gives affection, the gratification that the parent feels activates a response bond."[17]

One facet of the response bond is the general sensitivity, caring for, and responsiveness of the other member(s) in the relationship. When one's communication is accepted, and appreciation and feelings supported, this leads to a closeness and a desire to continue sharing together. Bonding may also exist because of special needs which one person meets for the other person. For instance, a dominant, controlling person may bond with a submissive type—with both their special needs being satisfied in the relationship.

Duration of close relationships is also a factor to be considered. Even though the bonding between newlyweds is intense, and the relationship between mother and a newborn child profound, loss of the newly-married mate or newborn will generally not be felt as severely as if the relationship had persisted for several years prior to the loss. As family members closely involved with each other continue their relationship, old bonds become intensified and new, stronger bonds emerge; and these stronger bonds unite these individuals together in a unique, sustaining relationship. These attachments are not substitutable—that is, no other person(s) can replace a particular member. Because these enduring bonds are not initially present, and grow through a close, sustained involvement, Turner terms these bonds *crescive bonds*.[18]

Although crescive bonding sounds like a natural phenomenon, it is not inevitable, and in some situations crescive bonds do not develop. Turner discusses two factors that inhibit their growth. First, bonds which are situationally based (based on the existence of certain specific needs or circumstances), such as those bonds which meet certain developmental needs which an individual will possibly outgrow, or task-oriented bonds, are far more vulnerable to weakening and eventual breakage. Second, bonding relationships based on contractual agreements, rather than sacred linkages, are also more vulnerable to dissolution, since contracts involve mutual obligations. In this case, if one partner fails to live up to his or her part of the contract, the contract can become invalid. In sacred linkages, the basis for staying together is felt to be God, family, tradition, and one's duty. The bond of parent–child is still seen in this light today (a case in point: States do not legally permit a parent the right to disown their minor children).[19]

Separateness and Connectedness

One of the central, overriding psychological issues involving family life is the way in which families meet their members' psychological needs, and how this affects the individual's identity and self-esteem. During the early years of socialization, families mold and program a child's behavior, thus forming his or her sense of identity. Minuchin explains further: "Human expe-

riences of identity have two elements—a sense of belonging and a sense of being separate. The laboratory in which these ingredients are mixed and dispensed with is the family, the matrix of identity."[20]

The child's sense of belonging comes from being a part of, or connected to, a specific family—playing the roles of child and sibling. The development of a sense of separateness and individuation occurs as a child participates in roles within the family and in different family events and situations, as well as through involvement in activities outside of the family. As a child grows the parents give him or her more autonomy to develop and to meet his or her own unique needs and interests.[21]

Thus in order to perceive and meet the psychological needs of family members, the family must achieve a satisfactory pattern of *separateness* and *connectedness*. Family members are both connected to and separate from one another. Each family handles the issues of separateness and connectedness in a unique fashion—some families placing much more emphasis on one facet than on the other.

Both conditions are basic and constitutive of family life. The young infant begins the separation process at about 6 months. Through the formative years, he or she forms an identity; but individuation and growth continue throughout his or her lifetime. Nonetheless, connectedness is equally basic, taking a variety of forms:

> Connectedness can range from physical proximity and rudimentary child care, to an intensity of mutual involvement which all but excludes all other interests, . . . In one family intense emotional exchange is sought; the members need to relax defenses and public facade, and they respond freely. In other families such confrontation is threatening, though the wish to feel themselves together in binding ties may be great. A family of this kind may be able to approach its desire only through much formalized action or ritualized action, such as giving gifts.[22]

The family needs to provide opportunities for the mastery of this duality. On the one hand, it must help its members want to be together and to develop and maintain cohesiveness or connectedness. On the other hand, it must gradually provide appropriate amounts of freedom and avenues of expression for members to individuate and become separate individuals.

How much of family life is regulated by power considerations is important to ponder. Parental authority—its scope and the manner of its exercise—is one of the forces shaping the patterns encouraging individuality (separateness) and cohesion (connectedness). Parents differ in how extensively they impose their image on their children. When parents expect children to do all the adapting, there is little room for negotiating, and the chances of promoting individuality are hampered.

Also, families vary in how fast they push their children to separateness and how intensively they encourage connectedness, i.e., how soon they expect their children to grow up and to separate from parents. Some parents encourage babyish, dependent behaviors in their children, while others pressure their children to act more adult at an early age. The pace set for their children's growing up is based on the parents' aims for themselves and their children. For example, if both parents are working and see dependency as a burden and frustrating to their goals, they will push their children at a faster pace to become self-sufficient and independent. As in other dimensions of family life, parental ideas about child growth and development and the acceptability of various behaviors are influenced by the family's culture and social class background.[23]

Need-Response Patterns

Parad and Caplan discuss the assessment of the *need–response patterns* in families. This concept is essentially synonymous with that of the family affective function. Mutual nurturance, respect, bonding, and separateness–connectedness aspects emerge as vital prerequisites or necessary corequisites to satisfactory need–response patterns in families. Parad and Caplan point out that family members' socioemotional needs include:

1. love for one's own sake;
2. a balance between support and independence with respect to tasks;
3. a balance between freedom and control with respect to instinctual expression; and
4. the availability of suitable role models.[24]

Three separate and interlocking phases are inherent in a family's affective response to these needs. First, family members must perceive the needs of the other individuals, within the constraints of the family's culture. Next, these needs must be viewed with respect and seen to be worthy of attention (as discussed under mutual respect balance). And lastly, these recognized and respected needs must be satisfied to the extent possible in light of family resources. It is especially propitious if family members each have confidants within the family with whom they can unburden themselves. This triad of perception, respect, and satisfacton of family members' needs is very much influenced by our sociocultural perspectives which view individuals as separate persons, meritorious of recognition and respect in

their own right, as well as a fair share in the family's resources.[25]

In working with families it has observed that the family's sensitivity to, and thus perception of the individual member's actions and needs, varies greatly. Most families usually fall somewhere between being extremely sensitive, and thus responsive to an individual member's input, and being extremely insensitive and unresponsive to individual members' inputs.

The extent to which basic psychological or socioemotional needs are met also varies depending on the family's social support system. Some families have a greater, more involved social network from which to draw support. In these families the meeting of family members' psychosocial needs can be accomplished by individuals both inside and outside of the family. In contrast, families which are truly isolated from social support systems—closed families—have limited outside resources and hence depend primarily, or solely, on family members to meet all their psychological needs. Naturally, this imposes a great burden on family relationships, since probably no one person, such as a mate, can meet all of the other person's needs. In fact, the advocates of alternative life styles and experimental family forms say that this is one of the serious weaknesses in the traditional nuclear family, i.e., that one's mate and children are unable to fulfill all of an individual's needs and that the nuclear family is too closed off and isolated from other necessary social support systems.[26]

The Therapeutic Role

In Chapter 11 the therapeutic role of spouses was discussed as one of the emergent roles increasingly expected of mates entering into marital and family life from all social classes—not just the middle class. This role is quite similar to the mates' role in meeting the affective needs of their mates. Hence there is a close relationship between the affective function and the spousal therapeutic role. While the affective function describes the broad mental health function of the family—as a group designed to meet the psychological needs of its members—the therapeutic role describes an important socioemotional role within the marital subsystem. This role has been explained by Nye: "The behavior . . . is therapeutic in assisting the spouse to cope with and, hopefully, dispose of a problem with which he is confronted."[27] When this role is extended to include the rest of the family, children and adults alike, some very important elements of family behavior come to light. Nye continues: "Listening and giving the family member an opportunity to verbalize, acting as a 'sounding board' for the ideas or reactions of the other, supplying additional information, concepts, or insights, and taking concrete actions in sharing the solution of the problem are all involved."[28] Some of these behaviors, of course, would not be appropriate (therapeutic) in relating to a young child or infant, but with older children, much of the same therapeutic, assistive relating can occur.

Primarily, the therapeutic role which spouses play is problem oriented. It involves listening to the problem, sympathizing, giving reassurance and affection, and offering help in solving the problem. In Nye's study of spousal roles, he reported that over 60 percent of both husbands and wives indicated that mates have the duty to enact this role, the remainder indicating the desirability of this role in marriage. Moreover, Nye found that 63 percent of wives usually engage in this role. More women than men enacted this role well, and also valued it highly.[29]

THE AFFECTIVE FUNCTION IN ENERGIZED FAMILIES

It is important to know how healthy, functional, or, as Pratt calls them, "energized" families achieve their affective function, since this will give us an optimal standard to use for comparative purposes.

A feature of energized family structure . . . is the tendency to provide autonomy and to be responsive to the particular interests and needs of individual family members. . . . This includes the tendency not only to accept, but to prize individuality and uniqueness, and to tolerate disagreement and deviance. Respect and acceptance are given unconditionally, without continuous comparison of the person to others or to prescribed standards. . . . The family members are encouraged in their various endeavors, especially in seeking new areas of growth and in developing their creativity, imagination, and independent thinking.[30]

ASSESSMENT QUESTIONS

The following questions have been included to assist the assessor in appraising the affective function.

FAMILY NEED-RESPONSE PATTERNS

1. Do family members perceive the needs of the other individuals in the family? Are the parents and spouses able to describe their children's and mate's needs and concerns? How sensitive are family members in picking up cues regarding other's feelings and needs? Do family members each have someone they can go to, within the family, to unburden themselves, i.e., a confidant?
2. Are each member's needs, interests, and differentness respected by the other family members? Does a mutual respect balance exist? Do they show mutual respect toward each other? How sensitive is the family to each individual's actions and concerns?
3. Are the recongized needs of family members being met by the family, and if so, to what extent?

For questions 1 through 3 it is suggested that a list of the family members be included with their needs identified (as perceived by family members) and the extent to which these needs are being met.

MUTUAL NURTURANCE, CLOSENESS, AND IDENTIFICATION

4. To what extent do family members provide mutual nurturance to each other? How supportive of each other are they?
5. Is a sense of closeness and intimacy present among the sets of relationships within the family? How well do family members get along with each other? Do they show affection toward each other?
6. Does mutual identification, bonding, or attachment appear to be present? Empathetic statements, concerns about others' feelings, experiences, and hardships are all indications of this being present.

SEPARATENESS AND CONNECTEDNESS

7. How does the family deal with the issues of separateness and connectedness? How does the family help its members want to be together and maintain cohesiveness (connectedness)? Are opportunities for developing separateness stressed adequately and are they appropraite for the age and needs of each of the family members?

REFERENCES

1. MacElveen PM: Social networks. In Longo DC, Williams RA (eds): Clinical Practice in Psychosocial Nursing: Assessment and Intervention. New York, Appleton, 1978, p 319
2. Satir V: Peoplemaking. Palo Alto, California, Science and Behavior Books, 1972
3. Adams BN: The American Family. Chicago, Markham, 1971, p 92
4. Ibid., p 92
5. Brown SL: Functions, tasks, and stresses of parenting: Implications for guidance. In Arnold LE (ed): Helping Parents Help Their Children. New York, Brunner/Mazel, 1978, p 25
6. Andrews E: The Emotionally Disturbed Family. New York, Aronson, 1974
7. Paul W, Paul B: A Marital Puzzle. New York, Norton, 1975
8. Satir, op. cit.
9. Brown, op. cit., p 25
10. Parad HJ, Caplan G: A framework for studying families in crisis. In Parad HJ: Crisis Intervention: Selected Readings. New York, Family Service Association of America, 1965, p 61
11. Colley KD: Growing up together: The mutual respect balance. In Arnold LE (ed): Helping Parents Help Their Children. New York, Brunner/Mazel, 1978, p 46
12. Ibid.
13. Ibid., p 47
14. Turner RH: Family Interaction. New York, Wiley, 1970, pp 51–55
15. Ibid., p 66
16. Ibid., pp 65–66
17. Ibid., p 72
18. Ibid., p 80
19. Ibid., pp 89–92
20. Minuchin S: Families and Family Therapy. Cambridge, Mass, Harvard University Press, 1974, p 47
21. Ibid., pp 47–48
22. Handel G: The Psychosocial Interior of the Family, 2nd ed. Chicago, Aldine Atherton, 1972, p 13
23. Ibid., p 16
24. Parad, Caplan, op. cit., p 60
25. Ibid., p 60
26. Lantz JE: Family and Marital Therapy: A Transactional Approach. New York, Appleton, 1978, p 3
27. Nye FI: The therapeutic role. In Nye FI (ed): Role Structure and Analysis of the Family. Beverly Hills, Calif, Sage, 1976, p 111
28. Ibid., p 115
29. Ibid., pp 121–129
30. Pratt L: Family Structure and Effective Health Behavior. Boston, Houghton Mifflin, 1976, pp 84–85

STUDY QUESTIONS

1. Give three reasons why the affective function is so important.

2. In order for families to adequately function in the need–response pattern area, the family members would need to demonstrate (name the three components in sequence):

Choose the correct answers to the following questions.

3. The spiral phenomenon relative to the generation and continuance of emotional support and warmth among family members can be explained as (select the best answer):
   a. Hate begets hate; love begets love.
   b. I'm okay, you're okay principle.
   c. Self-fulfilling prophesy.
   d. Marital role modeling, plus mutual nurturance.

4. The results and goals of achieving a balance in familial mutual respect are (select appropriate answers):
   a. Members of the family do not encroach on the rights of the other individuals in the family.
   b. No family members are expected to cater to the whims of other family members.
   c. Parents treat children as persons, not "inferiors" (objects to be manipulated and dominated).

d. Children do not develop "brat" syndrome, where they seek and receive gratification for their needs, but consider the needs, rights, and responsibilities of parents.

5. Match the four terms and/or concepts in right-hand column with definitions and descriptions in left-hand column.

Definitions/Descriptions	*Terms/Concepts*
a. Responsiveness of other member(s) to a family's positive feelings toward them.	1. Bonding or attachment.
b. Empathy or role taking.	2. Identification.
c. Sustaining force behind perception and satisfaction of family members' needs.	3. Crescive bonds.
d. Develops in familial relationships where there is continuity and positive interaction.	4. A response bond.
e. Grows in intensity with time.	
f. Identification precedes it.	
g. Parents obtain referent power when this is present.	
h. Receiver's reaction to sender's affection and warmth.	

6. Answer briefly: What is the parental task relative to dealing with connectedness and separateness?

7. The spousal therapeutic role differs from the family affective function in that (select all appropriate answers):
   a. They do not differ; both are synonymous terms.
   b. The spousal therapeutic role deals in a subsystem rather than entire family system.
   c. The therapeutic role is largely problem focused, whereas the affective function covers therapeutic aspects and other supportive and nurturing elements.
   d. The family affective function deals only with being sensitive to family members' feelings, while the therapeutic role suggests more skilled assistance.

8. Pratt describes energized families and how they can achieve their affective function. From her description, list two salient values or priorities which energized families display relative to this area.

FAMILY CASE STUDY

A family case study is presented with the study questions of Chapter 16. From this family study, answer the following questions concerning the assessment of the family's affective functioning.

9. To what extent do family members perceive and meet the needs of other family members?

10. Does a mutual respect balance exist, where each member shows respect for the other's feelings and needs?

11. To what extent do family members provide mutual nurturance to each other? How supportive of each other are they?

12. Is a sense of closeness and intimacy present among the sets of relationships within the family? How compatible and affectionate are family members toward each other?

14. Does mutual identification and bonding appear to be present?

15. How does the family deal with the issues of separateness and connectedness?

STUDY ANSWERS

1. a. Provides matrix necessary for individuals to grow and develop into healthy, functional, satisfied persons.
   b. This function is central to the formation and continuity of the family unit (without this function being met, the basis for continuing as a family would become tenuous).
   c. No other societal system (institution) is sufficiently involved in fulfilling this task.
   or
   d. Through fulfillment of this function, the family teaches growing individuals how to relate warmly and closely to others.

2. a. Perception of family members' needs.
   b. Mutual respect for needs and concerns of family members.
   c. Meeting of individual's needs in family.

3. c

4. All (a–d)

5. a. 4   e. 3
   b. 2   f. 1
   c. 1   g. 1 and 2
   d. 1, 2, and 3   h. 4

6. The parental task relative to connectedness and separateness is to (1) provide opportunities for family and children to be together, (2) have a sense of belonging and familial cohesiveness, and (3) identification so that the children will want to continue to be together and relate as a family. Concomitantly, the parents must provide opportunities for child to progressively have the freedom and autonomy to individuate, become self-directed, competent, and independent outside the family. The family, via parents, must achieve a satis-

factory pattern of separateness and connectedness, with both being present and properly emphasized.

7. b and c

8. Values or priorities (any two):
   a. They are responsive to particular interests and needs of individual family members.
   b. They prize individuality and uniqueness.
   c. They give respect and acceptance to members unconditionally.
   d. Members are encouraged to be independent, creative, and innovative.
   e. Family emphasizes separateness more than most families do.

FAMILY STUDY

Affective Area:
9. To what extent do family members perceive and meet needs of other family members? This involves an analysis of need–response patterns of family.

Family Member	Perceived Need by Parents	Extent Being Met
John (father)	Did not discuss in the vignette.	From study, no evidence that his socioemotional needs are being met; behavioral evidence is that family is not meeting his needs (avoidance behaviors—staying away and drinking excessively).
Ruby (mother)	No family recognition of her feelings of loss and depression or needs (to be able to be good parent) evidenced.	No data implying that family is meeting her needs; in fact, there is evidence that her emotional needs are not being met (physical illness, depression, and suicidal thoughts). Priscilla, her former confidant, is focused on her own needs and is unable to meet Ruby's relational needs.
Priscilla (age 13)	Parents recognize her needs to take on mother role and to be independent.	Since Ruby feels threatened by Priscilla's successful management of the younger siblings while she was gone, she is not able to positively reinforce her parenting efforts now. Neither parent encourages and/or facilitates Priscilla's separating efforts (becoming less involved with the family and more involved with her peer group).
Cindy (age 10)	None expressed.	Obviously, she likes being industrious and involved in projects and social activities outside of the home, which she is able to do. Family is not meeting this need, and behavior, especially staying away from the home for long periods of time, may be because of the family's inability to meet her socioemotional needs. Priscilla does serve as Cindy's confidant, which provides a vehicle for meeting some of her emotional needs.

Family Member	Perceived Need by Parents	Extent Being Met
John Jr. (age 6)	Only need expressed was that Ann's leaving might threaten younger children and make them feel that if they misbehave, they may be taken away from family.	No evidence that John's socioemotional needs are being met; in fact, there is behavioral evidence (school phobia, clinging to mother, poor school work) that his needs are not being attended to adequately.
Lisa (age 4)	Parents are aware of her problem with separation anxiety and the threatening effect Ann's loss may have.	Both parents evidently spend more time with Lisa, or are planning to give her more attention. She presently has behavioral manifestations of unmet needs; clingingness, frightened when mother leaves, and enuresis, but seems to be the child that is attended to affectively by the parents.

10. *Mutual respect existent?*

There is no direct evidence concerning whether mutual respect exists, but one can infer that there is substantial insensitivity and thus very limited respect accorded to each other's needs, since there is so little perception or recognition of individual needs in the family.

11. *Mutual nurturance provided?*

Again, seems to be limited. It was twice noted that the family did not share their feelings with each other in the face of present difficulties (this is a primary means of emotional support). Lisa seems to be comforted and nurtured more by the parents than the other family members are. Priscilla also provides nurturance to Cindy.

12. *Closeness and intimacy present among family members?*

There appear to be only three sets of relationships in the family that show these traits: between Cindy and Priscilla, Lisa and Ruby, and Lisa and John. Also, Priscilla and Ruby used to have closer relationship in past. Affectionate feelings, according to the parents, are and should be expressed only to the two younger children. The degree of compatibility is difficult to evaluate from this vignette. No open conflict was described between the children and parents except for the arguments between Priscilla and Ruby. John and Ruby show signs of incompatibility, handling it by withdrawal (John staying away and drinking, and both of them not discussing important issues). Part of lack of spousal discussion of important issues and feelings, however, maybe due to social class and cultural role expectations, i.e., they do not see this as one of the expected roles in marriage.

13. *Mutual identification and bonding?*

There is evidence that this is present: (1) spouses are staying together (although marital bonds need to be strengthened); (2) Priscilla's emulation of mother's mothering behaviors and role; and (3) separation anxiety of the two younger childen when mother leaves.

14. *Issues of separateness and connectedness.*
    The information in this area is limited. However, more emphasis is placed on the togetherness aspects with Priscilla and the other children. Parents do not stress individuality and personal growth (which is more of a middle-class phenomenon and luxury).

It is generally accepted that the family is more specialized in its function today than it has ever been, and although the family performs many functions that have changed over time, one vital responsibility has remained a primary focus of the family: socialization or the rearing of children. The nurse is frequently in a position to influence, support, and assist the socialization process in families. In an attempt to provide the knowledge needed for these interventions, this chapter will define and identify tasks of socialization, discuss the influence of culture on parenting patterns, review some contemporary trends in child-rearing practices, and examine socialization theory and its implications for nursing practice.

SOCIALIZATION: A FAMILY AFFAIR

Definition of Socialization

Socialization begins at birth and ends only at death. It is a lifelong process by which individuals continually modify their behavior in response to the socially patterned circumstances they experience. The concept of patterning is a general notion that conveys the fact that, with time, objects, traits, or personalities take on features that reflect the culture in which they exist. Socialization, on the other hand, is one means of patterning. It embraces all those processes in a specific community or group whereby human nature, by virtue of its profound plasticity, through significant experiences that individuals encounter in their lifetime, acquires socially patterned characteristics.[1] Simply stated, socialization refers to training for a social environment and involves the social and psychological development of the child.

Most often, socialization proceeds informally and inexplicitly, so that its changing emphasis in response to altering cultural and environmental conditions goes quite unnoticed. Through socialization, people learn to live with others in groups and come to play appropriate sex- and age-linked roles. This occurs within the larger context or process of development.

Under the rubric of socialization, child-rearing practices are subsumed as the primary focus of attention. However, according to Eshleman, socialization should not be thought of as pertaining only to child-rearing practices during infancy and early childhood, but as a lifelong process that includes internalizing the appropriate sets of norms and values for the teenager of 14, the bride of 20, the parent of 24, the grandparent of 50, and the retired person of 65.[2]

The term socialization most often refers to the myriad of learning experiences provided within the family. These experiences are aimed at teaching children how to function and assume adult roles in society such as

Chapter 14 was written by Maxene Johnston, R.N., M.A., Director of Nursing, Ambulatory Services, Children's Hospital of Los Angeles, Los Angeles, California.

14

The Socialization Function

LEARNING OBJECTIVES

1. Define and identify the tasks of socialization.
2. Explain how the family's involvement in socialization changes during the life cycle of the child-rearing family.
3. Discuss the role culture plays in socialization patterns, particularly child-rearing practices.
4. Describe the findings of McClelland et al. relative to their study of child-rearing patterns.
5. Explain the role which social class plays in socialization and give some broad differences which are found between working-class and middle-class parents.
6. Explicate the relationship between a society's value system and that society's child-rearing and socialization patterns.
7. Identify several important issues and/or changes in modern society which have directly affected socialization patterns.
8. Correlate the stage of child development with the stage of parent development and parent tasks according to Friedman's model.
9. Explain one's own biases regarding child-rearing practices and socialization patterns.
10. Utilizing the socialization assessment questions, assess a hypothetical family's fulfillment of the socialization function.

those mentioned above. Reiss points out that although other functions such as reproduction are deemed necessary to, and performed in, all societies, the nurturant socialization of children is found universally only within the nuclear family structure.[3]

Since this function is now shared with other institutions and is influenced by many extrinsic factors, the family has a reduced role in socialization. Although the family has never had complete and total control over the socialization of children and despite the fact that parents still try, and do, transmit their cultural knowledge to the next generation, contemporary changes in the level of shared responsibility are such as to render the situation qualitatively different. And so today, the outside influences may even negate the primary value system of the family.

What has not changed is the fact that the family continues to have the primary responsibility of transforming an infant, in a score of years, into a social being capable of full participation in society. The child has to be taught language, the roles he or she is expected to take at various stages of life, sociocultural norms and expectations of what is right and wrong, and relevant cognitive structures. Additionally, the socialization process includes the patterning of sexual roles and the cultivation of an individual's initiative and creativity.

One aspect of the socialization process of particular relevance for the nurse involves the acquisition of health concepts, attitudes, and behaviors. In most cultures and social classes, the mother has been and continues to be the family's primary health educator. She is responsible for teaching her children basic health habits and, as they get older, how to care for themselves. Also, she generally has more health knowledge than any other family member.

Another important and integral task of socialization is the inculcation of controls and values—giving the growing child (and adult) a sense of what is right and wrong. The development of morality has been described by Kohlberg as a developmental process similar to the stages of emotional and cognitive development of Erikson and Piaget, respectively.[4] By identifying with parental figures and being consistently reinforced both negatively and positively for their behavior, children develop a personal value system which is greatly influenced by the family's value system.

Socialization also involves learning, and with learning usually comes enforcement or discipline. The use of discipline as a means of socializing children includes both positive and negative sanctions. Positive discipline encourages a person to exploit his or her resources for growth and serves as a positive reinforcer of behavior. Most communities have their own values regulating what sanctions to employ. For example, middle-class mothers in a New England town in the

United States preferred incentives like praise to that of rewarding children materially with candy or prizes for being good.[5] Many American mothers present themselves as models to their children to illustrate what they want them to be and not to be.

Negative sanctions, on the other hand, imply punishment and involve a great variety of methods. Some European Americans favor techniques of distraction, chastisement, ridicule, and isolation by withdrawal of affection to indicate displeasure with a child's behavior. Although we know that punishment often succeeds in eliminating children's undesirable behavior, in itself it lacks direction and does not teach alternative behavior; in fact, it may result in creating some interference with the child's learning of acceptable behaviors that could successfully integrate him or her into the larger society.

One way to measure family success in the past has been to evaluate the outcome of the socialization process. Not only are there comparative standards by which we measure a child's progress and hence the family's, but there are also age-related standards, that is, we expect certain socialization skills will be learned at particular ages. Today this measure is no doubt biased and inaccurate, since parents share the socialization function with the school system, peers, other reference groups, and the wider community. Woodward states that parents today often feel powerless in the face of institutional interferences: "The growth of social services, health care, and public education has robbed them of their traditional roles as job trainers, teachers, nurses, and nurturers. And their control over their children's lives is threatened by the pervasive, and increasingly authoritative, influence of television, schools and peer groups."[6] He also believes that in turning to outside counselors to help solve family problems, parents lose even more of their parental authority and confidence in their ability to parent.

From another perspective, it has also been suggested that institutional "overseeing" of the training needs of children has resulted from a disenchantment with traditional family roles, as well as waning commitment to child rearing. Part of this decline in enthusiasm for raising children stems from the difficulties parents feel in trying to fulfill their primary roles due to increased economic and daily living pressures and increased personal needs for their own development and socialization.

Despite these changes, the mother usually has the primary responsibility for socializing the child through the preschool years. Traditionally, the siblings and the father often have supportive roles during this time. The responsibility is later shared among schools, parents, peer groups, and, to a lesser degree, religious institutions. In the United States today, socialization may also be shared with day-care nurseries, nursery schools, and organized after-school programs, which remove parents from and dilute their involvement in their child's socialization experiences at earlier and earlier stages of child and family development.

Changes in traditional socialization patterns, responsibilities, and time-honored methods are now occurring at a greater rate than ever before. The dilemma of who will teach children important sociocultural traditions, how and where these are to be learned, and at what age and stage, are the questions we have struggled with in the past and will continue to debate into the future.

INFLUENCE OF CULTURE ON PARENTING PATTERNS

Cultural factors in socialization are exceedingly difficult to disentangle from environmental, social, and psychological considerations. In fact, the relative influence of each is often a matter of conjecture and speculation. Over the years, however, specific cultural responses have been studied and have added to our understanding of the variety of socialization patterns among various ethnic and culturally divergent groups.

Cultural Conditioning

The context in which child-rearing and socialization patterns occur was identified by Kardiner and follows some basic postulates:

1. [The] techniques which the members of any society employ in the care and rearing of children are culturally patterned and will tend to be similar, although never identical, for various families within the society.
2. [The] culturally patterned techniques for the care and rearing of children differ from one society to another.[7]

It is Kardiner's contention that if these postulates are correct, and there is a wealth of evidence to support them, it follows

that since the early experience of individuals differs from one society to another, the personality norms for various societies will also differ.[8]

This concept has added to our understanding of the influence of culture on the behavior and personality of individuals and the significance of the child-rearing patterns of parents.

Because the process of child rearing is so intricate, professionals have specialized in different ages, with some interested scholars conducting longitudinal studies. Recent work in this area has revealed that despite individual variation, children demonstrate patterned behavior that is linked to the culturally patterned behavior of their caretakers.

Cross-cultural Comparisons

Caudill's work with middle-class families in Japan and with similar American families is one example of the studies done in this area. He found that mothers in the two cultures engage in subtly different styles of caretaking that have, however, strikingly different effects. Generally, the American mother seems to encourage her baby to be active and respond vocally, whereas the Japanese mother acts in ways that she believes will soothe and quiet her child.[9] By the age of three to four months, the infants of both cultures seem to have already learned responses appropriate to these different patterns. The striking discovery, however, is in noting the fact that the responses of the infants are in line with certain broad expectations for behavior in the two cultures: in America the expectation that the individual should be physically and verbally assertive, and in Japan that he or she should be physically and verbally restrained.

In America, the mothers perceive their babies as separate and autonomous beings who are expected to learn to do and think for themselves. The baby is seen as a distinct personality with his or her own needs and desires which the mother must learn to recognize and care for. She does this by helping her infant learn to express these needs through her emphasis on vocal communication; the baby can thus "tell" her what he or she wants so that the mother can respond appropriately. In contrast, the Japanese mother views her baby much more as an extension of herself, and psychologically the boundaries between mother and infant are blurred. As a result of this emphasis on close attachment, the mother is likely to feel that she knows what is best for the baby, and there is no perceived need for the infant to tell the mother what he or she wants. Because of this orientation, the Japanese mother does not place much importance on vocal communication and instead stresses physical contact.

Although there are few such cross-cultural observational studies on infants reported in the literature, it should be noted that Reblesky obtained similar results in her study of Dutch and American infants.[10] The Dutch mothers were like the Japanese mothers in that they engaged in less talking to and stimulation of their infants. In either case, however, these studies should be evaluated carefully before making any sweeping generalizations. For example, cross-class studies of infants in the United States have often found that middle-class mothers do more talking to their infants than mothers in lower socioeconomic groups. Therefore, the results of the cross-cultural studies may not apply to the child-rearing techniques of mothers in different socioeconomic groups within various cultures.

All cultures must deal in one way or another with the cycle of growth from infancy to adulthood. From a comparative point of view, Benedict has described the extreme contrast Western culture has given to definitions of the child and adult.[11] Children are considered to be sexless, whereas adult vitality is measured in terms of sexual activity; the child must be protected from the ugly facts of life, while the adult is expected to meet them without disruption; the child must be obedient, the adult must command. In our society the transition and the conditioning of children to assume adult roles takes place primarily during the short period of time between the late school-age and adolescent years.

Thus in Western cultures, a real difficulty in employing our cultural norms in training children stems from the fact that an individual conditioned to one set of behaviors in childhood must adopt the opposite as an adult. In other cultures, family practices allow the child to engage in some of the same forms of behavior which he or she will rely on as an adult. Benedict, for example, sees this as one major discontinuity in Western child-rearing practices. A child who is at one point a son must later be a father, or a daughter later a mother. In many cultures, behavior is not polarized into this general expectation of submission for the child and dominance for the adult. The child is conditioned to a responsible status role by a variety of child-rearing techniques that depend chiefly on arousing the child's desire to share responsibility in adult life. To achieve this, praise and approval may be stressed, whereas the need for obedience would be given little attention.

It makes sense then that punishment is not often employed as an acceptable approach to training in some parts of the world. And from this perspective, it is not difficult to understand how people from other cultures might conclude from observing the usual disciplinary methods used in this country that "white parents do not love their children."[12] In any culture where children are not required to be submissive, many opportunities for punishment disappear. Many American Indian tribes are especially explicit in rejecting the idea that a child's submissive or obedient behavior is valuable. For example, if a child is seen as docile, he or she is thought to eventually become a docile adult, an undesirable characteristic. An example of this belief was observed many years ago when a Crow Indian father was heard boasting about his son's obstinate behavior even though it was the father himself who was the target. The father, in commenting on this, remarked that there was no need to be concerned as his son's behavior was proof that "he will be a man."

These examples have indicated the need for a cross-cultural and ethnic-oriented approach to our understanding of families and their child-rearing patterns. We are only beginning to learn about the pluralistic aspects of our own society and the dominant values of white middle-class life on our socialization styles.

It has been years now since Sears et al. completed one of the most thorough studies of child rearing ever done in the United States.[13] They were particularly interested in how a mother handled a range of developmental problems. Did she cope with these problems by physical punishment, by withdrawing her love, or by depriving her child of privileges? Perhaps more importantly, they began to probe the crucial question in socialization: Did the way the mother treat the child really make a difference in adulthood? What was the impact of whether or not the mother had breast fed, punished, rejected, or smothered her child with love?

Despite all the attention given them over the past years, many of these questions remain unanswered today. Most recently, however, after reviewing much of this data, several psychologists have argued that parents have very little control over the formation of their child's personality and character and contend that most adult behavior is not determined by specific techniques of child rearing in the first five years. What they suggest instead is that the way parents *feel* about their children does have a substantial impact on their future development.

In their study of child rearing, McClelland and colleagues found that when parents, particularly mothers, "really" love their children, they were likely to achieve the highest levels of social and moral maturity.[14] The other dimension that was significant for later social adaptation was how strictly the parents controlled their children's expressive behavior. In other words, a child was less apt to become socially and morally mature when his parents tolerated no noise, mess, or roughhousing in the home, and when they reacted unkindly to the child's aggressiveness toward them, sex play, or expressions of dependency needs. When parents were concerned with using their power to maintain an adult-centered home, the child was not as likely to become a mature adult. All in all, it appears that mothers' affection relates to more adult outcomes, while physical punishment does not seem to be significantly related to any of the outcomes examined. Thus a mother's affectionate demonstrativeness or warmth toward the child was found to be a crucial determinant of adult maturity.

Such revisions of the traditional outlook, along with rapid social change, the diversity of cultural backgrounds, and the nomadism of contemporary life styles leads to increased confusion among parents since there is no longer an approved way of "parenting." Many modern parents have never been taught as children how to care for infants and other small children. Whiting notes that in traditional societies where women have important roles in the subsistence economy, children are required to act as nurses to their younger siblings.[15] In all the agricultural societies she studied, mothers designate a child, usually between seven and eight years of age, to be their assistant.

Ideas and beliefs about the capabilities of children are also part of a parent's culture. For example, mothers in these same subsistence cultures need to be freed to return to work in the fields and therefore believe that seven- or eight-year-old children can be trained to be capable caretakers for younger children. The opposite has been observed in mothers who have leisure time. They have been reported to underestimate the capabilities of their children. Whiting reports that Indian mothers in Khalapur, Uttar Pradesh, or Bubeneshaw in Orissa have been observed bathing and feeding their children beyond the age when societies with working mothers have long since taught their children to care for their own hygiene activities.[16] She points out that at one extreme is an Okinawa child of four, who was observed washing her own hair and clothes; at the other, the Indian mother who was seen hand-feeding a child of eight and bathing a son of nine.

There appears to be a new interest in using the young to help in day-care centers to prepare them in the physical, social, and developmental aspects of child care. Cross-cultural work has demonstrated the usefulness of this approach. This holds true even in the context of a rapidly changing world of information. Some of what we know today may no longer be relevant in the near future; but overall, because of the universal nature of the problems of infancy, childhood, and parenthood, it is worthy of transmission to the next generation.

Social Class and Child Rearing

Although it is now well accepted that a child's socialization is influenced by the social class position of his or her family, most of us have only a superficial acquaintance with the distinctions that exist between the classes in child-rearing practices, patterns of consumption, education, moral values, and sexual conduct. We often develop ethnocentric or stereotyped notions about the differences that exist between class definitions of goals and aspirations, and about attitudes toward responsibility, independence, authority, work, and success. The importance of understanding these differences, however, is particularly pertinent to the therapeutic relationship in a health or community setting.

It is not uncommon to find that in dealing with families in a health setting, variations from a white middle-class standard are often seen as deviant, interpreted as pathology, or treated as deprived. Acceptable child-rearing practices and parent behavior by lower- and upper-class standards are seldom taken into account,

since most practitioners continue to evaluate others in terms of their own middle-class standards. Nurses are often bothered, uncomfortable, or shocked by behavior which they perceive as shiftless, overdependent, aggressive, pretentious, or uninhibited. Class differences in definitions of what is considered to be good or bad child rearing, normal or abnormal, acceptable or deplorable also present possible barriers to the therapeutic relationship between the nurse and the family.

Research dealing with social class differences in the style of socialization continues to show that parents from middle- and lower-class social structures, by virtue of experiencing different conditions of life, go about rearing their children with different conceptions of social reality, different aspirations, and different conceptions of what is desirable. Gecas has reported on the investigations that have identified ways in which middle-class occupations (white-collar) differ from lower-class occupations (blue-collar).[17] One study found that white-collar workers are more likely to enunciate values dealing with self-direction (freedom, individualism, initiative, creativity, and self-actualization), while blue-collar parents are more likely to stress values of conformity to external standards such as orderliness, neatness, and obedience. These values are reflected in the style or type of parental discipline. Because of their emphasis on self-direction, white-collar parents are more likely to discipline the child on the basis of their interpretation of the child's intent or motive for acting as he or she does. On the other hand, blue-collar parents are more likely to react on the basis of the consequences of the child's behavior. In other words, they are more likely to punish the child when his or her behavior is annoying, destructive, or disobedient.

These findings should be treated with the eye of a professional skeptic. Social class is not a determinant of behavior, but merely a statement of probability that a type of behavior is likely to occur. We should also consider that parental behavior and socialization techniques are influenced by the amount of stress and strain parents experience, their learned methods of coping and adapting, and the resources available to assist, counsel, and support them. A great deal of parents' child-rearing behavior will have resulted from their socialization experiences as children and may or may not reflect their current occupational status. We are constantly faced with a variety of life styles and value systems that are frequently different from those we have experienced as children ourselves.

Cultural Influences

When an individual grows up in a particular section of this country, in a neighborhood where almost everyone has a similar background, origin, or nationality, and where there are not many others who differ in physical type or social class, one tends to think of people who are different as strange, their behavior as irrational, and their life styles as a product of ignorance. Mead has reviewed the relationship of this form of cultural conditioning and differences in social class status and its relationship to nursing practice:

> This way of looking at difference becomes all the sharper if it is mixed, as it so often is, with the questions of economic level, or of class difference. In a culture like ours in which what is "American," "right," and "modern" is so firmly tied up with a high standard of living—milk for the children, plenty of clothes kept very clean, separate beds in separate rooms—there are bound to be differences between those who, because they are recent arrivals from other countries or come from parts of the United States or Canada where very little education was available, make a poor living and must live in wretched housing, and those who, with knowledge of the country or a better education, have a higher standard. But because so many of us recognize that other people's differences are tied in with matters of hygiene, nutrition, privacy (matters on which all Americans, and especially those concerned with health and illness, make judgements), nurses may be less willing than most Americans to think and talk about differences. Almost always, these differences seem to mean that someone is being regarded as in some way ignorant, or superstitious, or inferior when compared with the American standard.[18]

In all nursing care, assessments and interventions based on appropriate sociocultural data are important, whether counseling a mother, teaching a child, supervising a medical therapy, or coordinating community resources to resolve identified problems. In each case the nurse should focus on the relevance to the family and not on his or her own values. For example, some families can accept and respond to instructions for improving the diet of their children if these are given the explanation that if the children are fed better, they will behave better and the family will be happier. In other families, however, having well-nourished children is valued in and of itself.

In our society, the fact that good health is very often interpreted as a virtue and illness is seen as punishment can have profound effects on the child-rearing practices of many families. For example, Murphree reports the following case of a black family in the South. It was winter, and the children in the home had colds and symptoms of other infectious diseases. During the visit, the mother escorted the interviewer to a nearby room and proudly displayed the baby of the family and announced that he was well. She explained that she felt the need to "always have one well child—the baby." As long as the child remained an infant and could be kept relatively isolated from older children and their frequent infections, she could keep the baby

well. This woman indicated that she felt a certain sense of virtue in being able to keep at least the youngest child well. Murphree believes that this situation offers a possible explanation for some of the resistance encountered in trying to implement family-planning programs in this area. This woman seemed to feel that by having a baby in the house, she could insure one well child in her family, and therefore demonstrate her mothering ability and deservingness.[19]

It is also in the context of the family that a child learns what steps are taken at times of illness. Typically, the women have the responsibility for deciding who is sick, whether or not to initiate treatment, and what kind it should be. In many Western cultures, for example, the mother begins treatment at home with over-the-counter medicines, remnants of previously prescribed medications, or a folk remedy. She may seek advice from older women, either within or outside the extended family, and may willingly follow such advice.

One example of the deeply rooted patterns of childhood training affecting adult health and illness behavior are feelings grouped around modesty. This occurs immediately at birth and with economy of training. Benedict has observed that

> we waste no time in clothing the baby, . . . in contrast to many societies where the child runs naked until it is ceremoniously given its skirt or its pubic sheath at adolescence. The child's training fits it precisely for adult convention.[20]

We are rarely aware of how deep and with what precision feelings of modesty are embedded in our culture until we see and feel the response of medical staff and patients dealing with this issue. For example, modesty may be one of the key factors in resistance to cervical examination in cancer detection programs.[21]

Perhaps the influence of socialization for adult life can be made more relevant by examining a habit we talk about more than modesty: eating three meals a day. By two years of age, a child is usually on an adult feeding schedule. By the time the child reaches adolescence, he or she is frequently eating six meals a day, since the snack or break-time has become a national institution. What is more talked about, complained over, and reported than what and how and why we eat? And yet we face a time in which the problems of obesity, hypertension, and other nutrition-related diseases are affecting a greater number of people.

TRENDS IN CHILD-REARING PRACTICES: A MATTER OF VALUES

No matter which society we observe, the attitudes and approaches to the care and rearing of children will be congruent with the social, moral, religious, and economic values of that society. Over time, the place of children in society changed, and the twentieth century has come to be known as the century of the child. Extraordinary gains have been made in the understanding and care of children. But along with such advances, new social and economic pressures and realities have introduced other attitudes and concerns.

Goodman's observations of these current events suggest that we are witnessing warnings that something is changing in the most basic relationship in any society: the relationship between its adults and its children, between its present and its future.[22] Goodman has commented on the reemergence of a hostile relationship between adults and children and expresses a concern for the untoward effects of this generational conflict:

> Now, increasingly, parenthood is regarded as a personal, individual decision—a "lifestyle," whatever that may be—made apart from community interests. Kids are listed not as economic assets, but as financial liabilities. Each year, someone tallies up the cost of raising them as if they were sides of beef. And each year, someone else tallies up their cost to the local town or city and wonders if they are worth it. In many places, the voters are saying "no."
>
> There are, of course, adults and parents who lavish enormous, even excessive, concern on children. They support an industry of advisers, consultants and authors. But they exist in a commitment to children, and, therefore, to the future. Having confused permissiveness with neglect, and authority with abuse, the generations now splinter into hostile camps. The adults often try to protect themselves with zoning laws, spiteful votes and rattans. They threaten us with a retreat to the darkest age of society; to a history of childhood which is too monstrous ever to be repeated.[23]

An examination of the various historical and contemporary attitudes and approaches to children illuminates the obvious; children have always generated an "air of ambivalence" that permeates society and influences its values and beliefs in the care and rearing of its young. Certainly the ambivalence that exists regarding children extends throughout society. Still, in the middle of conflicting values and beliefs about children and their place in society, an attempt is also being made to adapt to such ambivalence, change, and conflict by emphasizing the importance of the family in child rearing and "revaluing" the mother–child dyad relationship. Counter trends are emerging as a reaction to the increased extrinsic influences over the family's role in rearing their children. Families are demanding and increasingly using alternative methods for childbirth (home births, prepared childbirth, alternative birthing centers), pediatric care (emergency rooms for

primary care services), and primary education (private schools and alternative school programs).

Amidst these changes, there will always be families who will need more assistance and support in their socialization function than others. This is a fact that has not changed and is not likely to change in the future. Despite the specific issues and controversies which have arisen throughout history, the consistent and central dilemma has involved and will continue to involve the child's place and perceived role in society.

SOCIALIZATION IN A CHANGING WORLD

No sooner did we begin adjusting to the importance of mother–child relationships than the definition of the mother–child relationship specifically, and the nuclear family in general, as the crucial socializing agent became open to the challenges of contemporary change. The variety and degree of social change that is occurring in the world has laid these concepts open for criticism and investigation.

There is a real need to assess the changes that have occurred in the environment. Single-parent families, fathers as primary caretaker, working mothers, families migrating to new cultures, and a host of other social changes have given rise to many concerns and calls for a dynamic and flexible approach to our traditional notions of socialization. We do not yet know the long-term effects of these new social relationships and arrangements. Nor can we say with certainty what the impact will be of increased equity in parenting roles, reassignment of traditional male–female parenting practices, fragmentation of the family into single-parent–child units with the possibility of several nuclear configurations, or realignment of traditional cultural values with those of new host cultures. These changes suggest issues that we will inevitably face in caring for today's children and the emerging families of the future.

Postindustrial Issues of Child Rearing

Many of today's mothers, confronted not only with the complexities of how to raise their children but also faced with the economic and social realities of living in a highly industrialized and mobile country are forced to decide who can assist them. Just at the time when mother–child attachments are seen as highly valuable, mothers have to deal with the issue of the need for day care. Kagan proposes that this is a problem area, since many modern mothers now believe that a mother should not give her infant to a substitute caretaker.[24] In violating what she believes to be her natural obligation, it is felt that she is not only placing her child's development at risk, but also increasing the likelihood that doing so will produce a socially disruptive adult. This concern is common, despite the fact that new studies reviewing this issue have found that there are no important differences between day-care and home-reared children.[25]

Many scholars, as early as Plato and as recent as Bowlby, have remarked that the infant and young child is best prepared for adulthood by sustained contact with a mother. On the other hand, there are societies in which children are given over to one or a small number of surrogate caretakers on a regular and frequent basis with no evidence that they develop into more anxious, hostile, or nonadaptive adults.

Another complex child-rearing issue is the problem of the one-parent family in a changing two-parent society. Some single-parent families have been associated with negative characteristics such as poverty, abandonment, marital violence, child abuse and neglect, and parental depression and dissatisfaction. However, in one study of one-parent families in Britain, the influence of the family situation on the overall development of children was reported to be much weaker than that of other factors such as low social class, large family size, and limited parental aspirations.[26] The absence of a mother, regardless of the reason, was shown to have a more adverse effect on children's development than the absence of the father.

Another point to consider here is that social change which is seen as radical, untraditional, or frightening often generates a negative and ambivalent attitude on the part of the general community or society. In the case of single-parent families, the community's stigmatizing attitudes may be reflected by the inadequate health and social services provided for them. This may set into motion a vicious cycle of intolerable burdens leading a single parent to disengage from her children or, worse yet, to abandon them.

Turning to another problem area, the recent attention given to child abuse has resulted in conflicting opinions on child-care needs, the rights and responsibilities of parents, and the rights of children. We are still debating the best way of providing help to families, i.e., either working within the family to keep it intact or using external legislative and legal intervention to separate the child from parents. These quandaries go on in the background, while health professionals continue to be involved in a series of assessments, judgments, and discussions on the clinical and social problems involved in such instances.

The issues surrounding legislation and children are perhaps the least remembered but the most influential in terms of their impact on child rearing. There have been dramatic changes in this century in the laws concerning child care and protection, as well as numerous changes in the concepts of children's rights, parental rights, duties, and responsibilities. The legal system presents a sometimes contradictory picture of our expectations of parenting. Based on earlier patriarchal patterns of family organization, the father was regarded as the "natural guardian" of the child and was free to punish his child within reasonable boundaries. Loss of parents' rights over the care and discipline of their children could occur only in extreme cases when a "fit person" order was made by the Court. Our laws have evolved considerably from these earlier notions, so much so that the recent Children's Act of 1975 evidenced the present disenchantment with the natural family as inevitably providing the best care for the child. This change was brought about following the death of a child after being returned to her natural mother and served to strengthen the rights of foster parents, as well as directing the appointment in appropriate circumstances of a person to act as guardian *ad litem* of the child or young person in order to safeguard his or her interests.

The range of contemporary issues in the care and rearing of children is great. However, the most important socialization task is fairly straightforward. As socializing agents, parents need to motivate the succeeding generation to go on, guiding their children to realize the human need for continuity. Erikson's concept of generativity demonstrates an understanding of the importance of socializing for continuity. In his discussion of generativity versus stagnation, he describes the mature man's need of and dependence on the younger generation. The primary concern in this stage is in "establishing and guiding the next generation. . . . Where such enrichment fails altogether, regression to an obsessive need for pseudo-intimacy takes place, often with a pervading sense of stagnation and personal impoverishment."[27]

Bronfenbrenner reflects this concept in his expression of concern for achieving this developmental stage in the comment, "We must bring adults back into the lives of children and children back into the lives of adults."[28]

Achieving this motivation has become something of a dilemma. It is difficult to foster the concept of continuity in a time of discontinuity and change. Past traditions, values, and social norms are emptied of their utility for the day-to-day functioning of the family. This is neither to suggest that this type of social housecleaning is not necessary nor to imply that this type of separation from prior expectations may not ultimately be more adaptive to the current heterogeneous society. Rather, it is to suggest that the effects of a lack of traditions and continuity on children and families need to be examined as to their possibly subtle and disruptive nature.

Discontinuity with prior practices is evident in many aspects of child rearing. But perhaps one change that has the most profound impact on socialization patterns is that of sex-role behavior and expectations. Most parents today are being encouraged to socialize their children in an androgynous fashion, that is, not identified with a specific gender. Traditional sex-linked roles have taken on taboo-like connotations. Previous values supporting traditional masculine and feminine roles are still alive, however, and serve to create the current divergence between what may be regarded at one level as an ideal value that remains to be achieved in observed behavior. There is a question, however, as to whether the current push for a "unisex" upbringing may not also cause some problems.[29] Whatever the ultimate adaptive value, our children may be getting inappropriate preparation for an adult world that may remain sexist.

As much as we may hope for the realization of non-sexist attitudes in preparing children for changing adult roles, it will be delayed so long as parents hold disparate sets of expectations for their boys and for their girls. In a recent, multiethnic study of parental expectations of the jobs their children would have when they grew up, most parents believed that their girls could enter positions traditionally considered as male, such as policeman, doctor, engineer, or banker. On the other hand, they did not see their boys occupying traditionally female jobs such as model, typist, social worker, or librarian.[30]

The force of popular culture pulling at the bonds between children and parents is stronger than ever. But our new fascination with the notion of parenting, proclaimed in a flood of handbooks, implies a new formula for a scientific recipe to raising children. The word parenting itself reflects a substitution, a replacement, and serves as another example of the modern assumption that all of nature, including human nature, is raw material for transformation according to scientific principles.[31] In other words, it often appears that it takes a professional to know the right way to do things.

Today's parents tend to be overwhelmed with these issues, as well as with advice from many sources. The nurse will often be called on to understand, interpret, and consider the developmental stage of the parents as well as that of the child in helping parents cope with such contemporary stresses.

SOCIALIZATION THEORY AND CLINICAL PRACTICE: A DYNAMIC PROCESS

Education in child-rearing patterns and family problems is a major component of family health care. It begins with genetic and reproductive counseling, continues through prenatal/child care, and extends throughout the life cycle of the family. In order to lend direction to a parent and a family, however, we must be aware of the various aspects of the growth and development of children and the socialization patterns of families. How can we help a family, parent, or child achieve or maintain optimum functioning if we are not aware of what is considered normal or optimum?

It is no surprise that today's parents tend to be overwhelmed with the variety of child-rearing advice they receive from numerous sources. There are the scientific advisors: the researchers, developmental specialists, nurses, physicians, psychologists, and educators. And there are also the "folk" advisors: the friend, family and neighbor networks, herbalists, curanderos, clergy, authors, television and movie writers, and other commentators giving advice on the family and approaches to the care of children.

Using a Developmental Approach

In light of the array of available information on child rearing, the nurse will frequently be the health professional looked to in assisting parents to sort out and understand their children's needs and their own responsibilities. In this regard, Friedman has suggested five definitive stages through which parents progress and the appropriate child rearing task for the period.[32] Each stage reflects the major problems in the child's development with which the parent is grappling. These stages have been observed in a wide variety of socio-cultural settings and ethnic groups, as well as in single-parent families, and the basic concept appears to be universal. The five stages of parent development are outlined in Table 14.1.

Just as our knowledge of human growth and development has changed over the years, so has the professional advice given to parents. This often resulted from having increased information on children or may, in fact, be a reflection of the child's changing status in a particular time in society. When one examines the shifts in the advice given to parents over the past 60 years, the fluctuating philosophies and anxieties of a highly industrialized society appear evident:

1910—Spank them
1920—Deprive them
1930—Ignore them
1940—Reason with them
1950—Love them
1960—Spank them lovingly
1970—The hell with them!

The sarcasm expressed in the 1970 attitude may indeed be an expression of the despair and depression parents feel when they have lost confidence in their ability to

TABLE 14.1
Stages of Parent Development

Stage of Child Development	Stage of Parent Development	Parental Task
I. Infant	Learning the cues.	To interpret infant needs.
II. Toddler	Learning to accept growth and development.	To accept some control while maintaining necessary limits.
III. Preschooler	Learning to separate.	To allow independent development while modeling necessary standards.
IV. School-ager	Learning to accept rejection without deserting.	To be there when needed without intruding unnecessarily.
V. Teenager	Learning to build a new life—having been thoroughly discredited by one's teenager.	To adjust to changing family roles and relationships during and after the teenager's struggle to establish an identity.

Adapted from Friedman DB: Parent development. Calif Med 86:25, January 1957

succeed as parents. Nonetheless, we know that when parents understand their own emotional states, they can better understand what to do and how to respond to their children.

This brings us to the topic of educating parents for their job. In the past, no profession identified "parent development" as one of its functions. Parents were supposed to know how to raise children, either intuitively or through their own growing up in large extended families. Today, however, advice, counseling, and teaching about parenting is considered to be the responsibility of pediatricians, nurses, child development specialists, and other health professionals. It is not unusual to find "socialization failure" or "defective mother crafting skills" used as fairly common diagnoses today. Often an attempt is made to involve parents in some type of parenting program in order to assist them in dealing with their children.

Smoyak has identified three different parenting programs that have become familiar avenues of advice to parents on child rearing.[33] One program aims at helping parents accept their role with less anxiety and guilt. This is known as the parent-effectiveness approach. Another program focuses more directly on improving specific parenting skills. The third program supports a family therapy approach, assuming that after disturbing relationships in the total family system are eliminated, parents can go on with their work.

By discussing parents' expectations of their role, the family nurse may identify sources of frustration, confusion, and gaps in their information. By initiating parent education programs, conducting parent groups and client education sessions, and providing support and encouragement, parental role transition and improved confidence can be facilitated.

In considering nursing practice and socialization therapy, perhaps the most relevant question concerns how often we focus on the child's growth and developmental problems to the exclusion of the parents and how they are managing. The well-conducted Attitude Study Project, reported in 1964, evaluated the health supervision of children in child health conferences within the New York City Health Department.[34] Project staff who were well qualified in mental health worked with physicians and nurses to increase their communication skills and sensitivity. The results of this intervention demonstrated that after completing the series of mental health meetings, both nurses and physicians became more mother-centered and were thus better able to discuss and help mothers with concerns about their children.

Another issue to consider in working with parents and children is the possibility of role confusion. Taylor reminds us that most adults are protective toward children[35] and that all adults feel some responsibility for children, particularly the very young. It is therefore difficult for most adults not to interfere when a mother or family seem to be mishandling or abusing a child. This response has tremendous survival value for the species but does pose a problem for the nurse. In one instance, such feelings make it possible to work with families and children who are personally unattractive to the nurse, while on the other hand making it difficult to remain detached enough to function in the public and social capacity of the nursing role.

As stated previously, children come from families with diverse sociocultural backgrounds. Some families have child-rearing styles that the nurse has been conditioned, socialized, and taught to recognize as "good." Current attitudes place the responsibility for successful child rearing on a child's parents, while at the same time suggesting that most parents are not experts about their own children's idiosyncrasies. As a result, most health specialists who deal with the pediatric client tend to assume that the parents are somehow at fault because their child is sick. This covert attitude makes it difficult for the nurse to sustain an objective role. The nurse often does things for his or her clients that a mother does for a child. It is tremendously important for the nurse to remember the public and social capacity of the nursing role. This is important because it helps avoid replacing the mother, as well as helps the nurse to avoid displacing his or her own childhood frustrations on the mother and blaming the mother for the child's condition. The nurse's ability to support the mother without becoming a surrogate for her is critical for the child, as well as for the self-esteem and potential growth of the parent.

ASSESSMENT QUESTIONS

Ultimately, we must all examine our own attitudes, expectations, and biases regarding child-rearing practices and socialization patterns. How do you see the way you were raised and the way the families you work with are raising their children? How reasonable are your expectations of parents? For example, is it reasonable to expect a mother of five children never to prop a bottle? In determining the appropriateness of a particular family's child-rearing methods, it is helpful to ask yourself how functional the approach is for the particular family being considered. Another example would be to ask yourself how adaptive the family's form of discipline is for their particular situation.

Question your expectations of compliance with the advice and instructions given. Are they real or ideal? How should you adapt your routines and nursing methods to achieve a successful outcome with a particular family?

In your assessment of families, the following questions will provide useful data from which to identify potential or actual problems and plan care accordingly.

1. What are the family's child-rearing practices in the following areas?
   a. discipline
   b. reward
   c. punishment
   d. autonomy and dependency
   e. giving and receiving of love
   f. training for age-appropriate behavior (social, physical, emotional, language, and intellectual development)
2. How adaptive are the family's child-rearing practices for their particular situation?
3. Who assumes responsibility for the child-care role or socialization function? Is it shared? If so, how is this managed?
4. How are the children regarded in the family? What cultural beliefs are manifest in the child-rearing pattern?

We also need to examine the problems with which a family must cope in matters affecting their health care. On the other hand, we must not lose sight of the problems that nursing and health team members experience in providing care. These problems are often interrelated and mutually experienced and involve areas of communication and language barriers, broken or missed appointments, and a mismatched set of priorities between clients and practitioners.

Our unit of concern should be the ecological unit: the child in the family and the family in the social system. In the future we will increasingly meet with people who cannot be cured and who face a variety of social and environmental problems. The numbers of people who are able to live independently with chronic health conditions in their families have already pulled on the traditional cure-oriented strings of medicine. And their existence suggests that conventional treatment concepts are, in many instances, out of tune with people's needs. Families want more adaptive, creative, less costly, and more relevant methods and resources for their health and social problems. The nurse is most often the health professional in the position to investigate and initiate such measures.

The nurse is also an example of a competent, creative, and cost-effective resource for families. By providing appropriate health supervision, counseling, and referral, the nurse provides an opportunity for community-based care that is often both accessible and affordable. Working closely with the schools, health and other social agencies, the nurse coordinates a variety of resources and a wealth of necessary information and can assist families in coping with the complexities of raising children in a changing world of challenging expectations.

Considering the complexity of socializing children, Goode reflects an appreciation for the current state of the art in remarking that "we now at least know what are some of the worst ways of rearing a child, but we are much less sure of how to do it well."[36]

REFERENCES

1. Honigman JJ: Personality in Culture. New York, Harper & Row, 1967
2. Eshleman JR: The Family: An Introduction. Boston, Allyn and Bacon, 1974, p 38
3. Reiss IL: The universality of the family: A conceptual analysis. J Marriage Family 27:443, 1965
4. Kohlberg L: Education for justice: A modern statement of the Platonic view. In Moral Education: Five Lectures. Cambridge, Mass, Harvard University Press, 1970
5. Honigman, op. cit., p 183
6. Woodward KL et al.: Saving the Family. Newsweek, May 15, 1978, p 64
7. Kardiner A: The Psychological Frontiers of Society. New York, Columbia University Press, 1945
8. Ibid., pp vi–viii
9. Caudhill W: The individual and his nexus. In Nader L, Maretzi TW (eds): Cultural Illness and Health. Washington, DC, American Anthropological Association, 1975, p 70
10. Rebelsky FG: Infancy in Two Cultures. Psychologie. Ned Tydschr Psychol Grensgebieden 22:379, 1967
11. Benedict R: Continuities and discontinuities in cultural conditioning. In Brink PJ (ed): Transcultural Nursing, A Book of Readings. Englewood Cliffs, NJ, Prentice-Hall, 1976, p 83
12. Ibid., p 87
13. Sears R, Maccoby E, Levin H: Patterns of Child Rearing. New York, Harper & Row, 1957
14. McClelland D, Constantine CA, Regaldo D, Stone C: Making it to maturity. Psychology Today, June 1978, p 45
15. Whiting B: Folk wisdom and child rearing. Merrill-Palmer Quarterly 20(1):9, 1974
16. Ibid., p 14
17. Gecas V: The socialization and child care roles. In Nye FI (ed): Role Structure and Analysis of the Family. Beverly Hills, Calif, Sage Publications, 1976
18. Mead M: Cultural contexts of nursing problems. In MacGregor FC (ed): Social Science in Nursing. New York, Russell Sage, 1960
19. Murphree AH: Cultural influences on development. In Scipien G, Bernard M, Chard M, Howe J, Phillips P (eds): Comprehensive Pediatric Nursing. New York, McGraw Hill, 1975
20. Benedict R: Continuities and discontinuities in cultural conditioning. Psychiatry 1:161, 1938
21. Alpenfels EJ: Cancer in situ of the cervix: Cultural clues to reactions. In Lynch LR (ed): The Cross-Cultural Approach to Health Behavior. Cranbury, NJ, Fairleigh Dickinson University Press, 1969, p 75
22. Goodman E: America's war against its children makes monsters of us all. Los Angeles Times, June 25, 1978
23. Ibid.
24. Kagan J: The parental love trap. Psychology Today 12:3, August, 1978, p 58
25. Ibid., p 58
26. Hersov L: British Study Group Presentation. Paper delivered to the Ninth International Congress of the Association of Child Psychiatry and Allied Professions. Melbourne, Australia, August 1978
27. Erikson EH: Childhood and Society, 2nd ed. New York, Norton, 1963
28. Bronfenbrenner U: The origins of alienation. Sci Am 231:53, 1974
29. Johnston M, Sarty M: Ethnic differences in sex stereotyping by mothers: implications for health care. Paper presented to 1977 World Congress on Mental Health, Vancouver, BC, Canada, August 1977
30. Ibid.
31. Will GF: The cold war among women. Newsweek, June 26, 1978, p 100
32. Friedman DB: Parent development. Calif Med 86:25, 1957
33. Smoyak SA: Introduction: symposium on parenting. Nurs Clin North Am 12:447, 1977
34. Jacobziner H, Levy, DM, Suchman EA, O'Neil G: Mental Health in the Child Health Conference. U.S.D.H.E.W., Children's Bureau, Publication No. 407-1964, 1964
35. Taylor C: In Horizontal Orbit. New York, Holt, Rinehart and Winston, 1970
36. Goode WJ: Introduction to the Contemporary American Family. Chicago, Quadrangle, 1971

STUDY QUESTIONS

1. Which of the following is the *best* definition of socialization?
   a. The act of learning to relate to people.
   b. The training provided to function in a social environment.
   c. The social and psychological development of a child.
   d. Child-rearing practices.

2. The central task involved in socialization of children revolves around teaching them how to function and assume adult roles in a society. Subsumed under this main task are several more specific tasks. Name three of these.

3. American families have retained primary and almost exclusive responsibility for socializing their children during what life cycles of the family (select all appropriate answers):
   a. Stage of marriage.
   b. Childbearing (stage of expansion).

    c. Families with preschool children.

    d. Families with school-age children.

    e. Families with teenage children.

4. Culture plays a dominant role in socialization. Explain briefly.

Choose the correct answers to the following questions.

5. McClelland and his associates recently conducted a study of child-rearing patterns and their outcomes among American families. They found that (select the *best* answer):

    a. Strict limit setting and clear boundaries produced well-behaved, obedient children.

    b. No one approach to child rearing was superior over another approach.

    c. Parental love and acceptance was the crucial determinant in the child's acquisition of social and moral maturity.

    d. Parents have very little control over the formation of their child's personality and character.

6. Social class is another vital variable influencing a family's socialization patterns. Social class makes a difference because (select the *best* answer):

    a. By virtue of experiencing different life conditions, families from various social classes have varying conceptions of social reality and what is desirable, feasible, and most important.

    b. Social class determines how parents deal with the world and their children.

    c. Being in one social class or another gives a family a limited view of the world and consequently limits their child-rearing techniques to those with which they are familiar.

7. Research concerning social class differences in child-rearing patterns found that (answer *True* or *False*):

    a. The white-collar family stresses respect and obedience more than the blue-collar family does.

    b. Conformity and individualism are both emphasized more by middle-class families.

    c. Middle-class families are more concerned about the child's inner motives, while the lower-class families are more focused on the child's actual behavior.

8. The attitudes and approaches to the care and rearing of children in a society (select all appropriate answers):

    a. Will be congruent with the society's value system.

    b. May or may not be related.

    c. Will be positively associated with the society's value system.

    d. Will be related to the traditions but perhaps not the current values because of cultural lag.

9. Identify several important changes and/or issues affecting child rearing in our society.

10. Match the appropriate stage of parent development and parental tasks in the right column with the child's stage of development in the left column.

    a. Infant   1. To allow independence.

    b. Toddler   2. To accept rejection without deserting the child.

    c. Preschooler   3. Learning to build a new life for parents.

    d. School-ager   4. Learning the meaning of the cues.

    e. Teenager   5. Learning to accept child's growth and development.

                      6. Learning to master anger and frustration.

11. Self-examination of child-rearing biases: What particular beliefs and attitudes do you hold which might limit your effectiveness in working with parents and children in the area of parenting or child rearing?

FAMILY CASE STUDY

From the following family vignette assess the family's socialization function using the questions provided at the conclusion of the vignette as assessment guidelines.

Mr. and Mrs. Chin, ages 50 and 45, respectively, moved 10 years ago to San Francisco from Hong Kong. The Chins operate a small cleaners, and the family income has always been low despite the long, hard hours of work both parents engage in. They have four children: Harold, 23, who is at the California School of Technology studying engineering; Lee, 22, who is a registered nurse; John, 17, who is in high school and an excellent student; and Joe, 10, who is attending fifth grade. All the children (including the older ones) are always busy working. John and Joe work extremely hard on their studies, and with school work and home chores there is little time left over for playing or getting into "mischief." The parents have greatly encouraged their children on to higher education and academic achievement, and through their accomplishments, the Chins feel the children have brought honor to them.

During the home visit all the children were observed to be respectful of their parents' authority. In the presence of their parents, the two youngest were quiet and did not interject comments or express themselves until directly asked a question, at which time they answered quickly while looking to their mother for approval.

Mrs. Chin states that her husband is strict in child rearing and that if the two younger boys still living at home disobey, he administers immediate corporal punishment. Mrs. Chin relates that a misbehaving child in the Chinese community is considered "not trained," meaning that the parents are to blame; thus a child's wrongdoing brings shame and dishonor to the whole family.

When Mrs. Chin was asked how she raised her children, she related that she cuddled and fondled them a lot while they were little. But as soon as they became preschoolers she gradually withdrew her expressions of love and physical hugs and kisses. From school age on, she and her husband have pushed their children to become independent and responsible. Both parents said that they had emotionally removed themselves somewhat from their children lest their children might lose respect for them.

The parent–child relationships appear to be more restrained and formal than in most American families. However, though muted, one was still able to feel the obvious respect and caring they feel for each other.

12. Describe how the family dealt with the following areas of child rearing: discipline, reward, punishment, moral training, autonomy, initiative, creativity, dependency, giving and receiving of love, and training for age-appropriate behavior (social, physical, emotional, and language, and intellectual development).

13. How adaptive are the family's child-rearing practices for their particular situation (social class, culture, environment, etc.)

14. Who assumes responsibility for the child-care role or socialization function? Is it shared and if so, how?

15. How are children regarded in the family?

16. What cultural beliefs are operating in their child-rearing practices?

STUDY ANSWERS

1. b

2. Any three:
   a. Language development.
   b. Sociocultural norms and expectations (right and wrong).
   c. Sexual roles.
   d. Individual initiative and creativity.
   e. Acquisition of health concepts, attitudes, and behaviors.

3. b and c

4. The child-rearing techniques used in a society are culturally patterned, and hence there will be a tendency for various families within a particular society to rear their children similarly. These culturally patterned techniques for child rearing differ from society to society, as do the ideas and beliefs about the capabilities and needs of children during their stages of growth and development. Moreover, since socialization patterns differ from one society to the next, so will personality norms and broad expectations for personal behavior differ.

5. c

6. a

7. a. False
   b. False
   c. True

8. a or c

9. Several important societal changes/issues affecting child rearing (any three):
   a. Day care for children of working mothers and their feelings of guilt about working and dissatisfaction about the facilities available.

    b. The growing number of single-parent families and how well this type of family can fulfill the socialization function.

    c. The stigmatization which single-parent families and other variant family forms face in society and how this affects the ability of these families to rear their children.

    d. Methods or approaches for assisting families where child abuse or neglect exists.

    e. The emphasis on "unisex" upbringing and its consequences.

    f. Conflicting information from "experts" on how to raise children.

10. a. 4
    b. 5
    c. 1
    d. 2
    e. 3

11. Self-examination: Attitudes or beliefs which limit effectiveness include:

    a. Strong beliefs that orderliness, neatness, obedience, degree of restraint or assertiveness, etc., are desirable and should be important to everyone.

    b. Rigid values and beliefs that hold that there is a "right and proper" way to raise children.

    c. Religious convictions suggesting that certain customs and techniques are "good" and others "bad" or "sinful."

    d. The belief that the mother or parents are responsible for their children's behavior (blaming the parents).

    e. The attitude that the family's situation is not relevant, or is less significant, whereas what is *best* for the child is *the* focus (exclusion of the ecological unit and the constraints of the family's environment).

12. *Discipline and punishment.* Father administers punishment; uses physical (corporal) means. Parents consider a child's wrongdoing as a reflection of the parents' failure to train children adequately, and thus, they feel threatened and disgraced by their children's misbehavior. The children certainly feel shame for the "loss of face" they have brought to the family. Hence the punishment is more than corporal, since the child being punished also feels the interpersonal sanctions of rejection, disapproval, and withdrawal of acceptance and love.

    Rewards. Parents did not express how they reward children, except that Mrs. Chin verbally expressed (in front of children?) that her children, by virtue of their achievements, brought great honor to the family. This may indicate a pattern of verbal praise and acceptance.

    Moral training. Family is highly structured and has clear boundaries as to what is right and wrong. This is instilled through careful supervision when young (assumed) and strict discipline when children are assumed old enough to take on adult behaviors (responsibility, self-sufficiency). When children are young they are given much unconditional love and affection from parents.

    Autonomy and dependency. Children were pushed to be autonomous and responsible from school age on; conversely, dependency would not be reinforced positively during these same stages of development.

    Initiative and creativity. There was no mention of how parents handled the issues of creativity and taking initiative.

Giving and receiving of love. The mother mentioned the extensive expression of affection to children when they are young, but that from preschool age on (gradually) and especially beginning at school age, children were pushed away from parents' affectively. In fact, parents try to remove themselves to some extent, so that they can maintain the position of respect vis-à-vis their children.

Training for age-appropriate behaviors. Little is mentioned except that social responsibility (home chores) and school achievement (intellectual development) were stressed and promoted in this family.

13. The child-rearing approach is very adaptive for this family. The parents obviously desire their children to have a better life than they have had. Through their socialization patterns they are training children to be self-sufficient, productive, success-oriented, and independent.

14. The mother may have responsibility for the everyday matters, but the father definitely has ultimate responsibility to administer sanctions for misbehavior and thus ultimate responsibility for socialization. Socialization function is seen as the prime responsibility of this family.

15. There is little data from which to draw conclusions about how children are regarded in this family, but one senses that children are highly valued and are central to the aspirations and life goals of the parents.

16. The family is not acculturated to the dominant American culture. The parents are first-generation Chinese-American; they consider themselves part of the Chinese community, and the values and child-rearing practices they describe are congruent with the traditional values of the Chinese. In describing the Chinese child-rearing practices, Sung* verifies that the Chins' socialization patterns are indeed culturally patterned:

> Discipline is strict and punishment immediate in the Chinese household. . . . The Chinese child is taught that when he does wrong, it is not a personal matter between himself and his conscience; he brings disgrace and shame upon his family and loved one. . . . A Chinese baby may be cuddled and fondled, showered with kisses, and rocked to sleep in his mother's arms, but as the child grows older, the mother withdraws her expression of affection. . . . Chinese parents think they can maintain authority if they are careful to keep a certain distance from their children. . . . The father never tries to be a friend to his son, nor the mother a big sister to her daughter. . . . A parent is the authority that demands obedience, and authority must maintain its dignity.

---

* Sung BL: The Story of the Chinese in America. New York, Collier, 1967, pp 168–171.

For the family health professional, the health care function is a vital consideration in assessment. To place this function in perspective, it is a major component within the family function of provision of physical necessities: food, clothing, shelter, and health care. Shelter (housing and family's neighborhood and community) was discussed previously in Chapter 8 as part of environmental data. Dietary habits (food) are included in this chapter.

From the perspective of society, the family is the basic system in which health behavior and care are organized, performed, and secured. Families provide preventive health care and the major share of sick care for their members. Furthermore, families have the prime responsibility for initiating and coordinating health services rendered by health professionals.[1]

There has been a pervasive assumption that as the family has become more specialized in its functions, its health care function has been lost—being transferred to the doctor's office and hospital.[2,2a] And yet among health professionals, the tremendous role which families play in the provision of health care to family members is evident.* Therefore, it is the belief of this text, supported by Pratt[3] and others, that the provision of health care is indeed a vital and basic family function, and this fact should greatly influence health professionals in their delivery of services to both individuals and families.

FAMILY BEHAVIOR RELATED TO HEALTH AND ILLNESS

Health practices and the use of health care services vary tremendously from family to family. Family differences in both definitions and conceptualizations of what constitutes health and illness and the degree of motivation to seek health services and improve their health behavior constitute the main reasons for the observed diversity of health care practices.

Conceptualizations of Health and Illness

Conceptualizations of health and illness vary widely from culture to culture, region to region, and family to family, as well as among the several social classes and as a result of the degree of technological development that has occurred in a family's community.

Persons from the same cultural background and/or from similar socioeconomic status often share comparable attitudes, myths, and values concerning their health. This has been particularly documented in poor communities.[4] Some health problems endemic to whole communities or groups may be taken as a mat-

*The reader is referred back to Chapter 1, which discusses in depth the role of the family vis-à-vis the entire spectrum of health and illness concerns.

The Health Care Function

Learning Objectives

1. Recall the various ways in which the family carries out its health care function.
2. Identify three salient factors which influence a family's conceptualization or definition of health and illness, and whether they seek health care.
3. Discuss Baumann's study relative to the three diverse criteria (orientations) used to define health and illness, and the group differences found.
4. Explain Koos's central findings in terms of the influence of socioeconomic status on illness recognition and health-seeking behaviors.
5. Diagram the health belief model, explaining the several important components of the model and their relationships to each other.
6. Summarize Pratt's findings and conclusions concerning how adequately the American family performs its health care function.
7. Enumerate the basic aspects which need to be assessed when completing an appraisal of a family's (a) dietary practices, (b) sleeping and rest practices, (c) exercise and recreation practices, (d) drug practices, and (e) self-care practices.
8. Describe the basic specific preventive measures recommended for adults and children.
9. Discuss four health education areas families need to be cognizant of in order to provide adequate dental self-care.
10. Describe what is basically included in a family medical history.
11. Explain what effect poverty has on utilization of health services.
12. Pose several relevant questions which would be appropriate to ask related to a family's use of health services.

ter of course rather than defined as illness. Social customs and norms often determine whether particular behaviors are considered sick or healthy.[5]

It follows then that a family, neighborhood, community, or society must label a condition or certain behaviors as an illness or disability before it can be considered a health problem to that group. The frequency of a condition often influences whether the condition is labeled an illness or not. For instance, if practically everyone in a community is suffering from malnutrition, the associated fatigue will probably be considered normal. In America today we accept colds and dental caries as annoyances that are a part of normal living, and most sufferers of colds or toothaches do not consider themselves ill.

Kane et al. point out that the interpretation given to "health" by the poor is a natural consequence of the living conditions in which they find themselves.

> Their entire orientation is colored by the fact that they live with other poor people; they take on the perspectives of those around them and reinforce each other's beliefs and values. The way they cope with health problems is "traceable either to the material situation of poverty itself, to the social structure of poverty, or to the aspects of the life outlook of poverty—the ideals, values, and beliefs to which the poor man adheres."[6]

Hence people have different ways of defining whether they are sick or well. Some persons feel they are sick only when they can no longer work or carry on their usual daily activities and roles; others are very attuned to their physiological functioning and recognize even minor symptoms or signs as an indication of disease and illness; a third orientation of another group of people might be that they are sick when they are not feeling well.

Baumann[7] conducted a study of middle-aged and older chronically ill clinic patients from working-class and lower socioeconomic backgrounds and freshmen medical students in their first three years of medical school, who were generally from middle- and upper-middle-class backgrounds and in their early twenties, and she compared the two groups according to their definitions of health and illness. Baumann found the three prevailing basic orientations to wellness and illness alluded to above existed in the two groups: (1) a subjective feeling of well-being or ill health (the feeling-state orientation); (2) an absence or presence of general or specific symptoms (symptom orientation); and (3) a state of being able or unable to perform usual activities (a performance orientation). Consistent with the American society's productivity value orientation, both groups (representing both age and socioeconomic differences) mentioned an activity orientation in their conceptualization of health and illness. The clinic pa-

tients tended to identify subjective feelings as being a significant factor in their definition (supporting Koos's findings that the less educated were less articulate in their thoughts[8]), while the freshman medical students identified the presence or absence of symptoms as the second criterion in their definition of health and illness.

Koos, in a classic study, demonstrated that socioeconomic position greatly influenced an individual's interpretation of symptoms, i.e., whether symptoms were perceived as symptoms of illness or not, and when present, were indications that medical care should be sought. He found that as one descends the social class ladder, less symptom recognition and perceived need for medical services existed among the study population. Thus the middle-class worker was found to be much more knowledgeable about disease symptoms, while working-class and lower-class persons showed less recognition of symptoms as being signs of ill health and therefore did not view these symptoms as indicating a need for medical attention. Generally, the poor must reach a stage of being incapacitated before they define themselves as ill. Blatant symptoms of health problems such as loss of appetite, persistent coughing, shortness of breath, and the swelling of hands and feet were recognized by less than one-fourth of the lower-class participants in Koos's study.[9]

Social class differences are also quite pronounced relative to health priorities. In the lower class, health is found lower on the list of necessities unless a crisis is present. Jobs, food, and shelter are priorities for the poor.

Knowledge of Health

The family, as part of its task to protect the health of family members, sets up and carries out health maintenance activities based on what the parents or adult members believe to be healthy and what they feel is feasible. Families generally identify eating well and good nutrition as the most important methods of maintaining health.[10] Most families actively process and seek out information regarding health education, with a combination of mass media sources being most commonly cited. A considerable amount of health information is also shared among the family's social network of friends and relatives. Feldman found that the only health area a majority of parents did not cover with their children involved reproduction and sexuality.[11]

As illustrated by the previously mentioned studies of Baumann and Koos, the more educated a group or family is, the better the family's knowledge of health usually is. This expectation would have to be validated with a particular client. Also, certain family members, generally the mother, will be better informed. Women have consistently been found to have acquired more health education information due to their role responsibilities in the family.

Importance of Personal and Family Health Beliefs

What factors lead to the readiness and intention of an individual to seek health services or improve his or her life style, i.e., change personal health behaviors? Are the variables different for explaining preventive health actions (personal health practices and use of health services) versus explaining the seeking and receiving of curative health services or complying with the medical regimens? The most comprehensive scheme for looking at these important questions is the health belief model.[12] This model has been subjected to testing in a wide variety of preventive and curative health areas and, although modified since its inception, is felt to be the most efficacious tool for systematically analyzing personal health behavior, i.e., predicting such diverse activities as preventive health actions, medical care utilization, delay in seeking help, and compliance with medical regimens.[13]

The health belief model utilizes Lewin's theories stressing that it is the world of the perceiver that determines what he or she will do, not the physical environment, except as this environment is viewed by the individual. Lewin also identifies some aspects of life as having negative valence, some having positive valence,

and some a neutral one. Individuals seek to avoid the negatively valued aspects, whereas they incorporate the positive aspects into their lives. The original model dealt with explaining preventive health actions. In order for an individual to take preventive action to avoid disease, he or she would need to *believe* that (1) he or she was personally *susceptible* or *vulnerable* to the disease; (2) the illness was at least moderately *severe*, so the consequences of acquiring the disease would significantly disrupt that person's life; and (3) that taking a particular action would be *beneficial* (believing that effective and accessible health services exist) in that it would reduce susceptibility to or the severity of the disease; and (4) the *benefits outweighed the barriers* (costs, pain, time, convenience, and embarrassment). The susceptibility and seriousness of the disease again were perceived factors—not dependent on fact but on the person's personal beliefs. Both these individual perceptions become the "readiness" factors leading to the perceived threat of a disease. In the original model there were modifying factors (demographic, psychosocial, etc.) and cues to action. *Cues to action* refers to the immediate stimuli needed to trigger in the person's mind and recognition of the susceptibility and seriousness of a disease (the threat) and the need for taking action to reduce the threat.[14]

In newer, modified models (Fig. 15.1), the readiness factors have been extended to include both the perceived feelings of the susceptibility and seriousness of the health problem (the threat) and positive motivation to maintain, regain, or attain wellness. These motivations include concern about and the salience of health

FIGURE 15.1
Diagram of the (original) health belief model. *(From Rosenstock IM: Historical origins of the health belief model. In Becker MH (ed): The Health Belief Model and Personal Health Behavior. Thorofare, NJ, Charles B Slack, 1974, p 7)*

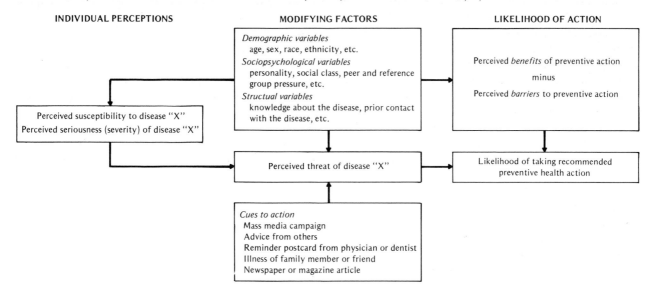

matters in general, willingness to seek and receive medical direction, plans to comply, and existence of positive health practices.[15]

In revised models used to explain sick-role behaviors and tested by a myriad of studies, additional modified and enabling factors have been inserted. These factors represent the variables identified as being significant in a multitude of compliance studies and include demographic, structural, attitudinal, and enabling factors.[16] These factors influence both the readiness to undertake recommended action and the likelihood that the appropriate actions will be taken.

In summary, the most important aspect to remember about this model is that it is a rational decision-making model, in which the occurrence of personal health behavior is influenced basically by several factors: (1) an individual's feelings of threat regarding a particular disease, consisting of perceptions of susceptibility and seriousness; (2) an individual's general positive motivation regarding health; and (3) an individual's belief regarding benefits minus barriers for seeking and accepting health care, with the above enabling and modifying variables affecting both the disposition to act and the actual outcome. The call to action—carrying out health behavior—is triggered by the presence of inner and outer environmental cues.

In regard to implications for family health care, this model was introduced at this point to emphasize the significance of the family's belief system (what they believe are serious health problems and what they believe in terms of their susceptibility to these health problems). If a family perceives a threat and if avenues are then presented to the family for reducing threat such as accessible and effective screening, health services, life-style improvements, and so on, the family will be more likely to act positively on their behalf. A health practitioner should not use the fear tactic, so as to build up anxiety and thus readiness, without offering an effective and accessible remedial action to handle and reduce threat, i.e., relating the dangers of lung cancer due to smoking and suggesting and referring to a health facility in the immediate future for chest x-rays. And needless to say, the emphasis in health education should be on the family's/individual's perceived benefits.

Langlie looked at social networks and their effects on personal health behavior, attempting to assess the ability of the health belief model to account for variation in preventive health behaviors. She found that the personal health behaviors were better when an individual had the perception of control over his or her health status and the benefits were seen as great and costs low, coupled with belonging to a social network characterized by middle and high socioeconomic class status and frequent interaction between nonkin that resulted in receiving "outside" information.[17]

HEALTH CARE FUNCTION

As elaborated in the introductory remarks, the health care function is not only a vital and basic family function, but also one which assumes a central focus in healthy, well-functioning families. Pratt underscores the significance of effective functioning in this area by stating, "The more numerous and vital the functions the family performs successfully for its members, the stronger the family system."[18] The focus of this section will be on exploring the question of how well a family fulfills its health care function.

Pratt assessed how well the contemporary American family is functioning as a personal health care system, examining the adequacy of health practices and home care for ill members, the use of professional health services, the level of health knowledge, and attitudes about good health.[19] Pratt found the family to be lacking. For instance, there is a serious breakdown between what should take place to maintain family members' health and what usually occurs. Significant indiscretions are present in the family's pattern of nutrition, exercising, rest, smoking, dental hygiene, communication, and self-care practices. Medication problems are commonplace. Care of dependent, sick, and/or disabled family members is often not possible or inadequately carried out. And a significant number of families either fail to utilize health services or use health services improperly, as in the misuse of emergency rooms for primary health services. Preventive health care is spotty, and although the level of health information is improving, it is still not sufficiently high to serve as a sound foundation in most families. Pratt concludes that "the composite picture is one of fundamental failure in caring for health."[20]

She suggests that the reasons for the ineffectiveness of families to provide health care for their members lies with both (1) the structure of the health care system and (2) the family structure.[21] Pratt found that when families had wide associations with organizations, engaged in common activities, and used community resources, they used health services more appropriately. Also, personal health practices were enhanced when husbands were actively involved in internal family affairs, including matters concerning the health care system. She identified certain basic problems with the structure of the medical care system that made it difficult for families to carry out their health care functions.

1. The health care system is organized predominantly around the interests and needs of health providers rather than consumers. This is operationalized by the preponderant control physicians have over their clients, hospitals, standard fees charged, and so forth. Professional auton-

omy is highly valued, resulting in inadequate re view and control over its members as professional organizations.

2. The hospital is organized bureaucratically, resulting in specialization of functions, rigidity of structure and roles, and depersonalization.[22]

In order for families to become a primary and effective health resource, they must become more involved in the health team and the total therapeutic process. This implies an equalitarian relationship with health providers in which both parties can openly express and negotiate in terms of their particular needs and interests. Pratt explains:

Families cannot become highly responsible about their health care duties if the professionals exclude them from participating in medical management. Nor can families provide good care for sickness at home unless provisions are made for the delivery of health services in the home.[23]

Such a partnership role is needed whether preventive health practices or curative and rehabilitative health needs are under consideration. People must be treated as responsible adults, not passive children, if health professionals wish them to assume self-responsibility.

Not only must the family be in partnership with health providers in directing and implementing their own health care, but clients should also be the ultimate decision makers and managers of those health issues affecting their welfare and lives. In order for clients to engage in effective self-care, they must have the knowledge and skills needed to provide good health care. This means that families need access to the primary sources of health information. Thus professionals must be willing to extend their role to include health education directed toward family self-care.

Most families appear to recognize the need to assume strong management of their own health care. However, both professionals and the health care industry—hospitals, pharmaceutical companies, supply companies, and health insurance industry—discourage it. Data from a study of family health behavior conducted by Pratt revealed that families who were most effective in obtaining appropriate medical services and who practiced a wellness life style on their own were the families referred to as "energized" families. These families assertively sought and verified information, made discriminating decisions, and negotiated aggressively with the health care system, rather than passively accepting and complying.[24]

HEALTH CARE PRACTICES

Promotion of health practices within the family is a basic goal of family-centered community health nurs-

ing. It becomes critical to gain information regarding the family's health practices to assist the family in health promotion and maintenance.

How well is a family performing the necessary health practices to protect and foster healthy growth and development? One often-used indication of the family's level of functioning is the overall level of health of its family members. This is often inferred by gathering information as to the incidence of disease per member in a specific period of time, realizing, of course, that the ages of individuals and their environment play major roles in the genesis and incidence of disease. Large families and families with young children, for example, have a greater incidence of disease per family. Troubled, problematic families are found to have less resistance to disease and thus have higher rates of disease than families who are functioning well.

In addition to looking at the overall health and illness patterns of family members, the presence or the absence of overt health practices are fruitful assessment areas, providing relevant areas for client education. Four primary areas of health practices will be explored in this section:

1. *Life-style practices*—diet, sleep and rest patterns, exercise and recreation, drug habits, and self-care.
2. *Environmental practices*—cleanliness and safety practices.
3. *Medically based preventive practices*—general physical examinations and more specifically, eye examinations and hearing examinations; immunizations; and record keeping.
4. *Dental health practices.*

Life-Style Practices

There are hundreds of thousands of Americans who die each year prematurely of diseases caused primarily by unhealthy life styles. These unnecessary mortalities result from heart disease, accidents, cirrhosis of the liver, suicide, homicide, and diabetes. Some 11.5 billion dollars are spent each year in the United States for health care associated with cigarette smoking, while at the same time the Federal Government provides subsidies to tobacco companies.[25] Nine million Americans are alcoholics or have serious problems with alcohol abuse.[26]

What we must realize, and this is supported by a myriad of articles and statistics, is that our overall health status is not related in any important degree to our health care systems and the differences in medical care provided. When differences among populations and their health status are examined at a specific point in time, other socioeconomic and cultural factors are found to be much more important than differences in the quantity and quality of health care. Fuchs, in his most recent book, *Who Shall Live?*, make this blatantly clear through a comparison of the states of Utah and Nevada in terms of their populations and health status:

> [These] contiguous states ... enjoy the same levels of income and medical care and are alike in many other respects but their levels of health differ enormously. The inhabitants of Utah are among the healthiest individuals in the United States, while the residents of Nevada are at the opposite end of the spectrum.... What, then, explains these huge differences? ... The answer almost surely lies in the different life styles of the residents of the two states.[27]

As a number of authors,[28-31] including Fuchs, have concluded, the greatest potential for improvement of both the overall and the individual's health status is through life-style improvement. Personal behavior changes are needed in the areas of diet, exercise, smoking, and alcohol consumption, which are critically important factors affecting health.*

Family Dietary Practices

The importance of nutritional awareness as a wellness strategy was explored in Chapter 2. In this section, specific assessment areas related to dietary practices are discussed. An assessment of the family's food practices will provide general information on (1) the adequacy of the family diet; (2) the function of mealtimes and the attitude toward food and mealtimes; (3) shopping practices; and (4) who is responsible for the planning, shopping, and preparation of meals.

The following specific assessment areas and questions are relevant here.

1. The adequacy of family's diet (the nutritional history):

    It is recommended for the nurse working with the family over any period of time that a 24-hour food history record (Fig. 15.2) of the family eating patterns during a typical day be completed, given the family's willingness and interest in this area. Needless to say, dietary variations exist among family members and must be considered. This record will serve as a valuable screening tool as well as provide specific data regarding what family members eat and where their dietary strengths and deficiencies lie. The 24-hour food history record is an excellent base for assisting families to assess their nutritional adequacy and nutritional goals. Having family members actively participate in the completion of the food

	Food Served	Quantity	Individual Differences. Everyone Eat?
Breakfast			
Snacks (between meals)			
Lunch			
Snacks (between meals)			
Dinner			
Snacks (between meals)			

FIGURE 15.2
The 24-hour food history record.

record, suggestions for improvement, and setting of goals for themselves is of the utmost importance in making this activity an effective one.

Using this record the nurse and family analyze the family's diet in terms of *caloric intake* (also observe family members' height and weight—the most valid index of caloric needs and status); the four food groups (the meats, milk, fruits and vegetables, and starches); critical vitamins and minerals not adequately assessed in the four food groups (vitamins A, C, and D, iron, calcium, and salt); amount and type of fat in diet (saturated versus unsaturated); and the amount of sucrose (refined sugar) in diet.* The amount of saccharin, sodium nitrates, coffee and tea consumed are recent nutritional concerns and should also be assessed.

Following from the 24-hour food record, the family nurse also needs to determine what the individual variances are. How does each person eat (types of food and quantity). His or her diet should be evaluated in relation to present nutritional status. This data would become part of the data on the individual health assessments. By learning about family food practices, preferences, and individual dietary habits, the nurse and family will gain a holistic picture of dietary patterns. For instance, is Johnnie's state of obesity and extensive tooth decay due to his eating excessive amounts of sugars and carbohydrates? If so, is this part of the family's customary diet, along with sedentary activities and poor dental hygiene? Or does the family serve well-

---

*Belloc and Breslow's study confirmed the importance of personal health habits.[32] See Chapter 2 for further information.

*For both assessment and intervention purposes, specific information is needed on the four food groups, number of servings needed for each of the various age groups, nutritious low-budget foods, and nutritional values of specific foods. Basic nutrition texts contain this information.

balanced meals and Johnnie's sweet intake is at school and/or a reflection of other problems?

Foods fads, special dietary beliefs or culturally based food patterns—such as dietary practices based on a traditional Jewish, Mexican, or Italian pattern, or special food practices based on a philosophic or health commitment such as held by many vegetarians—need to be appraised. Understanding the family's value system and beliefs underlying their food practices are also important and serve as a suitable foundation for later work with them on any modification which might be needed.

Obesity has been repeatedly demonstrated to be one of the key precursors to chronic illness (diabetes, arthritis, heart disease, back problems, etc.) and shortened longevity. Hence assessing the family's caloric intake and comparing this to their actual caloric need becomes germane to practice.

2. The function of mealtimes and the family's attitude toward food and mealtimes.

Does the family eat together (all meals, only dinner, etc.)? Is mealtime (when they are together) a social, pleasurable experience? How are the meals handled when the family doesn't eat together? When families are more atomistic or individualistic (each family member doing his/her own "thing"), junk foods and a less adequate diet are often found. In addition, it makes it difficult for the family to interact and share with each other, since mealtime is often the one opportunity families have to enjoy each other's company and share important and pleasurable experiences, thoughts, and feelings.

Do parents use the giving and withholding of food as reward and punishment? Where this occurs, the child learns to associate food with approval (love) and disapproval (rejection). Pairing food and social needs for love and acceptance is an unhealthy linkage, as counselors treating the obese will attest.

Shopping, Planning, and Preparation Practices. What are the shopping arrangements? Where is food purchased? Does the family plan for the week or several days at a time or do they operate on a meal-to-meal basis, shopping for each meal or one day at a time (this is certainly an inefficient means in terms of time and money)? What kind of budgetary limitations exist in their food shopping? If need is present, does family use food stamps? Is food storage and refrigeration adequate? What are usual ways in which food is prepared (fried, boiled, eaten cold, variety of means)?

Shopping, Preparation and Serving Responsibilities. Who is responsible for each of these tasks?

Although we generally assume that the mother-wife will be responsible, it is frequently otherwise.

Sleeping and Rest Practices

As reported by Belloc and Breslow, seven to eight hours of sleep on a regular basis for adults was found to be a health practice positively correlated with overall health status and increased longevity,[33] and regular, sufficient sleep patterns have been linked to improved mental status.[34] Every family has patterns for sleeping, even though in some families these patterns are erratic. The following assessment questions may be posed:

1. What are the usual sleeping habits of adults and children? Here one wants to know the number of hours of sleep per night. Are these suitable according to individual's age and health status?
2. Are there *regular* sleeping patterns, with regular hours for going to bed and getting up in the morning? Who decides when the children go to sleep?
3. Where do the family members sleep? In separate or shared beds? Are sleeping arrangements crowded?
4. Do any family members take naps or have any other regular means of resting or relaxing?

Under individual assessments relevant to sleep patterns, the nurse would want to find out if any individual had trouble sleeping (insomnia), what kind of trouble (i.e., falling to sleep, awakening early without being able to resume sleeping), and its recency (is the insomnia more frequent or severe than it used to be). Often, sleeping difficulties are due to housing and sleeping arrangements in the home.

Exercise and Recreation

Since regular exercise was found to be a pertinent health habit related positively to overall health, longevity, and improved mental outlook (see Chapter 2), the family nurse should include exercise patterns of family in her appraisal of family health habits. Specific assessment questions suggested are the following:

1. What types of family recreational pursuits (i.e., jogging, bicycling, swimming, dancing, tennis, etc.) are engaged in? How often?
2. Does everyone participate?
3. Does the family believe regular exercise and physical fitness are necessary for good health?
4. Do everyday activities involve any exercise?

Family's Drug Habits

As we know, taking medications is a ubiquitous activity of Americans, with over-the-counter drugs most often used (60 to 70 percent of the time). A significant amount of medication use by families is carried on as an alternative to professional care, since generally the health problems being treated are seen as too trivial to seek medical care or as conditions which the family can adequately handle. A national survey discovered that one-half of those sampled undertook self-medication for sore throats, coughs, colds, and upset and acid stomachs. Home over-the-counter medication was found not to be limited to gastrointestinal and upper respiratory complaints, but also covered other body system problems, including the central nervous system, urogenital tract, and skin.[35] Home medication is also frequently used as a supplement to professional treatment. Professional treatments are often altered or modified by patients, as seen in the extensive modifications made to diet and insulin regimen by diabetic patients. Prescribed medication, furthermore, is often rejected by patients. One study reported a rejection rate of 50 percent.[36]

Assessment of the family's use of over-the-counter and prescription drugs is obviously most important. What drugs does the family take and for what purposes? Are they over-the-counter drugs or prescription drugs? Drug abuse involves the regular taking of a deleterious or noxious quantity of any drug over a period of time. In a society where pills are regarded as a panacea for everything from sexual problems to headaches, it is no wonder that major community health problems exist in this area. By identifying drugs commonly used by the family, the assessor can look for possible side effects or harmful interactive effects. Also, drug usage can tell the nurse something about how the family and/or the family members cope with life events and health problems, as well as how they define health and illness.

Some over-the-counter drugs commonly taken by Americans are potentially harmful, or at best, unnecessary. The regular use of laxatives is an example. Although most of the fatal medication poisonings are caused by prescribed medications (with barbiturates heading the list), 20 percent are caused by over-the-counter drugs. Of the nonfatal drug poisonings, aspirin is the leading offender, primarily because of its tendency to produce gastrointestinal bleeding.

In homes where young children are present, storage of drugs and other hazardous substances in safe, child-proof containers and cupboards is imperative, as the incidence of poisoning among children is very high.

One important factor leading to medication poisonings is the tendency of older families to save and reuse medicines years later. Any nurse who has cared for older patients in their homes will attest to the fact that families will hoard medications prescribed many years ago and that many of these containers do not even contain the name and dosage of the drug. Such medications undergo change over time and, at best, become ineffective. Often families end up using their old medicines to treat a family member who they perceive to be experiencing the same or similar symptoms as the person for whom the drug was originally prescribed, and misdiagnosis by the family thus presents itself as a potential hazard.

In assessing the drug use of an older family, as part of a home health agency visit, it is suggested that the nurse both review with the family the medications in present use and make some attempt to convince them to properly dispose of drugs which are old, not marked, or not needed.

In considering drug habits, one should assess not only the use of medications, but also alcohol intake, smoking, and the use of caffeine and other stimulants. Smoking and alcohol intake should be assessed in terms of who uses either substance, and how much, when, and under what situations or circumstances. Is the use of tobacco or alcohol by a family member(s) perceived as a problem by that person or other family members? Does the use of alcohol interfere with their capacity to carry out their usual activities? How long has the present use of alcohol continued? What was the pattern of drinking in the past?

Smoking is included here as a "drug" to be assessed. This inhaled substance not only causes great harm but is also a most preventable habit. Some health authorities interpret the decline in mortality rates due to heart disease—beginning in 1975—to be primarily attributed to a decline in smoking in men 35 years of age and over.[37] However, the group that health professionals need to be most concerned with helping is the teenage population, since smoking often begins during these years, with 31 percent of teenage boys and 26 percent of teenage girls smoking regularly according to a nationwide survey conducted in 1974.[38]

Family's Self-care Practices

When assessing a family, a determination is needed of both the family's ability to provide self-care and their actual competence in health matters. Self-care practices involve not only the preventive practices just described, diagnosis, and home treatment of common and minor ambulatory health problems, but also include all the procedures and treatments prescribed for the care of illness of a family member, such as giving medications, using special appliances, dressings, exercises, and special diets. How adequately is the family able to handle the responsibilities of these therapies?

Estimates from the literature report that 75 to 85

percent of all health care is provided by self or family. These percentages hold for both populations who have and do not have access to professional health services.[39] There is no firm data demonstrating that lay-initiated self-care is any less effective than professional care (which is about 35 percent effective), or less dangerous (which involves 20 percent iatrogenic ill effects and 4 to 11 percent complications from nosocomial infections).[40] The authors Elliott-Binns in Britain and Poul Pedersen in Denmark found that 90 percent of self-care procedures taken prior to professional intervention were appropriate and helpful.[41, 42]

An assessment of a family's ability and use of self-care provides the foundation for our nursing intervention in that it identifies the family's strengths, resources, and potentials, in addition to the family's willingness to accept help. In evaluating the family's level of competence in handling health problems, we may find that a family or one of its members may be experiencing severe health problems, but if they are competently managing or coping with these, there may be no further nursing action indicated, except perhaps to provide support.

Environmental Practices

Environmental practices consist of habits or patterns which positively or negatively affect the family's or its members' health status. Smoking can be included here, although already covered elsewhere. It should be noted that smoking affects the health of other members of the family as well as that of the smoker. Respiratory infections are more frequent in the children of smokers than in those of nonsmokers. Air pollution in home and neighborhood can be caused by other pollutants beside tobacco smoke. How close does the family live to the nearest factory (and what kind of factory is it)? Is the family regularly exposed to smoke, herbicides, asbestos, or other harmful substances at work? Noise pollution may also be harmful, as well as water pollution and radiation exposure. More and more evidence demonstrates the adverse effects of long-term, low-level exposure to noise and to chemicals in our air, water, and food.

The family's hygiene and cleanliness practices may also be considered as environmental practices. Although cleanliness is not "next to Godliness," there are several general health habits which reduce the possibility of infection and its spread:

1. Washing before meals and after toileting.
2. Using separate towels. When an infectious skin condition such as scabies or impetigo is present, sharing towels can be a real problem.
3. Drinking from separate cups and glasses which are clean. In families with several children and an overworked and overwhelmed mother, you may see after the baby finishes his or her bottle or cup of milk that it sits a long time and is later drunk by the same or another child. A mother may not realize how rapidly milk spoils.
4. Bathing and cleanliness. As community health workers, we must realize our biases here. Most health workers have been found to be overly critical of families that they serve in terms of degree of family cleanliness. We need to carefully differentiate between family hygiene practices which are, in fact, deleterious to health and those which are contrary to our own habits and customs but are *not* harmful in terms of health.

Safety practices could also be included here, but have already been included in Chapter 8 as part of environmental data.

Medically Based Preventive Measures

In Chapter 2 the issue of whether annual physical examinations should be recommended to well (asymptomatic) clients was discussed. As mentioned, complete annual physical examinations for such populations are cost-ineffective and a waste of our precious health resources. On the other side, a selective preventive-oriented physical examination on a regular periodic basis is cost-effective and able to screen for and educate clients about the major health hazards for which they are at risk.

Annual health assessments (physical examination, history, and diagnostic tests) tailored to the client's age, race, and sex are vital and serve several purposes. They provide the necessary information to jointly establish with the client a health maintenance plan. The preventive health assessment identifies risk factors particular to an individual; for example, an adult who smokes and whose father died of heart disease has twice the risk of incurring heart disease as an individual who does not smoke and has no family history of disease. Health assessments can also detect unnoticed or covert signs and symptoms crucial for case finding (early detection and treatment).

Major risk factors are related to heredity, sex, race, and age. For instance, individuals whose families have had heart disease, diabetes, or cancer have an increased likelihood of inheriting a predisposition toward those diseases. Thanks to their sex hormones, premenopausal women are less likely to have myocardial infarctions than men of the same age group. Blacks have more than twice the chance of developing hypertension than whites. And generally, the older one gets, the greater the chance of developing a chronic illness.

This does not imply, however, that the above risk factors are inevitable harbingers of future events. In fact, susceptibility to some diseases can actually be reduced if an attempt is made to attenuate risk factors by improving one's life style and seeking routine, preventive health care.

What should be included in the annual health assessment of the well adult? Again, opinion varies. The minimum should probably be a general history (review of the systems and any present complaints), blood pressure, vital signs, weight, and urinalysis; for women, a pap smear and breast and pelvic examinations are indicated; for men older than 30 to 35 years of age, an electrocardiogram, heart auscultation, rectal examination, and lipid panel (serum cholesterol and triglycerides) should be performed. Middle-aged men should also have a protoscopy or sigmoidoscopy of the rectum done for detection of cancerous polyps, and blacks should be tested for sickle-cell anemia.

What are the family's feelings about having a "physical" when they are well? Past practices of the family may be a gauge to their feelings; nevertheless, a lack of periodic well-care may also be a function of inaccessibility to, ignorance about, and/or costs of such services, so that in order to ascertain the reasons behind not receiving health examinations, more direct questions may be warranted. In 1971 the National Center for Health Statistics reported that racial minorities and low-income groups were less likely to have a general checkup than whites and higher-income groups. Moreover, the difference between the highest and lowest socioeconomic groups was two to one.[43]

Vision and Hearing Examinations

Health assessments should be supplemented by vision and hearing examinations. This is particularly important, since glaucoma and hearing loss can be detected and can usually be treated effectively or prevented.

Children should have periodic vision and hearing examinations done as part of their well-baby and preschool care. During the school years children are periodically given Snellen tests, a rough screen for common vision problems.

Adults who wear glasses need an eye examination annually, unless visual changes are noted sooner. For others, every other year is adequate. The eye examination should include tonometry testing for detection of glaucoma, which is recommended on a yearly basis for all adults over 40 years of age.

If families do not know of an eye specialist to call, the nurse will need to review with the family the difference in training and focus of an optician, optometrist, and ophthalmologist. If while eliciting a family medical history, the nurse finds a history of glaucoma in the family, he or she should stress an annual eye examination even more vigorously, as there is now an overwhelming evidence of a higher incidence of glaucoma among siblings and offspring of patients with the disease than among the rest of the population.[44]

Since hearing difficulties can lead to serious behavioral and learning problems in school, children should be routinely given an audiometric test during the early school years. Primary care practitioners should also complete rough screening for hearing during well child care visits.

Although asymptomatic adults may not need annual audiometric testing, if hearing difficulties are noted or an individual is at high risk, testing is indicated. Progressive hearing loss can occur from exposure to certain types of noise. If a client is exposed to a high level of noise at work or home, the nurse should inquire into his or her use of ear protectors and hearing examinations. Hearing loss can also occur with age, due to vascular insufficiency of the cochlea. Smokers have greater hearing loss than nonsmokers, as smoking reduces the blood supply by vasospasm induced by nicotine, by atherosclerotic narrowing of the vessels, and by formation of thrombi in the vessels.[45]

Immunization Status

The most important specific preventive measure is that of immunization. At least 75 to 80 percent of susceptible children must be immunized to effectively protect a community from preventable communicable diseases.[46] Hence promotion of immunization services is a vital and integral part of family health care. For infants and children the need for being adequately protected against tetanus, diphtheria, pertussis (whooping cough), polio, mumps, rubella (German measles), and rubeola (measles) is crucial. Smallpox vaccinations are no longer advised, since the risk of untoward reactions to the vaccine are now greater than the risk of contracting the disease. Flu vaccines and tuberculin skin tests are also recommended for certain age groups and under certain situations. (The conditions and age of the person and the community incidence and exposure risk are important variables here.) Booster shots of diphtheria and tetanus are recommended for adults every 7 to 10 years, since both of these diseases are serious and still extant throughout the United States today.

When completing an assessment of the immunization status of family members, record the types of immunizations received, dates, and any adverse reactions to immunization.

Dental Health Care Practices

Dental health practices are vital in maintaining good teeth throughout an individual's life span. The prevalence of dental ill health is great, especially among the poor of our country.

Dental health care has been separated from preventive care and health practices, since it includes both of these elements. In order to maintain high-level dental health, a combination of personal habits or practices, as well as preventive care by dentist and/or dental hygienist, should be carried out. The four vital elements consist of (1) regular preventive dental services (dental examination, x-rays, cleaning, education, and for children topical fluoride treatments when indicated); (2) use of fluoridated water if available; (3) regular brushing of teeth after meals as well as flossing; and (4) reduced amounts of certain types of carbohydrates in the diet.

Although dental caries (commonly known as cavities) are the most prevalent dental disease, gum diseases are widely seen among adults. Periodontal disease is also common in adults and is the primary cause of loss of teeth in adults over 40 years old.

Dental caries are said to be one of the most prevalent diseases in man.[47] In the past the only way to handle this disease was to repair the lesions through dental restorations (fillings). Now through dissemination of research findings regarding the nature and course of caries formation, new methods of prevention and treatment are being utilized, including topical application of fluorides and oral hygiene.

Dental caries result from the interaction of several processes, primarily the amount and type of carbohydrates in the diet, the amount of plaque buildup, and the resistance of the teeth. Reduction in the amount of carbohydrate available in the mouth results in a less favorable environment for plaque formation, the precursor to dental caries and periodontal disease. Sugar clearance of carbohydrates (the length of time it takes the carbohydrate or sugars to disappear from the saliva) is an important element to consider; it is largely influenced by the type of carbohydrates ingested. It has been found that the sugar clearance of confectionary products (candies) is less than that of several breads (rye and white breads) with the exception of candies such as caramels which stick to the teeth. This is because bread can be retained on the teeth, retarding its clearance from the saliva and the mouth. A slow clearance means that carbohydrate is available to the oral bacteria for a longer time and the client is subject to greater risk of developing caries. Chewing gum is also quite poor in terms of sugar clearance due to the long period of time the sugar in the gum takes to dissolve.[48]

In order to control the plaque formation, which in turn controls the bacterial levels involved in dental caries, proper dental hygiene is needed. Kleinberg reports that

> there is no question that bacteria in the form of an adhering plaque are necessary for the formation of the caries lesion. In the most inaccessible regions of the human dentition . . . the plaque is seldom disturbed and there caries occur most frequently. The toothbrush is only partly effective in cleaning these sites. As a result, other devices such as dental floss have become popular. Only

recently has a study indicated that flossing of the approximating surfaces is of benefit in reducing approximal caries.[49]

Few persons know how to remove plaque effectively from their teeth and the surrounding gingivae according to Kleinberg. He suggests that learning how to brush teeth properly to remove plaque would probably be one of the best investments that a person could make in preserving his or her own dental health. Disclosing solutions are helpful in locating plaque buildup on the teeth.[50]

The United States Department of Health, Education, and Welfare in 1972 published the results of a large national health survey of periodontal disease and oral hygiene among children. They reported that many families were found to brush their teeth inadequately or not after meals and to use defective equipment (toothbrushes). Two-thirds of the children in the national survey were discovered to have moderate to large amounts of plaque loosely attached to teeth, showing that their dental hygiene practices were insufficient.[51]

The family health nurse, in teaching families dental health and hygiene, may wish to check the mouths of some of the children or adults for plaque buildup or bring some disclosing solution which they can use to detect plaque themselves. Teeth should be brushed after meals, and the sooner the better, to prevent sugars from remaining in the mouth. The object of brushing is to remove plaque and food particles from the teeth, which is done by effective friction of the toothbrush (a soft-bristled one) against the surface of the teeth. It is important to use dental floss once a day to supplement brushing, since some surfaces of the teeth and teeth–gum junctions are inaccessible by brushing alone.

Families (both children and adults) need thorough demonstrations of an effective method for brushing teeth. There are several acceptable ways to brush one's teeth; newer methods are much more effective than the older vertical (from gum line or down) method taught in the past. Regular, after-meal brushing and flossing teeth is considered a vital aspect in the prevention of dental caries, gum disease, and periodontal disease.

Routine dental examinations, including periodic x-rays, and cleaning of teeth are needed, minimally once a year, although this varies with each individual and his or her rate of plaque formation. Many dentists advise preventive care every six months. Dental checkups should begin at an early age, preferably preschool, and continue throughout one's lifetime, since doing so is extremely important in preventing the development of serious dental problems in the adult years.

Diekelmann, in describing primary health care for the well adult, remarks that even well-educated young adults do not know that loss of teeth with aging is not inevitable. Though every middle or older adult in the family may wear dentures, there is no reason why the young adult must anticipate the same for himself. Certainly there is an inherited trend; but the determining factor is often the degree and extent of routine dental care and dental hygiene. There is another very strong motive for care of the teeth at this age which the nurse should emphasize: the loss of teeth in itself accelerates aging and is often the cause of gastrointestinal problems in old age.[52]

The greatest success in curtailing the formation of dental caries has been achieved through the methods of increasing the resistance of the teeth to the acid generated by the plaque bacteria during the fermentation of dietary carbohydrate. The most acclaimed and widely used method is that of application or ingestion of fluoride.[53]

Systemic use of fluoride through the water supply has proven most effective—preventing nearly two out of three caries in children. Moreover, children are not the only ones to benefit from fluoridated water. Adults who have consumed fluoridated water throughout their lives can expect less decay, fewer extractions, and fewer dentures at age 65.[54] Less but still effective are the various means of applying fluoride topically, including application of solutions by a dentist or self-administration by the client.

Treatment of dental problems has not been mentioned except in passing, but is also of vital import. Although prevention has been stressed, early detection and treatment of dental and gum problems will certainly keep more serious problems from developing. Malposition problems—over- and underbites, unequal exertion of pressure on teeth—are targets for early detection in children. Orthodontia may be needed to correct these problems, which if untreated could later cause periodontal disease and speech problems, as well as resulting in cosmetic ill effects.

FAMILY MEDICAL HISTORY

This area is of great importance for several reasons: first, family histories will often identify familial risk factors of family members; second, the family's experience with certain diseases will possibly have resulted in fears, myths, or misconceptions about these illnesses, and the health worker should be sensitive to them; and third, through eliciting a family medical history, the assessor will learn more about both families of orientation and thus gain a better understanding of the family's past.

The family medical history consists of an identification of past and present environmentally and genetically related diseases of the family of orientation —going back to maternal and paternal grandparents

and including aunts and uncles and their children. Besides ascertaining the general health status of all these individuals, the family-centered health worker should specifically inquire about the presence of the following diseases, since people often forget important familial diseases:

1. Environmentally related diseases (to which family member might be or have been exposed)
   a. Psychosocial problems: mental illness and obesity.
   b. Infectious diseases: typhoid fever, tuberculosis, venereal disease, hepatitis, diarrheas (dysenteries), skin diseases (scabies, lice, impetigo)
2. Genetically linked diseases
   Epilepsy, diabetes, cystic fibrosis, mental retardation, sickle-cell anemia, kidney disease, hypertension, heart disease, cancer, leukemia, vision and hearing defects, hemophilia, and allergies, including asthma.

Some practitioners suggest drawing a family tree, including the ages of members, whether the individual is living or deceased, the cause of death, level of general health, and presence of chronic disease. Diekelmann, in describing elements within a family history, recommends using the family tree shown in Figure 15.3 for assessment.

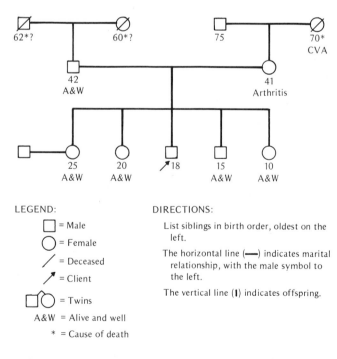

LEGEND:

☐ = Male
○ = Female
╱ = Deceased
↗ = Client
☐○ = Twins
A&W = Alive and well
  * = Cause of death

DIRECTIONS:

List siblings in birth order, oldest on the left.

The horizontal line (—) indicates marital relationship, with the male symbol to the left.

The vertical line (I) indicates offspring.

FIGURE 15.3
Family health tree for use in assessment. Directions for use are as follows: list siblings in birth order, starting from the left; the horizontal line indicates a marital relationship, with the male symbol at the left; the vertical line indicates offspring. *(From: Diekelmann N: Primary Health Care of the Well Adult. New York, McGraw-Hill, 1977, p 225)*

FAMILY HEALTH RECORDS

Families change physicians, are seen at several agencies or different specialists for different diseases, the years pass, and memories fade. All these factors underscore the need for families to keep records of the year-by-year medical events of each of the family members.*

Educating families about the importance of maintaining family medical records is an important health education area and critical for assisting families to become responsible for their health care. The data the family maintains will aid the family when new doctors are visited and may also obviate the need for expensive and time-consuming laboratory and diagnostic tests. And facts given in the record may assist a family in obtaining faster and more accurate diagnoses.

When there are young children in the family or adult members, especially oldsters, who have several illnesses and are seeing more than one physician concurrently, it is especially critical to have medical record information. For children, immunization records are important; for adults, diagnostic and laboratory tests, diagnoses, medications taken, and any adverse reactions to them should be carefully recorded.

The following broad areas of health information need to be included:

    family medical history (see previous section);
    maternity record;
    children's heights and weights;
    adults' weight records;
    childhood diseases (of children);
    accident records;
    major surgeries, illnesses, and hospitalizations;
    immunization records;
    allergies;
    corrective devices (glasses, hearing aids, dental plates, and special shoes are examples);
    blood groups and Rh factors;
    blood pressure; and other laboratory tests performed.†

FAMILY'S UTILIZATION OF HEALTH SERVICES

One of the central responsibilities of the family fulfilling the health care function is making appropriate use of health services to meet the on-going health needs of each family member. Health providers have long been concerned about the inadequate utilization of health resources by many families. Delays in seeking or returning for professional care are also cited as problems, as is the widespread problem of noncompliance among patients. Noncompliance ranges from 40 to 96 percent in a variety of recent studies, with noncompliance increasing where duration of medical regimen is prolonged or complicated or involves behavioral changes such as modifications in diet, exercise, and/or smoking.

Of course, many barriers are responsible for this sorry state of affairs. Tinkham and Voorhies comment that

> families today are victims of a maze of health care services and facilities. The specialism in medicine makes it virtually impossible to obtain a family physician, and patients are shuttled back and forth from one specialist to another. One of the ironies of this affluent country in the latter third of the twentieth century is that hospital emergency rooms are replacing the family physician. The high cost of medical and dental care is also one of the deterrents to seeking help.[55]

Throughout the discussion that follows concerning pertinent studies and statistics on family utilization of health and dental services, utilization will be referred to as the degree to which individuals use various types of medical services and facilities in seeking help for, or in preventing, health-related problems.[56]

Number of Medical Visits

The average number of visits the American family makes to physicians, laboratories, and dentists is greater than expected. Families consisting of husband, wife, and one or more children under 17 years of age averaged approximately 20 per year[57, 58] or 5.8 visits per person.[59] Men are found to use medical services less frequently and have fewer disability days than women, and parents make fewer visits than children.[60]

The National Center for Health Statistics reports that primarily due to Medicare, Medicaid, and the growth of health insurance coverage during the past 15 years, obtaining medical care has become less of a problem for certain segments of the population. Such barriers as cost and transportation still exist, but family income no longer accounts for a substantial difference in the percentage of people who visit a physician at least once during the year. Since the need for medical care is greater among low-income families, they should probably be seeing a physician more often than higher-income groups. The differences in income groups and their utilization patterns of medical services is greatest in services received by children. In

---

* The Department of Health, Education, and Welfare publishes a free booklet for families titled, "How to Keep Your Family's Health Records," DHEW Publication Number HRA 77-634. The American Medical Association (535 North Dearborn Street, Chicago, Illinois 60601) also issues an inexpensive pamphlet, "Family Health Record," which is an excellent guide for assisting a family in keeping complete and accurate medical histories.

† These areas are well explained, including format in which information should be recorded, in DHEW Publication Number HRA 77-634.

1975, 93 percent of children under five years in families who made $15,000 per year or more, saw a physician at least once during that year, while 86 percent of these children in families who made $5,000 or less did so.[61]

Generally, preventive health services are not well utilized by families, irrespective of all socioeconomic strata. In one of Pratt's studies she found that 50 percent of the family members had not had a physical examination in the past three years and 60 percent had not had a preventive dental check or cleaning of teeth during the same period.[62]

Utilization Patterns and Family Life Cycle

McEwan and Bruce have described the important role the family life cycle may play in determining the use of health services within a family.[63,64] On the whole, families tend to exhibit considerable variation in their needs and use of health services over the course of the life cycle. Thus the young and healthy childless couple tends to use relatively few health services, whereas families in the reproductive years are likely to make significant use of hospital and physician services, largely those associated with maternal and child care. When the size of the family begins to decline as children leave home, there is a concomitant reduction in the total amount of medical care received, offset in part by a rise in use per family member associated with the increased incidence of chronic illness from the middle years on.[65]

Utilization Patterns and Accessibility

A family's response to the onset of the health problems of one of its members is determined by several factors. Foremost, the family must recognize that the particular health problem requires medical attention. After this stage, pragmatic accessibility factors become paramount, that is, is there a physician or health agency which is available to the family? Accessibility means not only that the health resource exists, but also that the family can afford it financially, its hours of operation are amenable to the family's schedule, transportation to it is convenient, and, most important, the family has this information.

One index of accessibility is the determination of how adequate the numbers of health providers, physicians primarily, are to individuals living within the community. As has long been known, there are more physicians, both in absolute numbers and on a per capita basis, in and near metropolitan areas than in rural areas. Doctors in urban areas are more often specialists, while doctors located in rural areas or in small communities tend to be generalists. The concentration of physicians makes a difference in the number of visits made to physicians yearly; thus in the metropolitan areas the number of visits was significantly greater than rural areas.[66]

In 1978, Kronenfeld reported a study which identified the factors influencing the use of ambulatory health services. He found four patterns to be the key predictors of utilization. These included the following: (1) the more providers an individual saw the more visits were made; (2) utilization increases with the number of health conditions present and the number of disability days accrued in a year; (3) if a person has government insurance (Medicaid and/or Medicare) his or her use was greater; and (4) the lower the income level the greater the utilization. The increased utilization observed when multiple affiliations with providers existed was felt to result from the lack of coordination between specialists and generalists as the patient moved through the system.[67]

Utilization Patterns and Socioeconomic Status

Does being poor influence the utilization of health services? Since the enactment of Medicare and Medicaid, the poor actually visit doctors more often than the nonpoor. In addition to having more illnesses and more severe health problems, the poor use general practitioners more than specialists and seek medical care when health conditions have become more severe and difficult to treat, often seeking care in emergency rooms.[68] As with Kronenfeld's study, Galvin's utilization study also found that the poor visited physicians more frequently than the nonpoor (as shown in Fig. 15.4).[69, 70]

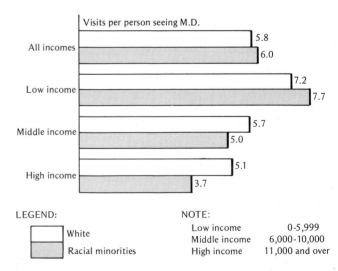

FIGURE 15.4
Mean number of physician visits per person by family income and race in the United States during 1970. (From: US Department of Health, Education, and Welfare: Health of the Disadvantaged Chartbook, DHEW Publication No. HRA 77–628, September 1977, p 37)

Poverty definitely makes a difference as to who receives dental care. The National Center for Health Statistics reports the following information:

Family income makes a significant difference in determining who will see a dentist at least once during the year. In 1975, in every age group, the proportion of people who saw a dentist was smaller in families of lower income than in families with higher incomes. Generally, Medicare offers no coverage, and Medicaid and private health insurance plans offer only limited coverage for dental services.

Among children ages 5–14, who should be seeing a dentist at least once a year, only 48 percent of the children from low income families and 78 percent of those from families with incomes of $15,000 or more saw a dentist even once during the year. At older ages the differences were as great.[71]

A determination of a family's actual use of health resources and an interpretation of whether this use is appropriate (based on family's needs) is the focus of this part of the assessment. Otto, the author of the family strengths approach to family analysis, identifies the appropriate use of community resources as a strength, while inappropriate use of community resources is a weakness.[72] Examples of insufficient and inappropriate use of available resources include the family that does not avail itself of food stamps, although their diet is sorely in need of nutritional supplementation; or the case of the low-income family who does not use the free pediatric clinic at the health department when one of the children is ill, but waits until the child's condition deteriorates and then rushes the child to a private hospital's emergency room (both a misuse of emergency rooms and also a terrible expense to the family and to the child's health).

As many health providers would attest, inadequately functioning families will often have hostility, bitterness, or apathy toward available health resources to the extent that serious health problems of their children go unattended or that health needs of parents prevent them from adequately caring for children.[73]

ASSESSMENT QUESTIONS

The following areas and questions are germane relative to the family's health care function.

1. Family's definition of health/illness and their level of knowledge:

   How does the family decide on who is sick or ill, what clues give them this impression, and who decides?

   Does the family know the pertinent information about health promotion, disease, treatment, and hazards?

   Can the family observe and report significant symptoms and changes?

   What serious health problems do family members perceive themselves susceptible or vulnerable to and what are their beliefs about the effectiveness and appropriateness of health actions to resolve these problems?

2. Family dietary practices:

   Is the family diet adequate? (A 24-hour food history record of family eating patterns is recommended.)

   What is the function of mealtimes and the family's attitude toward food and mealtimes?

   Shopping practices.

   Budgeting limitations (use of food stamps).

   Adequacy of storage and refrigeration. Ways food is prepared.

   Who is responsible for the planning, shopping, and preparation of meals?

3. Sleep and rest habits:

   What are the usual sleeping habits of family members? Are they appropriate to age and health status? Are regular hours established for sleeping? Who decides when children go to sleep?

   Where do family members sleep?

   Do family members take naps or have other regular means of resting or relaxing?

4. Exercise and recreation (duplicative of identifying data except for):

   Does the family believe regular exercise and physical fitness are necessary for good health?

   Do daily (work) activities allow for exercise?

5. Family's drug habits:

   What is the use of alcohol, tobacco, coffee, cola, or tea (caffeine and theobromine are stimulants)?

   Is the use of tobacco or alcohol by family members perceived as a problem?

   Does the use of alcohol interfere with the capacity to carry out usual activities? How long has family member been using alcohol?

   Family's use of over-the-counter and prescription drugs:

   Does family save drugs over long periods of time and reuse?

   Are drugs properly labeled and in safe place, away from children?

6. Family's role in self-care practices:

   Who is (are) health leader(s) in the family? Who

makes the health decisions in the family?

How competent is the family in self-care relative to recognition of signs and symptoms, diagnosis, and home treatment of common, simple health problems?

7. Environmental practices:

How exposed to air and/or noise pollution are family members?

What are the family's hygiene and cleanliness practices?

8. Medically based preventive measures:

Are periodic physical examinations appropriate for age, sex, and health status?

What are the family's feelings about having physicals when well?

When were last eye and hearing examinations?

What is the immunization status of the family?

9. Dental health practices:

What are the family's nutritional habits? (Include the amounts and types of starches and sugars consumed by the family.)

Brushing of teeth after meals.

Use of topical fluoride, fluoride tablets, or rinses if water supply not fluoridated.

Regular dental checkups, cleaning, and repair.

10. Family medical history: (Question regarding overall health of grandparents and aunts and uncles and if specific diseases have been present.)

Identification of past and present environmentally related diseases of the family of orientation of parents (and parents' siblings).

Identification of past and present genetically related diseases of family of orientation of parents (and parents' siblings).

11. Health services received:

What physician and/or health agency does the family receive care from?

Does this source see all members of the family and take care of all their health needs?

12. Feelings and perceptions regarding health services:

What are the family's feelings and perceptions regarding the health services they receive?

Is the family comfortable and satisfied with the care they receive and their relationships with their physician(s), family health nurse, school nurse, and/or the other health providers they are currently seeing?

Do they have confidence in their doctor, nurse(s), and social worker?

How do they perceive of the role of the various health providers?

If you are the community health nurse visiting the home, how does the family see your role?

What has been the family's past experience with the community health nurse?

13. Emergency health services:

Does the agency or physician the family receives care from have an emergency service?

Are medical services by current health providers available if an emergency occurs?

If emergency services are not available, does the family know where the closest available (according to their eligibility) emergency services are for both the children and the adult members of the family?

Does the family know how to call for an ambulance and paramedic services?

Does family have an emergency health plan?

14. Dental health services:

What dental health services are/have been received by members of the family?

15. Source of payment:

How will the family pay for services it receives or might receive?

Does the family have a private health insurance plan, Medicare, or Medicaid; or must the family pay for services in full or partially?

Does the family receive any free services (or know about those available to them)?

What effect does the cost of health care have on the utilization of health services?

If the family has health insurance (either private, Medicare, or Medicaid), is the family informed about what services are covered, such as preventive services, special medical equipment, home visits, and so forth?

16. Logistics of receiving care:

How far away are health care facilities from the family's home?

What modes of transportation does the family use to get to them?

If the family must depend on public transportation, what problems exist in regard to hours of service and travel time to health facilities?

REFERENCES

1. Pratt L: Changes in health care ideology in relation to self-care by families. Health Educ Monog 5(2):121–122, 1977
2. Leslie GR: The Family in Social Context. New York, Oxford University Press, 1976, p 233
2a. Adams BN: The American Family: A Sociological Interpretation. Chicago, Markham, 1971, p 84
3. Pratt L: Family Structure and Effective Health Behavior: The Energized Family. Boston, Houghton Mifflin, 1976
4. McLachlan JM: Cultural factors in health and disease. In

Jaco EG (ed): Patients, Physicians, and Illness. New York, Free Press, 1958, pp 94–105

5. Jahoda M: Current Concepts of Postitive Mental Health. Joint Commission on Mental Illness and Health, Monograph No. 1. New York, Basic, 1958

6. Irelan LM (ed): Low-Income Life Styles. US Department of Health, Education, and Welfare, Social and Rehabilitation Services. Washington DC, Government Printing Office, 1972, pp 56–57 (See also, Kane RL, Kasteler JM, Gray RM (eds): The Health Gap. New York, Springer, 1976)

7. Baumann B: Diversities in conceptions of health and physical fitness. J Health Hum Behav 2(1):40, 1961

8. Koos EL: The Health of Regionville. New York, Columbia University Press, 1954

9. Ibid.

10. Pratt, op. cit., p 21

11. Feldman JJ: The Dissemination of Health Information. Chicago, Aldine, 1966. Reported in Pratt L, p 21

12. Berkanovic E: Behavioral science and prevention. Prev Med 5:93, 1976

13. Becker MH (ed): The Health Belief Model and Personal Health Behavior. Thorofare, NJ, Charles B. Slack, 1974, p v

14. Rosenstock IM: Historical origins of the health belief model. In Becker, op. cit., pp 1–8

15. Becker MH: The health belief model and sick role behavior. In Becker, op. cit., p 89

16. Ibid.

17. Langlie JK: Social networks, health beliefs, and preventive health behavior. J Health Soc Behav 18:258, 1977

18. Pratt, op. cit., p 122

19. Ibid., p 33

20. Ibid., pp 45–46

21. Ibid., pp 45–46

22. Ibid., pp 49–56, 56–68

23. Ibid., p 171

24. Ibid., pp 106–123

25. Walker WJ: Government subsidized death and disability. JAMA 20:1530, 1974

26. ———. Alcoholism in the United States. Statistical Bulletin, Metropolitan Life Insurance Company, July 1974, p 3

27. Fuchs VR: Who Shall Live?—Health, Economics, and Social Choice. New York, Basic, 1974, pp 52–53

28. Ardell DB, Newman AB: Health promotion: Strategies for planning. Health Values: Achieving High-Level Wellness 1(3):100, 1977

29. Fuchs, op. cit.

30. Somers AR (ed): Promoting Health. Germantown, Md, Aspen Publication, 1976

31. Berkanovic, op. cit.

32. Belloc NB: Relationship of health practices and mortality. Prev Med 2:67–81, 1973

33. Ibid.

34. Berkman PL: Measurement of mental health in a general population survey. Am J Epidemiol 94(2):105, 1971

35. Roney TG, Nall ML: Medication Practices in a Community: An Exploratory Study. Menlo Park, California, Stanford Research Institute, 1966

36. Linnett M: Prescribing habits in general practice. Proceedings of the Royal Society of Medicine 61:613–615, 1970

37. United States Department of Health, Education, and Welfare: Health, United States Chartbook, 1976–1977. US Public Health Services, Publication No. HRA 77–1233, 1977, p 18

38. Ibid., p 17

39. Levin LS: Forces and issues in the revival of interest in self-care: impetus for reduction in health. In Fonaroff A, Levin LS: Issues in self-care. Health Educat Monogr 5(2):116, 1977

40. Ibid., p 116

41. Elliott-Binns CP: An analysis of lay medicine. J R Coll Gen Pract 23:255, 1973

42. Pedersen P: Varighed fra sygdoms begyndelse til henvendelse til prakliserende laege. Ugeskr Laeg 138:32, August 2, 1976. Reported in Levin LS, p 116

43. United States Department of Health, Education, and Welfare: Health of the Disadvantaged Chartbook. US Public Health Services, Publication No. HRA 77–628, September 1977, p 41

44. Perkins EJ: Screening for ophthalmic conditions. Practitioner 211:171–177, 1973

45. Diekelmann N: Primary Health Care of the Well Adult. New York, McGraw-Hill, 1977, p 234

46. Garner MK: Our values are showing: Inadequate childhood immunization. Health Values: Achieving High Level Wellness 2(3):129, 1978

47. Kleinberg I: Prevention and dental caries. J Prev Dent 5(3):9, 1978

48. Ibid., p 12

49. Ibid., p 14

50. Ibid.

51. United States Department of Health, Education, and Welfare: Periodontal Disease and Oral Hygiene Among Children. US Public Health Services, Series 11, No. 117, June 1972

52. Diekelmann, op. cit., p 235

53. Kleinberg, op. cit., p 15

54. United States Department of Health, Education, and Welfare: Fluoridation is for Everyone. US Public Health Services, Publication No. EDC 77-8834, 1977

55. Tinkham CW, Voorhies EF: Community Health Nursing: Evolution and Process, 2nd ed. New York, Appleton, 1977, p 142

56. Kane RL, Kasteler JM, Gray RM (eds): The Health Gap. New York, Springer, 1976, p 8

57. United States Department of Health, Education, and Welfare: Physician Visits, United States, 1969. US Public Health Services, Series 10, No. 75, 1972

58. Pratt L, op. cit., p 30

59. Anderson R, Lion J, Anderson O: Two Decades of Health Services. New York, Ballinger, 1976

60. Pratt, op. cit., p 24

61. USDHEW, HRA 77-1233, op. cit., p 21

62. Pratt, op. cit., p 40

63. McEwan PJM: The Social Approach. Working Paper, Consultation on Statistical Aspects of the Family as a Unit in Health Studies. World Health Organization, December 14–20, 1971

64. Bruce JA: Family practice and the family: A sociological view. J Comp Family Studies 4:10, 1973

65. Anderson R: A Behavioral Model of Families' Use of Health Services. Research Series No. 25. Chicago, University of Chicago Center for Health Administration Studies, 1968

66. USDHEW, HRA 77-1233, op. cit., p 24

67. Kronenfeld JJ: Provider variables and the utilization of ambulatory care services. J Health Soc Behav 19:68–76, March 1978

68. USDHEW, HRA 77-628, op. cit., pp 37–38

69. Galvin ME, Fan M: The utilization of physicians' services in L.A. County, 1973. J Health Soc Behav 16(1):74–94, March 1975

70. Monteiro LA: Expense is no object . . . Income and phy-

sician visits reconsidered. J Health Soc Behav 14:99–115, June 1973
71. USDHEW, HRA 77-1233, *op. cit.*, p 22
72. Otto HA: A framework for assessing family strengths. In Reinhardt AM, Quinn MD (eds): Family-Centered

Community Nursing: A Sociocultural Framework. St. Louis, Mosby, 1973, pp 87–93
73. Geismar LL, LaSorte MA: Understanding Multi-Problem Families. New York, Association Press, 1964, p 221

STUDY QUESTIONS

1. Which of the following are major ways which the family carries out its health care functions? (Select all appropriate answers.)
   a. Family provides preventive health care to its members at home.
   b. Family provides the major share of sick care to its members.
   c. Family pays for most health services received (directly or indirectly).
   d. Family has prime responsibility for initiating and coordinating health services.
   e. Family decides when and where to hospitalize its members.

2. List three primary factors which influence a family's conceptualizations of health and illness and whether they seek health services.

3. Name the three basic orientations used to define health and illness (according to Baumann). Keeping in mind the two groups studied, correlate the orientation(s) each group identified more frequently.

4. Describe what Koos's central research findings (or conclusions) were.

5. Fill in the missing components in this representation of the health belief model (original form).

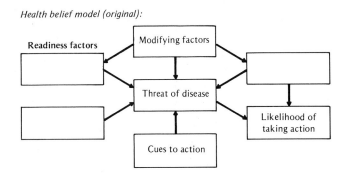

Health belief model (original):

6. Pratt found that on the whole most American families were not adequately performing their vital health care function. On what basis did she conclude this? And what are two basic reasons for this inadequacy?

7. In America, our overall health status is most closely related to (choose two):
   a. The quality and quantity of health services we receive.
   b. Our health care system.
   c. Socioeconomic and cultural factors.
   d. Personal health practices (life styles).

8. List four assessment areas to cover when appraising a family's dietary practices.

9. The following is a list of several areas that should be assessed under family's sleep and rest practices:

   Number of hours usually slept each night by family members.

   Who takes regular naps during day or what other rest techniques do family members use?

   Where do family members sleep?

   What important area(s) has (have) been omitted?

10. Formulate three basic questions to ask a family in relation to their exercise and recreational practices.

11. Which of the following substances constitute drugs which need to be assessed by the family completing a family health assessment? (Select all appropriate answers.)
    a. Coffee, tea, cola, and cocoa.
    b. Alcohol.
    c. Aspirin.
    d. Tobacco.
    e. Diazepam.

12. An appraisal of self-care practices involves an assessment of:
    a. Preventive practices.
    b. Diagnostic practices.
    c. Home treatment practices, including home care of sick or disabled members, and (fill in the missing item)
    d. _____ .

13. Cleanliness was the major area covered under environmental practices. Identify two general areas of concern related to family hygiene practices.

14. Name four salient general health education areas for families to learn about concerning dental health.

15. Which of the following measures are generally recommended for plaque control? (Select all appropriate answers.)
    a. After-meal toothbrushing.
    b. Reduction in dietary sucrose.
    c. Daily flossing of teeth.
    d. Use of an antiseptic mouthwash twice a day.

16. A family medical history consists basically of two parts. First, information would be elicited about each family member (going back to maternal and paternal grandparents) and their present and past health status. What would be the second area of assessment?

17. The poor differ from the nonpoor in their utilization of health services in which of the following ways:
    a. They use preventive services more.
    b. They use all health services less.
    c. They use emergency room inadequately.
    d. They often delay in seeking treatment.
    e. They present themselves to the health providers with more severe health problems.

18. A health assessor would want to learn not only about a family's source of medical care (who, when, and for what problems). Identify two other general areas he or she would want to gather information about.

STUDY ANSWERS

1. All but e. Physicians have virtually total control over when and where to hospitalize *their* patients.

2. a. Socioeconomic status (also can identify level of knowledge which is correlated with the educational status and socioeconomic status).
   b. Family's value system or priorities (is also related with socioeconomic status).
   c. Frequency of symptom or health problem in community (certain prevalent symptoms or problems are accepted as being part of living and thus viewed as inevitable, unavoidable, and "normal").

3. *Orientations*

	Groups Which Mentioned Orientation More Frequently
a. Feeling-state orientation.	Chronically ill clinic patients (lower socioeconomic group).
b. Performance orientation.	Both groups.
c. Symptom orientation.	Medical student group (younger, presumably well, and of middle- and upper-middle-class background).

4. Koos's study found that as one descends socioeconomic scale, a lack of recognition of and indifference to symptoms of illness increase. Also when these individuals failed to recognize behaviors as indicative of possible disease, they failed to see that medical care was indicated.

5.

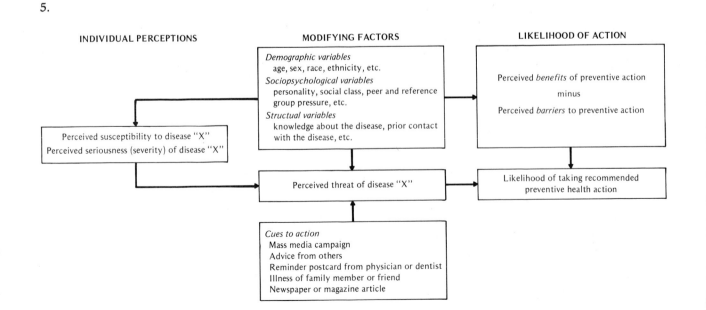

6. Pratt concluded that American families were generally inadequate in carrying out their health care function based on the following observations:

   Many homes are not suitable for maintaining health and controlling infectious disease and accidents (crowdedness, safety hazards, pollution, lack of infectious disease control).

   Widespread unhealthful personal and family health practices.

   Medication misuse is widespread.

   Dependent and/or disabled family members were not cared for or inadequately cared for.

   Use of health services (lack of use or inappropriate use) found frequently.

   Level of health knowledge insufficient.

   Family's self-care practices are inadequate.

   Reasons for this inadequacy:

   Basic structure of the health care system (health care provider dominated; bureaucratic structure).

   Family structure itself (family needs to be more widely involved with community and husbands-fathers need to be actively involved).

7. c and d

8. Any four of the following:
   a. Nutritional history (the 24-hour family food record).
   b. Observe the family members in terms of their heights and weights. Does visual inspection indicate normal limits?
   c. Identify any special dietary preferences (food fads, culturally or philosophically based dietary food patterns).
   d. Psychosocial aspects of mealtimes and eating (food used as a reward or punishment?).
   e. Shopping, planning, and food preparation practices.
   f. Shopping, planning, and food preparation responsibilities.

9. a. Are there regular times established for children to go to bed and get up? Who decides when children go to sleep?
   b. Do any members of family have sleeping problems? If so, what kind of problem?

10. a. What types of family recreation involving physical exercise does your family engage in?
    b. How frequently do you as a family go biking, swimming, etc., and does everyone participate?
    c. What effect do you think exercise has on your family's health?

11. All (a–e).

12. The determination of the family's ability to provide self-care (family's potentials).

13. a. Lack of washing hands after toileting and before meals.
    b. Sharing common dishes and/or utensils.

14. Four of the following:
    a. Importance of fluoride for increasing resistance of tooth to decay.
    b. Importance of brushing and flossing teeth (and use of an effective method of brushing).
    c. Role of carbohydrates (starches and sugars) in producing dental caries.
    d. Importance of regular dental examination and cleaning of teeth.
    e. Early treatment of dental caries and treatment of major orthodontic problems.

15. a, b, and c

16. Specific diseases (both genetically based and environmentally related diseases) family members might have had.

17. c, d, and e

18. Two of the following:
    a. Types of health care other than primary care (such as dental and emergency health services).
    b. Family's perceptions and feelings regarding receiving care.
    c. Logistics of receiving care (transportation, agency's hours, etc.).
    d. Source of payment for services.
    e. Family's social network (family's source of assistance other than health providers).

Families constantly face the need to modify their perceptions and lives. The stimulus for this change comes from within and without: the normal, continually evolving developmental needs of all the family members, in addition to the presence of unexpected situations involving family members, make up the inner demands for change, whereas the external stimuli come from the changing society as it interacts with the family during its life cycle. These continual demands force the family to adapt—in order for the family to survive, continue, and grow. Family adaptation, and more specifically family coping, is the essential process or function which makes this possible. A family's perceptions and handling of its problems through various coping mechanisms are crucial to the family's success or failure in dealing with these problems. Geismar and La Sorte, in writing about multiproblem families, confirm the vital nature of adequate family coping mechanisms during periods of stress or crisis, without which families are likely to become disorganized or dysfunctional.[1]

Most important, moreover, the family coping function serves as a vital process or mechanism through which all the other family functions are made possible. Without effective family coping, the affective, socialization, economic, and health care functions cannot be adequately achieved. Hence the family coping function is not only one of a set of crucial functions, but is *the* underlying process which enables the family to enact these necessary functions.

Assessing family coping patterns and capacities will provide the foundation for assisting families in their coping and adaptation, so that they will be better able to increase their level of functioning or achieve a higher level of wellness. Achieving this result is precisely the goal this text sees as the *raison d'être* of family-centered nursing practice—that of health promotion or assisting families and their members to reach a higher level of wellness. Strengthening and encouraging adequate adaptive responses and enhancing adaptive capacities, as well as reducing the actual and potential stressors from within and outside the family, are part of this broad and encompassing goal. Whether the family is essentially healthy or dysfunctional (at one or the other pole within the health–illness continuum), the family health worker is still dealing with the same issue: assisting families to help themselves achieve a higher level of functioning or wellness within the context of their particular aims, aspirations, and abilities.

Families have both great strengths and pervasive weaknesses, as the results of different studies make clear. In 1975 authors Yankelovitch, Skelley, and White summarized their findings from 2,194 interviews with 1,247 families selected by national probability sampling method. They concluded: "What does emerge as heartening news in the present study is a

16

The Family Coping Function

LEARNING OBJECTIVES

1. Describe the vital nature of the family coping function.
2. Present evidence of how adequately families are fulfilling this function.
3. Define and differentiate the meanings of these terms and concepts: stressor, stress, adaptation, coping, defense mechanisms, mastery, and crisis.
4. Identify four broad sources of family stressors.
5. Explain what coping tasks are appropriate for each of the three time phases of stress.
6. Explain the findings of Holmes and Rahe relative to the impact of stressors on individuals.
7. Compare and contrast the Social Readjustment Scale of Holmes and Rahe with the balancing of forces diagram presented here.
8. Trace the sequence of events which occur during a family crisis.
9. Relate several of the important findings from Pearlin and Schooler's study of normative coping tactics.
10. Identify two major variables involved in the development of crisis or successful resolution of the problem (non crisis).
11. Briefly describe four functional coping strategies used by families and four dysfunctional adaptive strategies utilized by families.
12. Differentiate whether specific coping strategies are functional, dysfunctional, or both (could be either healthy or unhealthy).
13. Recall the two basic purposes of social support systems and the three predominant social network styles.
14. Utilizing a family case example, assess the family in terms of the family coping function.

picture of the great strengths and adaptive capabilities of the American family—the flexibility, sturdiness, and vitality of the family."[2]

From community mental health literature on the other hand, we are reminded of the pervasiveness of mental illness in the community—a sign of the failure of families to cope. The two classic studies of the prevalence of mental disorders in North America attest to the situation. Conducted in the 1950s and 1960s, these studies were based on community surveys of the prevalence of mental disorders rather than on the number of psychiatric patients known to treatment agencies. One study was called the Mid-Manhattan Study and involved a sample of 1,660 men and women between the ages of 20 and 59 in an area of Manhattan, New York. The second is referred to as the Stirling County Study. This survey study consisted of 1,000 persons in a rural area of Nova Scotia. While the studies differed somewhat in how they defined mental illness, their estimates of the extent of mental illness in the general population were staggering. In the Stirling Country Study, it was concluded that at least half of all the adults in Stirling County, Nova Scotia, were currently suffering from some form of psychiatric disturbance. In the Mid-Manhattan Study, which used a narrower definition of mental illness, investigators found nearly one-quarter of the respondents to be significantly psychiatrically impaired.

What are some of the major stressors leading to a greater prevalence of mental health problems? Poverty and marital disruption have both been linked with increased rates of mental illness. Families most exposed to hardship are also the least equipped to deal with these stressors.[3] Moreover, of all the social stressors studied relative to their correlation with mental illness, none has been more consistently and powerfully associated with mental illness—using criteria such as psychiatric hospitalizations, suicides, and homicides—as has marital disruption.[4] Marital disruption—divorce, desertion, or death of spouse—affects an enormous number of people yearly, and in many of these cases it can be assumed that a primary underlying problem was the existence of inadequate family coping patterns.

BASIC CONCEPTS AND DEFINITIONS

All of the concepts and terms defined below, with the exception of family coping function, are well established and their meanings fairly well agreed on. Family coping function is a new term created for this text, since it is felt that families have crucial coping patterns which need to be appreciated if we are to understand their impact on family life and assist families to stabilize and grow. In defining this new concept, definitions

of coping as applied to the individual have been adapted to the family.

Stressor refers to the initiating or the precipitating agent that activates the stress process.[5] These are tension-producing stimuli with the potential for causing family and personal disequilibrium, crisis, or the experience of stress.[6] Family stressors can be interpersonal (inside or outside of the family system), environmental, economic, or sociocultural. Perceptions color the nature and gravity of possible family stressors, since families react not only to the presence of actual stressors, but also to events they see as particularly threatening and dangerous. Thus the family's perceptions are of paramount importance. It is significant to note that families that are crisis-prone consistently tend to perceive events in a distorted, subjective manner. Events which the healthy family would look at objectively and be able to respond to effectively are viewed by the crisis-prone family as real threats to their survival. In these cases extensive stress is experienced by the family, since the family and its members are experiencing pressures which greatly tax their coping and adaptive capacities.

Stress is the end result of experiencing a stressor. Or conversely, stressors create stress. Stress is defined as the dynamic force that generates tension or strain within a social system (individual, family, etc.) and is a reaction to a pressure-producing situation.[7] People and families react to stress by use of both conscious and unconscious adaptive strategies.

Adaptation is a process of adjustment to change. The outcome is an altered state of equilibrium or homeostasis. Adaptation may be positive or negative, resulting in the increase or decrease of a family's state of wellness.[8] For example, seeking help from community agencies may be a very positive move when outside assistance is needed to help remedy a child with learning problems, but the same adaptive strategy may be negative if it becomes a predominant defensive pattern, since the family does not learn to utilize its own potential inner resources.

Strategies for Adaptation

White identifies three strategies for adaptation: defense mechanisms, coping, and mastery—these making up a whole "tapestry of living."[9]

Defense mechanisms, according to White, are learned, habitual, or automatic (built-in) ways of responding. They are usually tactics for avoiding the problems the stressor pose and are usually used when no apparent solution is known or accessible to a family. Denial of an important family issue is an example of such a defense mechanism and would be classified as dysfunctional if this is the *habitual* way in which the family deals with its problems. Because defensive mechanisms are largely avoidance behaviors, they are usually dysfunctional responses to problems.

Coping refers to efforts to deal with stressors and stress which are not adequately managed by the habitual defensive responses. Coping tactics are positive, problem-appropriate, active strategies[10] geared toward solving problems and "approaching" the problem. The coping patterns are used to master a task or to deal with life strains encountered. Families may use the same set of strategies fairly consistently over time or may change their coping methods when some new substantive developmental or situational demand is made on the family.[11]

Mastery is the end result of using effective coping resources or strategies. In this case, situations would be competently handled as a result of effective, well-practiced coping efforts. Mastery is very closely aligned with family competency. Just as individuals gain self-esteem and feelings of competency, so do families. Competence refers to the possessing of sufficient means to meet the exigencies of a situation or task.

The *family coping function* is one of the six basic functions which the family fulfills, involving efforts to combat family stressors and stress in a positive, problem-appropriate, and active manner.

In the presence of a stressor and stress, a *crisis* represents a failure or the ineffectiveness of the adaptive strategies a family is using. Thus crisis situations differ from stress situations in that the usual or known adaptive techniques (the family's repertoire of adaptive strategies) does not appropriately handle the stressor. Hence a family crisis refers to a disruptive period in the family's life when an extremely stressful event or series of events significantly taxes the family's coping abilities, with no resolution of the problem in sight. This results in familial instability and disorganization. At this time the family generally feels a greater need for help than during periods of normalcy and is more receptive to suggestions and information.[12]

There are two types of crises which families undergo: developmental and situational crises. Developmental or maturational crises are those stemming from the stressor events which families experience in the process of the psychosocial growth of its members. They are inherent within the stages of the normal life cycle of both the family and its members. Situational crises are events or stresses that are not common or normally expected, such as the death of a child or serious illness of one of the family members.

STRESSORS AND STRESS
Basic Sources of Family Stress

The many changes and stressors a family faces over time may be viewed, as Minuchin has done, as coming from four basic sources.[13]

Stressful Contact of One Member with Extrafamilial Forces

When one member of the family is stressed by extrafamilial stressors (e.g., loss of job, school problem, legal problem), other family members feel the need to accommodate to his or her changed circumstances. They do this by supporting—the functional way—or attacking the individual—the nonfunctional mode. They may also keep the problem contained within a subsystem, although if the extrafamilial stressor is prolonged and major, its effects "seep" into the other subsystems, thereby affecting the whole family. For example, a father stressed at work comes home and begins criticizing his wife and then redirects his hostility to a child. This reduces the danger to the spouse subsystem, but stresses the child. Or the husband may criticize the wife, who then turns to her daughter for solace and support, thereby creating an unhealthy coalition of mother and daughter against husband.

Stressful Contact of the Whole Family with Extrafamilial Forces

Economic hardships such as poverty and discrimination are two particularly threatening forces straining families today. Family coping mechanisms become overtaxed, as family resources are depleted. Another common stressor immigrant families face is the cultural shock and major adjustments to be made when migrating from one nation and culture to another.

Transitional Stressors

Problems of transition occur in a number of situations, the most common being produced by developmental changes in family members and by changes in family composition. Five of the most frequent transitions in which family nurses become involved are (1) the arrival of a new baby into a family; (2) the emergence of a child into adolescence; (3) the merging of two families through marriage of single parents; (4) the introduction of an older grandparent into the family due to infirmity or for financial reasons; and (5) loss of spouse during the last family-cycle stage.

Situational Stressors

This type of stressor is associated with unique idiosyncratic problems a family may be facing, such as the transitory problems which illness and hospitalization of one of the parents create for the family as a whole. These stressors are unanticipated and may tax a family's coping capacities. For instance, an overload in coping mechanisms may occur if the illness is serious and prolonged, since this represents a powerful, continuing negative force and creates a need for major change (the redistribution of roles and functions).

Time Phases of Stress and Coping Tasks

When nurses are working with families, they need to be aware of the time phase of the stress, as well as the coping tasks of the phase. Coping behaviors are divided into three phases: (1) ante-stress period; (2) the actual stress period; and (3) post-stress period.

Ante-stress Period

In the period before actually confronting the stress, if anticipation is possible, there is an awareness of danger or the perceived threat of the situation. If families or helping persons can identify a future stressor, anticipatory guidance as well as other coping tactics to weaken or reduce the impact of the stressor may be sought or provided. Also, in some situations, moves might be instituted to remove the impending stressor.

The Actual Stress Period

Coping strategies during the period of stress usually differ in intensity and kind from those tactics utilized prior to the onset of the stressor and stress. There may be very basic survival, defensive tactics used during this period if the stress in the family is extreme. With tremendous energy expended in coping with a stressor(s) and stress, many family functions (some which may be crucial to family health) are often temporarily set aside or are inadequately performed until the family has the resources to deal with them again.

Post-stress Period

The coping tactics following the stress period, termed the post-trauma phase, consist of strategies to return the family to a homeostatic, balanced state. To promote family wellness during this phase, the family needs to pull together, mutually express feelings and solve their problems,[14] and/or seek out and utilize familial supports for resolving their stressful situation. A family may also, unfortunately, go through the stressful period, ending up functioning at a lower level of wellness.

Impact of Stressors

Families daily are bombarded with tension-producing stimuli—some of which are only mildly irritating and hardly noticed, such as traffic noise and poor housing, and some of which are potentially or actually devastating to families, such as marital disruption or the loss of a child. Holmes and his associates realized the great quantitative and qualitative differences which stressors have on individuals, and as early as 1949 began to systematically study the quality and quantity of life changes observed, both desirable and undesirable,

which clustered at the time of the onset of an illness. From these data they were able to assign a weight to each of the 43 life events found to be associated with the onset of health problems (see Table 16.1). Other

TABLE 16.1
Social Readjustment Rating Scale of Holmes and Rahe

Rank	Life Event	Value*
1	Death of spouse	100
2	Divorce	73
3	Marital separation	65
4	Jail term	63
5	Death of close family member	63
6	Personal injury or illness	53
7	Marriage	50
8	Fired at work	47
9	Marital reconciliation	45
10	Retirement	45
11	Change in health of family member	44
12	Pregnancy	40
13	Sex difficulties	39
14	Gain of new family member	39
15	Business readjustment	39
16	Change in financial state	38
17	Death of close friend	37
18	Change to different line of work	36
19	Change in number of arguments with spouse	35
20	Mortgage over $10,000	31
21	Foreclosure of mortgage or loan	30
22	Change in responsibilities at work	29
23	Son or daughter leaving home	29
24	Trouble with in-laws	29
25	Outstanding personal achievement	28
26	Wife begins or stops work	26
27	Begin or end school	26
28	Change in living conditions	25
29	Revision of personal habits	24
30	Trouble with boss	23
31	Change in work hours or conditions	20
32	Change in residence	20
33	Change in school	20
34	Change in recreation	19
35	Change in church activities	19
36	Change in social activities	18
37	Mortgage or loan less than $10,000	17
38	Change in sleeping habits	16
39	Change in number of family get-togethers	15
40	Change in eating habits	15
41	Vacation	13
42	Christmas	12
43	Minor violations of the law	11

* *Social readjustment rating scale instructions:* Add up value of life crisis units for life events experienced in a two-year period:
Score of 0 to 150—No significant problems.
Score of 150 to 199—Mild life crisis and a 33 percent chance of illness.
Score of 200 to 299—Moderate life crisis and a 50 percent chance of illness.
Score of 300 or over—Major life crisis and an 80 percent chance of illness.
Adapted from: Holmes TH, Rahe RH: The social readjustment rating scale. J Psychosom Res 11:213, 1967.

investigations have generated similar lists, all verifying the temporal relationship of high life-change scores preceding illness.[15] Although these scales were developed for individuals, their applicability to families is significant. Families experience most of these same life crisis events and are also negatively affected by the onslaught of numerous stressors impacting on them within a short period of time. It needs to be emphasized that the three most stressful life events—death of a spouse, divorce, and marital separation—all involve a marital and/or family disruption. The next five events, in order of stressfulness, include a jail term, death of a close family member, personal injury or illness, marriage, and losing one's job. Again, these all can involve the family intimately and impact on it powerfully.

While the work of Holmes and Rahe identified and quantified stressors, epidemiologists have long used a multifactorial model, the epidemiologic triad, based on the interaction of the agent, host, and environment (in contrast to Holmes and Rahe's model, which looks at the "agent" or causative factors only), to explain the state of health, illness, or any point in between on the health–illness continuum. In this chapter, this triadic model has been adapted so that the agent, host, and environmental factors are visualized as weighted forces, both positive and negative, and so that it applies to the family rather than the individual. These weighted forces are balanced against one another, with the greater forces on either side creating an imbalance toward a higher or lower level of wellness in the family. Using this model, it can be seen that it is not just the magnitude of weighted life events within a specified period of time which causes a greater chance of illness, but that it is the imbalance of stressors vis-à-vis assets (with the negative forces offsetting the positive forces because of their greater weight). Moveover, environmental forces, both positive and negative, are considered an inherent facet to be assessed in each of the two sets of forces.

Studies have linked particular situational sets—stressors—with dysfunction in a cause-and-effect relationship. This finding suggests how difficult it is to assess families, since their problems stem from multiple factors. We have tended to think that in order to eliminate a problem one would need to find a way to eliminate or treat the particular causative factor, rather than view the situation more broadly. By assessing the balance between the stressors (their duration and strength) and the nature and strength of supportive or protective elements, one can either attempt to eliminate or reduce the potency of stressors or to build up and strengthen the family's resources (assets). Figure 16.1 illustrates this "balance" concept and how the family's level of wellness is affected.

Given an asssessment of the duration and strength of the family's stressors or current life stressors and other risk factors, on the one hand, and of their psychosocial, physical, and environmental assets, on the

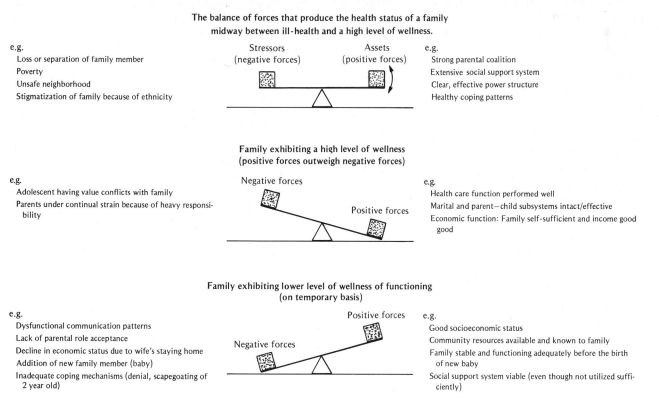

FIGURE 16.1
Impact of positive (assets) and negative (stressors) forces of the family health balance.

other, it will be easier to anticipate which families are truly at risk; and it may be possible to reduce or eliminate certain stressors, or conversely to strengthen or add certain assets or resources to modify the balancing of forces in favor of the family's greater health.* Furthermore, many of the most stressful life events that cannot be changed may have their impact weakened by preparing the family for the event (anticipatory counseling) or providing reality, present-oriented, short-term counseling such as crisis intervention during the time when the overwhelming stressors are being experienced.[16]

FUNCTIONAL COPING STRATEGIES

Normative Coping Responses

Pearlin and Schooler reported an extensive well-conducted study in which they interviewed a sample of 2,300 people, ages 18 to 65, representative of the population in the urbanized area of Chicago to determine the kinds of coping tactics which they used and how efficacious these were. Their analysis emphasized the normative coping responses being utilized in response to life strains in their major social roles (occupational, economic, parental, and marital). This study's significance is noteworthy because it is one of the few research studies which describe the everyday coping experiences of people. Past studies have been conducted in clinical situations where there has been a distinct tendency to regard coping as a highly individualistic defense aroused in very special situations.[17]

As just mentioned, healthy, functional families under stress tend to act in a direction which reduces the stress. Pearlin and Schooler used this social system characteristic to define the effective coping mechanisms, i.e., the coping strategies which led to a reduction in stress in the role being strained were deemed efficacious, whereas those responses which did not alleviate or attenuate stress were defined as ineffective.[18]

Pearlin and Schooler identify three types of coping tactics used extensively by individuals in their social functioning. Each of these types will be described briefly, with a comment as to their effectiveness in reducing stress. Much of this discussion has direct relevance for families and how they cope, since the coping mechanisms used by the adult family members may be taken as representative of those used within sets of family relationships or the family as a whole, if we assume that parents set the tone for how the family as a whole would respond.

The first type of coping responses are the tactics that

modify the stressful situation. These represent the most direct ways to cope with life strains, for they are geared toward altering or eliminating the stressor. Pearlin and Schooler included self-reliance and seeking help from others under this type of coping. Interestingly enough, they found that in parental and marital roles, self-reliance was reported to be more effective in attenuating stress than was the seeking of help and advice from others. Perhaps those that seek outside help are not the same persons as those who successfully receive help. The authors point out that as yet, we do not know the conditions under which help from others can be effective.[19]

The second type of coping strategy consists of those tactics that function to control the meaning of the problem. "The way an experience is recognized and the meaning that is attached to it determines to a large extent the threat posed by that experience."[20] Thus the same experience may be highly threatening to one family and innocuous to another, depending on family members' cognitive and perceptual evaluation of the event.[21] The following are examples of coping which cognitively neutralize the threats that are experineced in life: making positive comparisons ("count your blessings," etc.); selective ignoring (minimizing the negative elements and maximizing the positive facets); and substitution of rewards (making the most strain-producing experiences the least valued areas of one's life). A substitution of rewards was found to work well in both occupational and economic areas of a person's life. For example, in the economic area this usually involved the demeaning of the importance of money and elevating other aspects of one's life or work such as work hours or fringe benefits. However, in parental and marital roles, this type of coping was not found to be helpful, since one cannot easily relegate one's marriage or children to a less important place in one's list of priorities.[22] Conversely, the most efficacious types of coping tactics in both enactment of marital and parental roles were those that entailed involvement (the first coping tactic), not selective ignoring or manipulation of values.

The third type of coping tactic includes those mechanisms essentially utilized to help people accommodate to and manage existing stress, rather than deal with the problems or stressor itself. Six coping responses were listed in this category. In marriage, emotional discharge of feelings and controlled reflectiveness were identified, as well as passive forebearance and self-assertion. In parental roles, feelings of potency and helpless resignation were stated as examples. Pearlin and Schooler discovered that in marriage a reflective probing of problems was more effective than the open and emotional discharge of feelings. In parental areas, the conviction that one has

---

* Otto's list of family strengths or resources as reported in Chapter 3 may be helpful in recognizing family assets.

power (potency) to effect change and exert influence over one's children proved to be more helpful in stress management than helpless resignation.

Lastly, the authors point out that a variety of coping strategies is usually more effective than a limited repertoire of coping responses. The single coping tactic, regardless of its effectiveness, cannot possibly be appropriate for the wide range of life strains commonly experienced.[23]

Crisis-Prone and Non-Crisis-Prone Families

Now that the normative, common coping responses have been described, attention will be turned to some of the salient differences that have been observed in comparing crisis- and non-crisis-prone families. In assessing a family in trouble, it is important to be knowledgeable of these differences so that a judgment can be made as to whether (1) the family's problem is being adequately coped with by the family, (2) a crisis state exists, or (3) a chronic inability to solve existing problems is present. Nursing intervention would vary substantially in each of these cases. Moreover, in working with a family that is not presently having problems, but has had a history of being crisis-prone, a family worker would want to be more tuned-in to this tendency so that early problem recognition and assistance could take place.

Hill's description of the stages of crisis development serves as a clarifying review of the sequence and the interrelationship of the events involved in dealing with stress. Figure 16.2 presents a visual representation of the adaptation of Hill's model that is used in this text.

All families are continually subject to the effects of stressors requiring internal changes. What then precipitates a crisis in one family and not in another? As seen in Figure 16.2, there are two basic factors involved. The first and foremost is the family's perception and interpretation of the stressor (or stressor-event as Hill calls it). Families who consistently perceive and define events and changes as threatening rather than challenging, subjectively rather than objectively, and in a distorted fashion rather than in a realistic way, will most likely be crisis-prone if their orientation is combined with the use of ineffective coping responses. Hall and Weaver explain that

successful families have found ways to utilize certain crucial processes to facilitate all the growth-promoting potential in crisis-laden situations. The first of these processes is *cognitive mastery*. . . . A major task is to assist in the development of a cognitive map of what is happening, as a first step in achieving purposeful problem-solving.[24]

The second basic factor influencing the outcome—crisis or success—of dealing with a stressor is the family's use of coping mechanisms. Stressors often force families to use coping responses rather than habitual, stereotypic defenses. If the family does not make use of one of the effective coping mechanisms from its repertoire of possible responses, the result is the same as if the family did not possess a successful way of adapting. However, the intervention is easier in this case because it is less difficult to assist families to utilize past coping patterns than to help families learn new ways of responding. Family coping mechanisms or responses include both inner strengths and the resources of external social support systems.

Inner strengths or resources consist of the ability of the family to pull together to become cohesive and integrated. Family integration entails the control of sub-

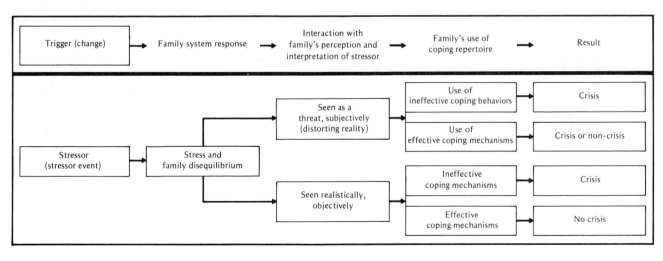

FIGURE 16.2
Factors leading to crisis and noncrisis states. *Adapted from Hill R: Generic features of families under stress. In Parad H (ed): Crisis Intervention: Selected Readings. New York, Family Service Association of America, 1965, p 4*

system components through bonds of unity. Families that deal most effectively with their problems are most often the families that are well integrated—where family members are highly committed to the group and its collective goals. Another inner resource is role flexibility—being able to modify family roles as needed.[25]

Externally, effective coping mechanisms deal with the family's use of social support systems (some authors call them adequate situational supports). Support systems will be elaborated on shortly. In looking at this aspect of outer resources, it is obvious that families differ in the extent to which they are able to obtain *compliance* from their environments to meet their needs for information, energy, matter, and services. The family must also be able to reduce some of the demands being made on it, as well as dispose of services, information, and energies. This is all accomplished through regulation of its family boundaries, as previously discussed. Without an adequate knowledge of or ability to secure environmental compliance through the effective regulation of family boundaries, the family will be more crisis-prone.

Hall and Weaver also emphasize that family communication patterns are of crucial importance in adaptive coping. Communication processes in the family greatly influence, if not determine, the quality of the family life. Moreover, in the last analysis, families must choose to grow and learn from their experiences. An element of choice exists,[26] i.e., between a set of alternatives, and these choices are usually conscious and voluntary, even though heavily influenced by cultural and personal values and norms. Lewis et al. noted optimally functioning families were found to excel in *choosing* growth-generating alternatives. In approaching problems, these families explored various options, and if one alternative did not work well, another was tried and evaluated.[27]

Inner Resources of Families

Functional coping mechanisms have been broadly identified. Starting with the two basic types of family resources—inner and outer resources—it is now helpful to look into each of these broad areas in more detail. Under family inner resources, five selected specific types of coping responses will be described. These are (1) self-reliance through greater family control, (2) the use of humor, (3) increased sharing together, (4) developing strong subsystems and family members (a long-term task); and (5) controlling the meaning of the problem.

Self-Reliance Through Greater Family Control

Certain families when under stress will cope by becoming more reliant on their own resources and ac-

complish this by providing greater structure and organization in the home and family. This is an attempt at a greater control over the subsystems and is comparable to the "tighter" regulation of troops in the military under combat conditions. This usually involves tighter scheduling of members' time, more tasks, a more close-knit organization, and a more rigid, prescribed routine. With the closing of family boundaries comes a call for greater family organization and discipline of members, coupled with the expectation that members will be more self-disciplined and conforming. Families utilizing greater control do this to achieve greater integration and cohesiveness. This type of family coping usually stems from the influence of the traditional Protestant ethic, which values self-control and self-sufficiency, seeing them as particularly necessary during hardship periods. Concomitant with structuring is a need for members to be "strong" and to learn to conceal feelings and master tension within themselves.

Burgess points out that this particular coping strategy, involving self-discipline for certain members of the families, may be very necessary in stressful situations such as when parents are confronted with a serious accident at home. They must maintain composure and the capacity to problem solve, since they then are responsible for their own lives and those of their children.[28] And, in fact, Pearlin and Schooler found that self-reliance was an efficacious coping response in the area of enacting one's marital and parental roles. Nonetheless, this strategy can also be dysfunctional if in certain circumstances outside help is needed but not sought or if it becomes an habitual, pervasive mode of adaptation.

Use of Humor

Hott points out that a sense of humor is an important family asset that contributes to improving the family's attitude toward its problems and health care.[29] Grojahn reiterates this contention further by stating, "Besides maturity, humor implies strength, superiority in face of danger and calamity, victory and triumph over defeat."[30] Although identified here as functional, if humor is used repeatedly to mask direct emotional expression and cover up and shun problems, its use is obviously dysfunctional.

Greater Sharing Together

One way of bringing the family closer together and maintaining and managing stress levels and the necessary family morale is by engaging in a greater sharing of feelings, thoughts, and joint family experiences or activities. An excellent cultural example of this coping is the traditional Jewish custom of sitting shivah—a seven-day period after a funeral in which relatives and close friends visit with the bereaved family and share their thoughts and feelings, providing mutual emotional support and nurturance.

Leisure-time family activities are especially important coping resources to rejuvenate a family's cohesiveness, morale, and satisfaction. The increasing importance of leisure-time activities has been verified in studies of marital satisfaction.[31-33] Like so many sayings, the adage, "A family that plays together, stays together," contains much truth in it. This coping strategy is ultimately aimed at building greater integration, cohesiveness, and resiliency in the family.

Development of Strong Subsystems and Family Members

This specific inner coping response is of a different nature than the three coping responses already described. It is included here as a reminder of the vital role that the sets of familial relationships and the persons in the family play. If the family subsystems (the critical relationships) and individuals in the family are both healthy and have a strong sense of self-esteem, then the basic foundations of the family are sturdy and resilient. Pratt discusses the importance of the individual in assisting the family to cope well. She states that providing freedom to each member and fostering individuality is a necessity for effective family coping efforts, as the effective functioning of individual members makes possible and enhances the family's ability to respond adaptively. Families must provide the opportunities for their members to learn to problem solve, take actions, and feel competent about their ability to do so.[34]

Rainwater alludes to the fact that poor families have less adequate health practices than families of higher socioeconomic status not only because of their lack of tangible resources, but also because of their limited sense of ability to affect significantly the course of events through problem solving and personal action. Thus a sense of fatalism and powerlessness is pervasive, and results in basic health care being neglected in favor of more pressing immediate concerns.[35]

Controlling the Meaning of the Problem

One of the primary means Pearlin and Schooler found to be effective in coping was by use of the mental mechanism—controlling the meaning of the problem—which ameliorates or cognitively neutralizes the threatening stimuli that are experienced in life. As mentioned earlier, the interpretation given to events can make the difference between hyperreacting to a situation, wherein the family experiences great stress; reacting in a realistic way, wherein the situation is seen objectively and appraised accurately; and underreacting, wherein an element of denial is present and the problem is not confronted adequately. Families which use this coping strategy, that is, controlling the meaning of the problem, tend to see the positive facets of life's stress-producing events, as exemplified by the making of positive comparisons ("count your blessings"; "it could have been worse"); selectively ignoring the negative aspects ("I've learned a lot from this negative experience"); and making the stressful events or experiences less important in terms of the family's hierarchy of values.

External Resources of Families

Although inner resources are crucial, most authors writing in this area today emphasize the necessity for families under stress to bring in or receive greater external information, tangible goods, services, and support—an aspect previously discussed in terms of the concept of boundaries in the system's framework. Most of the discussion here will deal with family support systems, since this is the major external resource; but the seeking of information, increased linkages with the broader community, and mastery as the end result of successful coping efforts will also be touched on.

Use of Knowledge

Particular families under stress who are more cognitively based respond by seeking knowledge and information concerning the stressor or potential stressor. This acts to reduce fear of the unknown and to appraise the stressor more accurately (its meaning), in addition to strengthening the family's means of preventing stressors from impinging on them.

Parents who actively cope with parenting by seeking out new information and other resources demonstrate positive results and feelings of coping well with parenting responsibilities.[36] For example, Hoeflin reports that parents who avail themselves of books and magazines and newspapers to aid them in parenting use significantly more functional child-rearing techniques than parents who do not seek out this type of information. When parents use this activist approach to child rearing, children will also learn to problem-solve in active, mastery-oriented ways.[37]

Increased Linkages with the Broader Community

This category differs from coping by use of the social support systems in that it is a continuing, long-term, and general family coping effort, not one which is geared to alleviate any one specific stressor. In this case, family members are active participants (as active members or in leadership positions) in clubs, organizations, and community groups. There is extensive use of the society's varied resources and exposure through travel to alternative ways to life.[38]

The rationale for the importance of this linkage as a coping technique is grounded in systems theory, which states that any social system must have a movement of information and activity across its boundaries if it is to perform its functions. Since the family alone cannot serve all its members' and group needs without enrichment from other sources, the initiation and promotion of growth-producing relationships within the neighborhood, town, and wider society is essential.[39] If, however, the family's boundaries are continually open and do not sufficiently allow for family integration and control over input, this strategy then would be dysfunctional.

Social Support Systems

Social support systems and the social network are the major external resources families draw on in coping. Between families and the whole network of professional services, experts, and bureaucracies there exists a great reservoir of potential help: kin, friends, neighbors, employers, fellow employees, classmates, teachers, groups, organizations, and communities of identity. Communities of identity are community groups with which a family shares common interests, goals, life styles, or social identity. Subcultural and reference groups have been discussed previously and are examples of the same type of group. These groups can be based on common professional interests, political goals, ethnic identity, and/or recreational involvements. Social networks serve as a third "set of players" for the family wrestling with making suitable arrangements in matters of education, child care, health and welfare services, and so forth.[40]

Hogue explains the concept of a support system further:

> A support system is a defined set of persons consisting of a focal or anchor person, all the family, all the friends and all the helping persons who stand ready to serve the anchor person, and the linkages or relationships among those people. Support systems are different from "expanded families" or "individuals and significant others," in that support systems have patterns and properties of their own.[41]

According to Caplan there are three general sources of social support. These consist of spontaneous, informal networks; organized supports not directed by professional health workers; and organized efforts by health professionals.[42] Of these, the informal social network (defined above as the social network) is viewed as the group providing the greatest amount of help in times of need.

The duration and permanency of support systems vary. Some family support systems are long-term or continuous sets of individuals and groups that assist the family in more general life issues such as developmental tasks and situational crisis, e.g., a loss of family member. Other support systems may be crisis-oriented, dealing with specific issues and are short-term in duration.[43]

A family copes with its problems within its social network; needless to say, it is impossible to survive if one is isolated from outer resources. Every family and person has a unique, special social network which provides important linkages, as well as being critically important to the family's and its members' self-image, sense of belonging, and feeling of group satisfaction.[44]

Hogue reports four studies showing that a substantial proportion of persons who are exposed to stressors and who are able to stay healthy are protected by the presence of psychosocial factors she and others term coping resources (composed of both personal characteristics, e.g., intelligence and motivation, and social characteristics—support systems). Thus she contends that "support systems are the powerful means people have for maintaining health, despite the pressures of society, and that nurses can strengthen and augment their care by understanding these systems."[45]

Purposes of Social Support Systems

Social networks of support systems have two primary coping purposes: emotional support and direct assistance. First, they provide nurturance and emotional support to family members.[46, 47] In these types of relationships the nurturing persons or groups care for, support, and emotionally meet some of the psychosocial needs of the family members. Support systems are concerned with the morale and welfare of the family as a group also and will work to sustain or improve the group's morale and positive motivation. In addition, the family's informal social network provides a family with opportunities for feedback about itself and validation about its expectations and perceptions of individuals and of groups which, in turn, may improve the family's communication with groups in the community with which it interacts.

Extended families or close friends encourage members to communicate freely about their personal difficulties. The family then shares its problems with this support system and is offered quite individualized advice and guidance—in keeping with the family's traditions and values. After all, who knows the family better than these supportive individuals? Can health professionals have the same keen sense of the uniqueness of a particular family such as close friends and family have? And who has the greater and more lasting interest in the family's welfare and happiness? The answers to the above speak for the vital nature of social networks.

The second primary purpose support systems achieve is that of task-oriented assistance. Extended family, friends, and neighbors may provide assistance to a family. An important element of this assistance is not only telling them how to find sources of care and assistance in the community, but also assisting them to make arrangements. In our society, usually only close relatives will provide extensive long-term help. Assistance from extended family also takes on the form of direct help, including continuing and intermittent financial aid, shopping, care of children, physical care of old people, performing household tasks, and practical assistance in times of crisis.[48] The absence of such assistive relationships can generate a sense of vulnerability.

Caplan, in explicating how social support systems help families and individuals communicate effectively with the external world, emphasizes that in times of illness or trouble, this system becomes crucial in assisting families to cope successfully.[49]

Inadequate Use of Social Networks

When families need help to whom do they turn? The evidence is that many persons do not seek external help.[50] Several factors inhibit families, especially those in the middle class, from fully utilizing these resources. First, there exists the belief that professional services are often best along with the feeling that only the best is worthwhile. (Though professional services may be best, they are less personalized and very costly and, hence, beyond the family's means in many instances.) Second, while the family is thought of as a place where families can let down defenses and receive and give support and care, some believe that in facing the outside world the family should exhibit independence and self-sufficiency. Despite the fact that family members often yearn to be interdependent, to be supportive of others outside of the family, and to receive support in return, there persists a feeling that this is a sign of weakness and fallibility. Thus, when a family "fails" to handle its own problems, some feel they "should" be prepared to turn to paid professionals to resolve the problem.[51]

Howell describes closed families as being the mythical standard or the "ideal" family for contemporary life:

> These families provide for their needs either by drawing on their own insular resources or by applying to agencies outside themselves. They are inward-looking units with tight boundaries. . . . For a large proportion of their needs as a group and as individuals, they are expected to be quietly self-sufficient and entirely competent.[52]

In cases of family "failure," that is, where the family is unable to succeed solely through its own means, society provides professional services, with sliding scales sometimes available for those middle-income groups who do not qualify for welfare and yet do not have the funds to cover expensive services. Although personal values and communities encourage use of professional services over accepting the advice and interest of interfering or uninformed friends and family, the services available to the lower-income family or to those who cannot pay full fees are often inadequate and/or inaccessible.

As alluded to above, professionals tend to overemphasize the self-reliant, closed, "ideal" nuclear family. Rather than encourage self-care and self-control, they often rob families of their control over their own problems and, ironically, because of their lack of real understanding and knowledge of the family, may very well provide unsatisfactory solutions.[53]

In contrast with closed families, it has been suggested that open families are able to define their boundaries more loosely and flexibly, according to the needs of its members and the group and according to outside demands and requests for help from their social network. Because such boundaries allow for a greater exchange of energy, matter, and information, these families are able to use that third "set of players," the family's informal social network.

A family's use of its social network as a resource for assistance will alter the use of professional services in a more appropriate direction, namely, for those specialized or complex needs which cannot be met by the social support system or self-care resources.

Mutual Aid or Self-help Groups

Mutual aid groups have become an increasingly important part of the social support system of many families,[54] as many family members find they need to share and seek help from others who have the same concerns and needs and discover that their usual support system does not adequately provide for these needs, which often are more specialized in nature. As an important coping strategy for many individuals and families, participating in one of these organizations can be seen as part of a search for a supportive and/or assistive system sufficiently sharing to meditate communication, guide action, and make personal experiences more bearable.[55]

Individuals and families join mutual aid groups as a coping strategy to meet a wide variety of special needs. Hence self-help groups include a wide gamut of groups established with varied purposes and processes. For instance, some self-care groups such as the Vietnam Veteran's rap groups are alternative care giving systems; some such as the ostomy clubs are adjuncts to the health professional's services; some are an expression of democratic, political ideals, such as women's groups; and some are vehicles for promoting individual change, such as TOPS, Recovery, and Alcoholics Anonymous.

DYSFUNCTIONAL ADAPTIVE STRATEGIES

Whereas functional families experiencing stress tend to act in a direction that reduces stress, dysfunctional families tend to utilize habitual defensive strategies which tend not to dissipate the stress and/or to eliminate or attenuate the stressor.[56] There are various specific dysfunctional strategies which families use to attempt to cope with their problems. In most cases these are selected unconsciously, often as responses which their families of origin used in attempting to cope.

As might be expected, the literature dealing with dysfunctional adaptive patterns is much more voluminous than the literature dealing with healthy ways of solving familial problems, having been generated primarily by family and other psychotherapists interested in family interaction and process among their clients.

Typology for Dysfunctional Family Adaptive Strategies

Since no all-encompassing typology or classification of family dysfunctional adaptive strategies exists in the literature, the following classification has been constructed to describe the familial dysfunctional adaptive (defensive) strategies:

I. Stress reduction achieved through *denial* of problems and *exploitation* of one or more family members.
   A. Nonphysical, but active emotional exploitation: scapegoating, use of threat.
   B. Nonphysical passive emotional exploitation: child neglect.
   C. Both physical and emotional exploitation employed: child abuse and spousal violence.
   D. Dysfunctional communication; *triangling*.
II. Stress reduction achieved through denial of problem. Adaptive mechanism impairs family's ability to meet affective function.
   A. Through family belief system: *family myth*, use of threat.
   B. Through establishment of emotional distancing, certain customs and traditions: *pseudomutuality* and *triangling*.
III. Stress reduction by means of separation or loss of family member(s): husband or wife abandonment, institutionalization, divorce, physical absences of

family members (alcoholism, physically absent husbands).
IV. Stress reduction by authoritarianism (submission to domination).

Denial and Exploitation

Now that a classification of some of the dysfunctional strategies has been presented, it will be easier to relate the discrete adaptive mechanisms to each other. This section will cover the several exploitative ways that families reduce tension for the family as a group, but do so at the emotional and perhaps physical expense of one or more individual members. Parad and Caplan explain that emotional exploitation can happen in two basic ways:

> . . . *passively*, by emotional neglect through concentrating family energies in such a way that the needs of an individual are not attended to, though the details of his own role may not be important in reducing tension; and *actively*, by the *emotional exploitation* of a family member through investing him with a role which does violence to his needs as an individual.[57]

Under this broad category of denial and exploitation, three familial dysfunctional patterns will be briefly discussed: marital and parental violence, scapegoating, and use of threat.

Spousal Violence. Although the use of physical force by husbands against their wives—wife beating—has recently been recognized by the mass media and health and welfare professional groups as a significant social problem, it has been a commonly used tactic for handling of frustration and stressors throughout our country's history and, as such, is practically societally sanctioned. Straus has undertaken a nationwide survey of marital violence. His preliminary studies in 1975 showed that 16 percent of middle-aged couples had violently and physically attacked one another.[58] Benedek reports that some studies have shown that there is a victim of spousal abuse in one of every two couples, with the women almost always being the victim.[59] Overwhelming statistics show homicides are not caused by strangers, but by intimates, in many instances mates. Husbands tend to murder wives with exceptional brutality, evidencing the enormous irrational rage present. Wives, on the other side, tend to murder their husbands quickly with a single knife wound or bullet and almost always do so out of self-defense. Straus believes that some dynamic is at work in the family that makes it an arena of physical violence—from slaps to murder. He suspects it is sexism, those beliefs that keep women subordinate, even through force if necessary. In some instances, the marriage license is viewed as legitimizing the husband's right to keep his wife in line, with violence if deemed necessary, despite the fact that similar acts against a person on the street would result in criminal sanctions. However, the legal system presently enforces this "right" to private violence with the doctrine of "spouse immunity" that prohibits a wife from suing her husband for assault and battery in many regions of the country or the widespread refusal of police to interfere in "family fights." This reluctance of police and prosecutors to punish wife-beaters stems from our society's traditional belief that husbands have the right to control their wives.[60]

Women who are beaten by their husbands often stay in the marriage with the hope that the husband will change, although statistics indicate he almost never does. Many of these women remain very passive and are unwilling to run away because they have often come from families where violence was customary and thus see their predicament as part of "normal" married life. In fact, many wives are unaware that it is illegal for their husband to beat them up. Moreover, many of the men are super-macho types who will not let their wives go out alone, and follow and harass them if they try to run away, leaving the wives with the idea that they will never be able to become free.[61]

Despite the vast numbers of wives who remain in marriages where spousal violence is present, increasingly wives and their children are leaving home. In response to this trend, shelters for battered women are being opened up in communities across the nation.

Child Abuse. The family provides the first initiation of individuals into uses made of physical force to control and socialize children. Straus reports that 93 percent of the parents in one survey of both the United States and England were found to use physical punishment as an important means of reinforcing and sanctioning children's behavior. To these children the message is clear: physical force as a means of imposing one's will on another is effective and is accepted (especially for male children). Boys are encouraged by parents to fight back if they are attacked at school by another child.[62]

Child abuse is a case in point of the ubiquitousness of physical violence committed by parents against their children carried to its ugly conclusion. *The Journal of the American Medical Association* stated that the assaults on children, if complete statistics were available, could turn out to be a more frequent cause of death than such diseases as leukemia, cystic fibrosis, and muscular dystrophy, and may even rank with automobile fatalities. The abusing parents frequently present a history of having been physically abused as children themselves, and so the physically violent behavior perpetuates itself from generation to generation. Divorce,

alcoholism, drug addiction, mental retardation, emotional illness, unemployment, and financial stressors all play major roles in leading the potentially abusive parent to strike out at a "special child."[63]

Scapegoating. Scapegoating is a dysfunctional adaptive mechanism because although it reduces the tension level of the family system and makes the continuance of family homeostasis possible, it does this at the expense of the emotional health of one of its members, i.e., the scapegoat or "the identified patient." The scapegoat's function is to effect a total clearance of the emotional ills that beset the family. This pattern is fairly common in troubled families and can be recognized when a family has achieved unity and cohesiveness while at the same time negatively labeling and stigmatizing one of its members. The identified patient or scapegoat is "selected" to be the focus of its difficulties, thus hiding the real problems within the family, e.g., the marital relationship. "Thus the deviant within the group may perform a valuable function for the group by channeling group tensions and providing a basis for solidarity."[64]

How is the scapegoat selected? First, the person must not be someone who has great significance for family survival; thus children are by far the most common choices of scapegoats. Children are in a relatively powerless position, cannot separate from family, are pliant to behavioral changes, and can adopt the roles parents assign to them. Usually the first child is more vulnerable, because in a faulty marriage which is further strained by the advent of a child, the stressful marital difficulties are quickly displaced onto the first available and "appropriate" object—the first child. A particular child may also be selected because of his or her age or sex, intelligence, health status, developmental stage, resemblance to another family member with negative attributes, or simple availability. Also, a family member who has already been negatively labeled is particularly vulnerable to scapegoating.[65, 66]

How does the scapegoating process start and continue? Bell and Vogel suggest that the family is initially faced with an unresolved marital stressor, with the mates having deep-seated fears about their relationship, and thus a need to deny the problem's existence.[67] The family's problem is perceived to be insoluble and beyond their coping resources. Because of this, the situation is felt to be a threat or danger to the family's survival and the life goals of its members. Concomitantly, the tension and stress levels rise and throw the family into a state of disequilibrium.

As a result of the increased stress level and precarious family stability, the family attempts to reduce the tension through the exploitation of one or more of its members. Scapegoating now reduces family tensions, since tensions, hostilities, and guilt can be directed toward (displaced onto) the identified problem member. Furthermore, the scapegoat begins taking on the assigned roles, which started as negative labeling and later became internalized, that is, into the role of the scapegoat.

When scapegoating has become an established family adaptive mechanism, family homeostasis is achieved. There is open acknowledgement and labeling of the identified patient or scapegoat. Psychic economy results as group tensions are attenuated by the displacement of anxieties, guilt, and hostility onto an object acceptable to the value system of the family.

Later, when the problem has been further walled off, the individual is reclassified in the family structure as a "problem member," different from all other family members. Eventually the outside world verifies the differentness by also labeling and stigmatizing him. Such labeling maintains the family system's dysfunctionality.

Why would the scapegoat maintain his or her unpleasant role? The answer lies in the self-fulfilling prophesy: a person does what is expected of him or her and responds to the reinforcement he or she receives to maintain this role. Reinforcement consists of secondary rewards of extra attention, even if negative, and exemption from responsibility.

If the scapegoat leaves the family, is removed by the community, or does not enact the proper role (because of psychiatric treatment), the family will face another homeostatic crisis. At this time the scapegoat may step back into the former role or a new scapegoat may be selected.

In summary, the scapegoating mechanism can be viewed as functional for the family, in that the scapegoat produces family equilibrium on a short-term basis, but in the long run is dysfunctional for the emotional health of the exploited member and, for that matter, the health of all family members.

Use of Threat. Threat is another dysfunctional coping technique used as a means of keeping the family together at the expense of the emotional health of its members. Smoyak views threat as a recurrent family dynamic in some troubled families. This technique is employed by the family to produce and maintain connectedness and discourage member's efforts to individuate and achieve separateness. The purpose of doing so is to ensure the survival of the family.[68]

Smoyak describes the control technique involved in using threat. The initial basis for needing this means of ensuring family survival is that the family system views its surrounding environment as hostile and threatening. The family feels the only way it can survive is to stick together as a closed family system. Family preservation then becomes emphasized over the individual needs of its members, and the family value

of connectedness becomes elevated to a place of high importance to maintain the family. When any one or more family members act in an autonomous, individualistic fashion, the other family members become threatened by the separating individual's impending breach with the family and thus take action to bring him or her back into the fold. They may do this either by themselves threatening to leave the family system—including threats of suicide or self-destructive acts; by threatening social ostracism—forbidding reentry into the family; threatening an aggressive act against the separating individual; or threatening emotional rejection—withdrawal of affection and support. These maneuvers may result in the "deviant" family member retreating from his or her separatist efforts and again conforming to the value of connectedness. Furthermore, once reintegrated, this individual will then usually take part in sanctioning another member who attempts to individuuate.

Forcing deviating members back into the family so that all members espouse connectedness restores the family's equilibrium. However, individuals from such families have severe adjustment problems when they leave the family environment, since they have not learned autonomy, self-directedness, and how to relate effectively with the outside community.[69]

Triangling

Another way of reducing stress within the family is through the use of triangling. This term applies to the reduction of tension in a dyadic relationship by adding a third member, who then absorbs and diffuses the ongoing tension in the dyadic relationship.[70] In other words, bringing in a third member relieves the emotionality between the original two by shifting the tension to the new dyadic member and making one of the initial partners into an "outsider." The balance of forces within the triangle are fluid and may shift either frequently or over long periods of time. In periods of very high stress, a system will triangle in more outsiders, again reducing the stress within the family.[71]

For instance, a husband and wife may be involved in an unsatisfactory, argument-laden relationship which results in neither of their needs being met. Triangling in a third person, one of the couple's children, say, reduces the marital relationship strain. Both mates begin to focus on the child, although one mate usually develops a dyadic relationship with him or her (in this case, most likely the mother) and the other mate becomes the third person—the outsider. This process forces the child to take sides: for one parent and against the other. The mother tries to fulfill her emotional needs through the parent–child relationship, putting new unrealistic demands on this relationship, so that often the newly formed dyad also becomes strained. As a result, the husband is again triangled in, resulting in a shift back to the marital dyad. "If a triangled person remains in this position for a period of time, it is quite possible he/she will develop some physical or emotional problem as an outlet for his/her anxiety."[72]

Triangling is included here as a dysfunctional coping strategy because it is a commonly used way in which to reduce interpersonal tension within the family without treating the underlying ills of the situation. Although triangling can be looked on as a phenomenon occurring to some extent in all emotionally laden interactions, and especially in dyadic ones under stress, the pervasive use of this stress-reducing mechanism over a long period of time may be considered to be dysfunctional because it does nothing to alleviate the stressor and is injurious to long-term emotional needs of family members.

The Family Myth

Through the family's belief system, myths can be created about one's family which obscure reality and deny some of the real issues and problems within the group, these problems being perceived as either too painful to be brought out in the open or as unnecessary to discuss since doing so will only make things worse. A family myth refers to a belief that is generated in response to the unfulfilled wishes and expectations of the family, instead of being based on a rational and objective appraisal of the situation.[73] Ferreira clarifies the concept of family myth further as being "a series of fairly well integrated beliefs shared by all family members, concerning each other and their mutual position in the family life, beliefs that go unchallenged by everyone involved, in spite of the reality distortions they may conspicuously imply."[74]

As wish-fulfillment fantasies, family myths are established early in the family cycle to serve as a defense against the limitations that the reality of family life imposes. Family myths thus tend to suspend reality. The more myths a family has, the less realistically a family can judge a situation and the fewer the alternatives they have to draw from. For instance, if a myth exists that the mother needs to be protected and helped, then during times of the father's absence, the family's role flexibility is diminished because the mother's ability to function in an instrumental role is stifled by the family myth.

Myths are inner images of the family group and not the facade which the family holds out to outsiders. Battiste cites some very good examples of family myths:

"We all like to do things together"; "We stay married only because of the children"; "Father is the strong one"; "We're a happy family."

She further explains when to suspect that family myths are operating: "When these inner images a family has of itself seem to not ring true to the outside observer, but when the family clings tenaciously to them, one is probably on the track of a family myth."[75]

As previously mentioned, most family myths begin in the early days of the family, when relationships are being formed and cemented. These formulas for togetherness are sought to promote closeness and set limits on possible untoward interpersonal reactions. Circular, repetitive communication patterns, roles, power, and value characteristics develop based on a myth, which, in turn, preserves the family unit.[76]

Occasionally, during a time of family crisis, a family myth will be used as a balancing mechanism. As a means of achieving homeostasis, the myth is called into play when a family experiences stress that threatens to disrupt family functioning. Thus the family myth functions as a defensive mechanism in that it prevents the family from destroying itself by maintaining, and sometimes even increasing, the level of family organization through the establishment of patterns set up as part of the family myth—a myth such as, "When in times of distress, we all help each other."[77]

On the surface, one might say that this "coping" tactic is functional—after all, it provides satisfaction for the family, automatic agreement, a common frame of reference, and stabilizing, reassuring rituals. However, it is a dysfunctional adaptive mechanism because it narrows the vision of reality and the choices or alternatives available. Members react to family issues in a stereotypical, nonindividualized way and become limited in their repertoire of responses used to deal with significant issues and life problems. Thus the growth of the family and its members is stifled because, in the presence of family myths, they will not acquire the feelings of confidence and growth which come from meeting life head-on and confronting the disappointments, problems, and broad range of possible solutions.[78]

Pseudomutuality

Pseudomutuality may be classified as a long-term dysfunctional adaptive strategy since it maintains family homeostasis at the expense of meeting the affective function: recognizing and responding to the socioemotional needs of its members. The real problem, the inability to foster and maintain intimate, close affective relationships, is covered up by a facade of solidarity and cohesiveness.

Wynne defines pseudomutuality as "a type of relatedness in which there is a preoccupation of family members with a fitting together into formal roles at the expense of individual identity."[79] As with use of threat, individual separateness or divergence is forbidden. Individual differentness or divergence is perceived as leading to disruption of the relationship and must therefore be avoided. The use of threat is sometimes used in families displaying pseudomutuality.

These families may desire closeness and intimacy but are afraid of it or are unable to reach one another on a feeling level. Affective communications are almost nil. Each family member strives for relatedness, but feels that other members block his or her efforts at closeness.

To the outside world these families usually present a picture of family solidarity, since their face-saving needs are great. However, they are able to approach this desire only through much formalized or ritualized action, such as giving gifts, celebrating birthdays, holidays, and so forth.

Pseudomutuality is a long-term adaptive strategy used by families. It presents "a stifling structure that constricts autonomy . . . consists of ambiguity, meaninglessness, and emptiness. . . . Individuality poses a great threat, especially with family members who have poor ego structures to begin with."[80]

Submission to Domination: Authoritarianism

Submission to marked domination is included in this section as a long-term dysfunctional adaptive strategy, since through the submission of family members to the dominant, ruling figure, usually the husband, family equilibrium is achieved, but again, at the emotional expense of the subordinates and, less obviously, the dominator. Peace and balance may be accomplished on either a short- or long-term basis, but when it is reluctant and forced, anger rages beneath the surface—to be either repressed, with conformity and dependence the outcome, or expressed as depression, somatization, and/or through acting out behaviors of defiance, antisocial acts, destructiveness, and so on.

Authoritarianism refers to the tendency to give up one's independence due to feelings of powerlessness and dependency and to fuse self with somebody or something outside one's self in order to acquire the power or strength felt lacking. In an authoritarian family, persons renounce their own personal integrity and become part of an unhealthy, submissive–dominance symbiosis. The submissive family members are very dependent on the dominant individual. Life as a whole is felt by the submissive members to be something overwhelming, all-powerful, and uncontrollable. Interestingly enough, the dominating member is also dependent on his or her subordinates, since the need for power and control is paramount. Along with having absolute power over the other family members and making them into instruments to be used and exploited is the feeling, "I rule you because I know what's best for you" and "I have done so much for you, now I expect something in return."

As with all the other dysfunctional adaptive strategies, all members in these families suffer. This authoritarian symbiosis curtails efforts of family members to individuate, grow, and become self-directed and independently proficient in life. Moreover, they learn only two ways of relating to people—either the ruler or the ruled—and with this background they perpetuate these roles in all their other relationships and transmit it to the next generation.

The types of families who fit into this category are those which display marked dominance, no negotiation of issues, and no input from others sought before decisions are made. Many families are mildly husband-dominated and function very effectively. It is only when this dominance pattern becomes exaggerated that it becomes a dysfunctional way to adapt to life's stressors. Cultural patterns must also be considered here. For instance, both the Hispanic and Asian families are traditionally patriarchal. However, even in these families marked domination is not salubrious and does not follow the current social mores of these cultures.

ASSESSMENT QUESTIONS

The following questions have been included to assist the assessor in appraising the family coping function.

1. What stressors (both long- and short-term) are impinging on the family? Refer to the Social Readjustment Scale of Holmes and Rahe, so that any of these factors will be identified. Also consider environmental and socioeconomic stressors. Is it possible to estimate the duration and strength of the family stressors? What strengths counterbalance them?

2. Is the family able to make decisions (adapt) based on a realistic and objective appraisal of the situation?

3. How does the family react to stressful situations? What functional strategies are used? What are the coping resources of the family? What coping strategies does the family use, or has it used, to deal with what types of problems?

4. Does the family have the following inner resources (integration and role flexibility resources)?
   Family group reliance via greater control.
   Use of a sense of humor.
   Sharing of feelings, thoughts, and activities.
   Development of strong subsystems and family members.

What are the problem-solving abilities of various family members?

Are they able to articulate their needs and concerns?

Can they outline ways of satisfying these needs, arrive at solutions, implement, and evaluate them?[81]

Controlling the meaning of the problem.

5. Can the family draw on any of the following external resources?

Use of knowledge.

Increased linkages with the broader community (general external involvement).

Social support systems.

Informal (friends, family, neighbors, employers, employees, organizations and groups, i.e., self-care or mutual aid groups and others, and communities of identity).

Formal support systems (professional services, both in health and health-related areas).

What support systems fulfill family's needs for support and assistance?

6. In what problem areas or situations has the family, in its dealings over time, achieved mastery?

7. Is the family able to meet the usual stresses and strains of daily family life?

8. How does the family react to stressful situations (dysfunctional strategies)? What dysfunctional adaptive strategies has the family used or is the family using? Are there signs of any of the dysfunctionalities listed below? If so, record the assessment data.

Spousal violence.

Child abuse.

Scapegoating.

Use of threat.

Child neglect.

Triangling.

Family myth.

Pseudomutuality.

Authoritarianism (submission to marked dominance).

REFERENCES

1. Geismar LL, La Sorte MA: Understanding the Multi-Problem Family: A Conceptual Analysis and Exploration in Early Identification. New York, Association Press, 1964
2. Yankelovitch, Skelley & White, Inc.: The American Family Report: A Study of the American Family and Money. Minneapolis, Minn, General Mills, Inc., 1975, p 13
3. Pearlin LI, Schooler C: The structure of coping. J Health Soc Behav 19:18, March 1978
4. Bloom BL: Community Mental Health: A General Introduction. Monterey, California, Brooks/Cole, 1977, pp 84–89
5. Chrisman M, Riehl J: The systems-developmental stress model. In Riehl J, Roy C (eds): Conceptual Models for Nursing Practice. New York, Appleton, 1974, p 251
6. Selye H: Stress. Montreal, Acta, 1950, pp 12–13
7. Burgess AW: Nursing: Levels of Intervention. Englewood Cliffs, NJ, Prentice-Hall, 1978, p 46
8. Ibid., p 50
9. White RW: Strategies of adaptation: An attempt at systematic description. Cited in Burgess, op. cit. pp 51–52
10. Oehrtman SE: Assessment and crisis intervention. In Hall JE, Weaver BR (eds): Nursing Families With Crisis. Philadelphia, Lippincott, 1974, p 139
11. Burgess, op. cit., p 52
12. Wallace AM: Typology of stressors: A developmental view. In Burgess, op. cit., pp 76–108
13. Minuchin A: Families and Family Therapy. Cambridge, Mass, Harvard University Press, 1974, pp 60–66
14. Burgess, op. cit., p 53
15. Nickolls K: Life crisis and psychosocial assets: Some clinical implications. In Kaplan BH, Cassell JC: Family and Health: An Epidemiological Approach. Chapel Hill, NC, 1975, p 40
16. Ibid., p 53
17. Pearlin, Schooler, op. cit., p 2
18. Ibid., p 8
19. Ibid., pp 6, 10
20. Ibid., p 6
21. Lazarus RS et al: The psychology of coping: Issues of research and assessment. In Coehlo GV, Hamburg DA, Adams JE (eds): Coping and Adaption. New York, Basic Books, 1966, pp 277–291
22. Pearlin, Schooler, op. cit., pp 10–11
23. Ibid., pp 7, 13–14, 18
24. Hall JE, Weaver BR: Crisis: A conceptual approach to family nursing. In Hall JE, Weaver BR (eds): Nursing Families With Crisis. Philadelphia, Lippincott, 1974, p 5
25. Ibid.
26. Ibid., p 7
27. Lewis J et al: No Single Thread—Psychological Health in Family Systems. New York, Brunner/Mazel, 1976, p 208
28. Burgess, op. cit., p 60
29. Hott JR: Mobilizing family strengths in health maintenance and coping with illness. In Reinhardt A, Quinn M: Current Practices in Family-Centered Community Nursing. St. Louis, Mosby, 1977, p 109
30. Wessel ML: Use of humor by an immobilized adolescent girl during hospitalization. Maternal Child Nurs J 4:35–48, Spring 1975
31. Orthner DK: Leisure activity patterns and marital satisfaction over the marital career. J Marriage Family 37(1):91–102, 1975
32. Rapoport R, Rapoport R, Thiessen V: Couple symmetry and enjoyment. J Marriage Family 36(3):588–591, 1974
33. West P, Merriam LC Jr: Outdoor recreation and family cohesiveness: A research approach. J Leisure Res 2:251–259, 1970
34. Pratt L: Family Structure and Effective Health Behavior. Boston, Houghton Mifflin 1976, pp 86–87
35. Rainwater L: The lower class: Health, illness, and medi-

cal institutions. In Deutscher L, Thompson EJ (eds): Among the People. New York, Basic, 1968. In Pratt, *op. cit.*, p 87

36. Pearlin, Schooler, *op. cit.*, p 18
37. Hoeflin R: Child rearing practices and child care resources used by Ohio farm families with pre-school children. Genet Psychol 84:271, 1954
38. Pratt, *op. cit.*, p 91
39. *Ibid.*
40. Howell MC: Helping Ourselves: Families and the Human Network. Boston, Beacon, 1975, p 70
41. Hogue CC: Support systems for health promotion. In Hall J, Weaver B (eds): Distributive Nursing Practice: A Systems Approach to Community Health. Philadelphia, Lippincott, 1977, p 68
42. Caplan G: Support Systems and Community Mental Health. New York, Behavioral Publications, 1974, p 7
43. Hogue, *op. cit.*, pp 68–69
44. MacElveen PM: Social networks. In Longo DC, Williams RA (eds): Clinical Practice in Psychosocial Nursing: Assessment and Intervention. New York, Appleton, 1978, p 319
45. Hogue, *op. cit.*, p 67
46. *Ibid.*, p 68
47. MacElveen, *op. cit.*, pp 319–338
48. Caplan, *op. cit.*, p 27
49. *Ibid.*, pp 4–7
50. Pearlin, Schooler, *op. cit.*, p 18
51. Howell, *op. cit.*, p 71
52. *Ibid.*, p 72
53. *Ibid.*, pp 72–74
54. Katz AH, Bender EI: The Strength Within Us. New York, Franklin Watts, 1976
55. Vickers G: Institutional and personal roles. Human Relations 24(5):433, 1971.
56. White, *op cit.*
57. Parad HJ, Caplan G: A framework for studying families in crisis. In Parad H (ed): Crisis Intervention: Selected Readings. New York, Family Service Association of America, 1965, p 59
58. Straus MA: Marital violence. Paper presented at American Psychological Association Convention, Chicago, 1975. Cited in Eldridge E, Meredith N: Environmental Issues: Family Impact. Minneapolis, Minn, Burgess, 1976, pp 177–178
59. Benedek E: Paper on "spousal abuse" presented to the 1978 Winter Scientific Session of the American Medical Association, Las Vegas, Nevada. Reported by Nelson H:

Abused Wives Cling to Hope, Doctors Say. Los Angeles Times, December 8, 1978, pp 1, 18
60. Straus, *op. cit.*, pp 177–178
61. Benedek, *op. cit.*, pp 1, 18
62. Straus, *op. cit.*, pp 177–178
63. Fontana VJ: To prevent the abuse of the future. In Eldridge E, Meredith N: Environmental Issues: Family Impact. Minneapolis, Minn, Burgess, 1976, pp 185–189
64. Bell NW, Vogel EF: A Modern Introduction to the Family. New York, Free Press, 1968, p 412
65. Goodspeed HE: Scapegoating: A process continuing when parents divorce. In Smoyak S (ed): The Psychiatric Nurse as a Family Therapist. New York, Wiley, 1975, pp 150–151
66. Roberts RH: Perceptual views of family members of the identified patient. In Smoyak S (ed): The Psychiatric Nurse as a Family Therapist. New York, Wiley, 1975, p 165
67. Bell NW, Vogel EF: The Family. New York, The Free Press, 1968, p 414
68. Smoyak SA: Threat: a recurring family dynamic. Perspect Psychiatr Care 7:267–268, 1969
69. *Ibid.*, pp 267–274.
70. Hallen LL: Family systems theory in psychiatric intervention. Am J Nurs 74(3):463, 1978
71. Anonymous: Toward the differentiation of a self in one's own family. In Framo JL (ed): Family Interaction: A Dialogue Between Family Researchers and Family Therapists. New York, Springer, 1972, pp 123–124
72. Francis GM, Munjas BA: Manual of Socialpsychological Assessment. New York, Appleton, 1976, p 38
73. Battiste HB: Family myths. In Smoyak, *op. cit.*, p 99
74. Ferreira AJ: Family myth and homeostasis. Arch Gen Psychiatry 9:457, 1963
75. Battiste, *op. cit.*, p 101
76. *Ibid.*, p 101
77. Peters LA: Family team or myth. In Hall JE, Weaver BR (eds): Nursing Families in Crisis. Philadelphia, Lippincott 1974, p 227
78. Battiste, *op. cit.*, pp 101–102
79. Wynne LG, et al: Pseudomutuality in the family relationships of schizophrenics. Psychiatry 21:205, 1958
80. Silver J: Solidarity versus pseudomutuality. In Smoyak, *op. cit.*, p 111
81. Robischon P, Smith JA: Family assessment. In Reinhardt AM, Quinn MD (eds): Current Practice in Family-Centered Community Nursing, Vol 1. St. Louis, Mosby, 1977, p 94

STUDY QUESTIONS

1. The family coping function is vitally important because (select *the best* answer):
   a. It is the mechanism through which all other family functions are made possible.
   b. It provides opportunities for family members to learn how to cope effectively.
   c. It leads to problem solving and mastery over family issues and stresses.
   d. It either eliminates stressors or leads to stress reduction activities.

2. In this chapter, one convincing piece of evidence that shows that many families are experiencing problems in adaptation (family coping) is:

a. Crisis intervention centers are springing up everywhere.
b. More money is being pumped into family counseling centers.
c. The pervasiveness of mental disorders in our communities.
d. Nursing is increasingly focusing on helping families cope with their health problems.

3. Match the definitions in the right-hand column with the concepts and terms in the left-hand column.

Concepts/Terms	Definitions
a. Crisis.	1. The end result of functional coping, where repeated successful problem-solving efforts have taken place.
b. Mastery.	
c. Defense mechanism.	
d. Stressors.	2. Active, effective adaptive efforts.
e. Stress.	3. The precipitating or initiating events or agents which generate stress.
f. Adaptation.	
g. Coping.	4. The general process of adjustment to change.
	5. The strain, disequilibrium produced by threat or actual existence of stressors.
	6. Habitual, stereotypic responses to threat or actual presence of stressors.
	7. In the presence of the stress and stressors, the family's failure in use of effective adaptive strategies.

4. Minuchin has identified four general sources of family stressors. What are they?

Are the following statements True *or* False?

5. In the ante-stress period, anticipatory guidance would be contraindicated.

6. Defensive tactics are often necessary adaptive responses during the actual stress period.

7. During the poststress period, coping tactics consist of strategies to return the family to a homeostatic state.

8. In their studies, Holmes and Rahe were able to demonstrate the following relationships (select *the best* answer):
   a. A positive correlation between stressor and stress.
   b. A sequential relationship in which high life change scores existed prior to the advent of illness.
   c. A cause-and-effect relationship between number of life change events and presence of illness.
   d. A negative correlation between stress and wellness.

9. The balancing of forces diagram given in Figure 16.2 extends the Holmes and Rahe model in these ways (select all appropriate answers):
   a. It includes environmental factors.
   b. It is adapted to fit the family system.
   c. It takes into account the family's assets or strengths.
   d. A higher level of wellness is seen as an "imbalance."

10. Pearlin and Schooler conducted a study of normative coping responses and found that in each of the following primary roles certain coping responses were perceived of as more effective by their respondents. Identify an effective coping response for each of the following roles.
    a. Occupational and economic role.
    b. Marital role.
    c. Parental role.

11. Which of the following are the *two* primary variables involved in whether crisis develops or not?
    a. Compliance with environment.
    b. Perception of event or change.
    c. Efficacy of coping or adaptive responses.
    d. Choice to grow or stagnate.
    e. Open or closed communications.

12. Select four functional family coping strategies (two inner coping resources and two external coping resources) and describe each of these briefly.

13. Select four dysfunctional family coping strategies and describe each of these briefly.

Choose the correct answers to the following questions.

14. The two prime purposes of social support systems are to:
    a. Provide direct assistance.
    b. Become a family advocate.
    c. Replace professional services.
    d. Provide emotional support.

15. Indicate which of the following are functional (F) or dysfunctional (D) or which could be either (E) depending on the situation.
    a. Family group reliance via greater control.
    b. Scapegoating.
    c. Pseudomutuality.
    d. Sense of humor.
    e. Increased linkage with community.
    f. Spousal violence.
    g. Child neglect.
    h. Triangling.
    i. Social support systems.
    j. Use of knowledge.
    k. Role flexibility.
    l. Controlling the meaning of the problem.

Choose the correct answer(s) to each of the following questions.

16. Functional coping by families usually occurs when:
    a. The family has adequate inner and outside resources.
    b. The crisis-provoking event is interpreted in an objective, realistic manner.

c. Family bonds and unity exists.

d. The family has the capacity to shift course and modify roles within the family.

17. The purpose(s) for families utilizing threat as a control mechanism is (are) to:
    a. Maintain authoritarian structure within the family.
    b. Maintain or reinstate connectedness within the family.
    c. Insure the survival of the family group.
    d. Decrease family members' attempts to behave in an autonomous, individualistic manner.

FAMILY CASE STUDY*

Read the following family study, then assess the family in the areas of affective functioning and family coping functioning of the family.

Mrs. Ruby Nichols, a 34-year-old obese woman, came to the mental health clinic because, she said, "I just don't know what to do." She was crying hysterically and unable to respond to further questioning. After remaining with her for an hour, the nurse was able to elicit that her 5-year-old foster daughter was being removed from the home per court order. Welfare funds, her only support for herself, her unemployed husband, and their five children, were being terminated in a week, leaving her unable to pay the bills or buy enough food for her family. Although Mrs. Nichols was still tearful and depressed, she was able to be driven home by a community worker.

The following day the nurse made a visit to the Nichols's home. Mrs. Nichols related the following history.

Ruby and John Nichols had been married 15 years. Four children were born of the marriage: Priscilla, 13; Cindy, 10; John Jr., 6; and Lisa, 4. Their foster daughter, Ann, was 5. The couple had known each other a year before their marriage in their home town of Smithfield, Louisiana. John was an unskilled laborer, but had always managed to be employed. Ruby had attended business school prior to the marriage and was employed as a bookkeeper until the first child was born. She described her early marriage as fine except for moving so many times, caused by John's "meddling mother." The family would move to get away from his mother, but she would always manage to locate them and appear on the scene. "We were a healthy, happy family and everything was fine as long as John's mother stayed away." Ruby related that this source of conflict between herself and John was resolved each time by a new move on their part. However, she and John never really discussed their mother-in-law problems according to Ruby. Following each new move, Ruby would join clubs and organizations to make new friends and John's work provided a similar opportunity for him. John also spent several evenings a week in the local bar, "shooting the bull" with the boys from work.

The last move was six months ago. After two months John lost his job and was unable to find another. This resulted in the family receiving welfare, which Ruby and John felt ashamed of, as they had always prided themselves on paying their own bills. Shortly after this, John's mother found the family and moved into town. When she came to visit, a bitter argument ensued regarding John's mother and since then John had been staying away from home and drinking a lot. Moreover, three months ago Ruby had abdominal surgery which

---

* Adapted with permission from Black BB: Families in Crisis: Assessment and Nursing Intervention. Los Angeles, Intercampus Nursing Project, California State University, Los Angeles, 1974.

was followed by complications and a prolonged hospitalization period. During her absence from home, the role of mother was assumed by Priscilla, who managed well with the help from the next door neighbor, Mrs. Law.

Ruby was released from the hospital three weeks ago as sufficiently recovered to stay at home. When she got home she perceived that the children had functioned "very well" in her absence; in fact, she felt that they did not need her and even seemed to resent her. John remained away most of the time and was minimally involved in family life during her hospitalization, as well as presently.

A week ago she learned of the court's decision to remove Ann from the home and the termination of welfare funds. Ruby felt herself becoming less and less able to manage and admitted to depression and suicidal thoughts. However, her concern for her children prevented her from doing anything self-destructive. The next-door-neighbor, Mrs. Law, realizing the gravity of the family's situation, told Ruby to go to the mental health clinic for help.

Subsequent visits to the family revealed that the children were having problems and that Ruby had difficulties relating to their problematic behaviors. It was observed that the children and parents did not discuss these problems or their concerns with each other, and that there was no movement toward sharing their feelings about Ann's leaving, the mother-in-law's disruptive influence, or Ruby's health problems.

Priscilla, age 13, seemed to resent Ruby's return, since it meant the loss of her mothering role. She and her mother have engaged in frequent arguments over the discipline of the younger children, what they should wear, and how they should act. The arguments usually ended with Priscilla leaving the house for long periods of time without telling Ruby where she was. This caused Ruby to worry. Priscilla was not interested in school, her main interest being to grow up as quickly as possible and emulate her mother. She also wanted desperately to be independent and make her own decisions in life. Ruby had "weaned" Priscilla early in terms of her being self-sufficient at home: from age 6 on, Priscilla was caring for her younger siblings and helping her mother out in the home.

Cindy, age 10, seemed unaffected by the situation. She was quite involved with her school activities and Campfire Girls and spent much time in these activities and at her friends' homes. Priscilla and Cindy evidently have a closer sibling relationship than the other siblings do. Cindy tells "all her secrets" to Priscilla when she is upset or worried or needs someone to talk to.

John Jr., a first grader, was refusing to go to school. Every morning it was now a struggle to get him off to school. He would cry and hang on to his mother. His teacher reported poor school work and lack of attentiveness when he was present.

Lisa, age 4, displayed similar clinging behaviors to that of John Jr. She seemed frightened when mother left the house and was wetting the bed again after having no problems in this area for two years. Both John Jr. and Lisa frequently questioned their mother about the recent absence of Ann. They asked if Ann went away because she was "bad."

On the third contact between the family (the parents) and the nurse at the mental health clinic, the nurse asked the parents to describe each child, what he or she was like, and what personal needs or problems they were trying to assist their children with at that time. It was noted that specific information on each child was difficult to obtain. For instance, these general statements were made: "Oh, he (she) is just the average 6 year old (or whatever age applied)," or "Priscilla's just like all other teenagers, wanting her way all the time," or "I treat all my children the same, regardless." They were able to recognize, though, Priscilla's need to care for her younger siblings and to be independent, but were not open to her staying away from the family very much, or developing a set of friends outside the family with whom she might have frequent social contact.

The mother also recognized that Lisa was very attached to and dependent on her, and needed reassurance that mother would be back when she left home. Additionally, both parents thought Ann's leaving was threatening to the younger children, who might think this might happen to them if they misbehaved. Ruby was trying to spend more time with Lisa to help her with her fears over the mother's separation and Ann's leaving. John showed interest in "comforting" and being involved with Lisa also, since Lisa always responded "in such a cute, loving way to her daddy," according to the mother.

Both parents are able to show affection and warmth to the younger children (John Jr. and Lisa), but do not feel that it is appropriate to be so "physical" when they get older. It was noted that the parents were not physically affectionate to each other and seemed emotionally distant during the interviews. Ruby says that they have never shared their personal concerns with each other much. "It takes another woman to understand my feelings. I used to confide in Priscilla a lot, but since she is upset with me, I haven't been able to talk with her."

18. What short- and long-terms stressors are impinging on the family? What strengths counterbalance these stressors?

19. Is the family able to make decisions based on a realistic and objective appraisal of the situation?

20. How does the family react to stressful situations—both functional and dysfunctional strategies should be described.

STUDY ANSWERS

1. a

2. c

3. a. 7   e. 5
   b. 1   f. 4
   c. 6   g. 2
   d. 3

4. a. Stressful contact of one member with extrafamilial forces.
   b. Stress contact of whole family with extrafamilial forces.
   c. Transitional stressors.
   d. Situational stressors.

5. False

6. True

7. True

8. b

9. b, c, and d

10. a. *Occupational and economic role.* Controlling the meaning of the problem, by minimizing the negative and substitution of other more accessible rewards.
    b. *Marital role.* Self-reliance and involvement (modifying stressful situation) and reflective probing of problems (stress management).
    c. *Parental role.* Self-reliance and involvement (modifying stressful situation) and conviction that one has power to effect change and exert influence (stress management).

11. b and c

12. *Inner Resources (two)*
    a. *Integration.* Control of subsystem through bonds of unity and cohesiveness.
    b. *Role flexibility.* Ability of family members to adapt by shifting roles as needed.
    c. *Family group reliance via family control.* The tighter structure and control over subsystems, greater degree of family organization.
    d. *Use of humor.* Improves attitude toward problems and gives some respite and lightness to a stressful situation.
    e. *Greater sharing together.* Increasing family efforts to converse about feelings and thoughts, participate in family activities.
    f. *Development of strong individuals and subsystems.* Strengthening subsystem; assisting members to become good problem solvers.
    g. *Controlling the meaning of the problem.* Interpreting or defining a change or event realistically, objectively (where cognitive mastery is involved).

    External Resources (two)
    a. *Use of knowledge.* Greater amount or pertinent information sought to deal with issue/problem at hand.
    b. *Increased linkages with broader community.* This is a more general life-style characterization, where family members have open boundaries and continually participate and involve themselves in community organizations and activities.
    c. *Social support systems.* Social support systems function to provide support and assistance either more generally or on an as-needed basis. These social support systems are composed of friends, extended family, employers, employees, neighbors, groups (including mutual aid groups), organizations, and professional persons and agencies.

13. Dysfunctional family coping strategies (any four):
    a. *Spousal violence.* In response to pent-up frustrations in marital relationship and hostility of marital partners, one spouse attacks other.
    b. *Child abuse.* Physical violence, usually by parents, against one or more of their children.
    c. *Scapegoating.* Selecting one or more family members to be the identified family problem. Negatively labeling and imposing unhealthy exploitative role onto the scapegoat.

d. *Use of threat.* By use of threat or ostracism, expulsion or self-destructive acts, family keeps all its members in conformity. "Separateness" acts by individuals are thus curtailed.

e. *Triangling.* Introduction of a third member into a stressful dyadic relationship when stress level reaches point where stress reduction is sought. This is exploitative of third member and does not confront problem in relationship.

f. *The family myth.* Beliefs developed in family about themselves which have themes of wish-fulfillment. These tend to hide real problems and limit family's alternatives and problem-solving resources.

g. *Pseudomutuality.* Maintaining pseudo or false closeness. Family members have difficulty in expressing affection and closeness. As a result, they build up all sorts of customs and rituals which structure family members' responses and establish a facade of closeness and solidarity.

h. *Authoritarianism.* Is a long-term adaptive response to deal with feelings of powerlessness and dependency. One member becomes the dominator and the others the subordinates. All "lose" in this type of family structure, since there is no opportunity provided to learn the value of negotiation, discussion, and how to relate effectively with others and be autonomous.

14. a and d

15.
a.	E	h.	E
b.	D	i.	F
c.	D	j.	F
d.	E	k.	F
e.	E	l.	E
f.	D		
g.	D		

16. all (a–d)

17. b, c, and d

FAMILY CASE STUDY

18. Short-term stressors impinging on the family:
   Husband's unemployment.
   Being on welfare and then the threat of termination.
   Ann's loss (removal from the home).
   Ruby's recent ill-health, hospitalization, and convalescence.
   Ruby's depression and suicidal thoughts.
   Long-term stressors impinging on the family:
   The perceived interference of John's mother.
   Emotional distance and lack of communication in family and especially within marital relationship.
   Continual geographic movement, from one community to the next, so that no stable and sufficient social network is established.
   Husband's minimal participation in family life and his excessive and frequent drinking activities.

Family strengths:

Presence of social support system, although small: receiving help from mental health clinic; Mrs. Law, neighbor.

Ruby's caring for and commitment to children.

Parents' staying together and father's interest in Lisa and potential of greater participation in family life.

Parents' motivation to find employment, be financially self-sufficient.

Priscilla's interest in and ability for child care.

19. The parents' ability to make decisions based on objective and realistic appraisal of a situation is limited. In terms of the interference of John's mother, they perceived events as a problem which they had no control over, i.e., seen as John's mother's behavior, rather than a situation in which they needed to communicate with each other and John's mother in order to define problems and identify a mutually satisfactory way of handling situation. Data does not reveal their perception of why Ann was removed or why welfare was terminated. Ruby personally distorted the parenting situation in feeling that her children did well without her and did not wish her back.

20. 1. No evidence for the use of some of the functional coping strategies related to family's inner resources such as greater family reliance on themselves; increased sharing of feelings and thoughts; shared activities; and controlling the meaning of the stressors.

  2. Family (Ruby and then family) did seek one support system when problems reached crisis proportions, i.e., the mental health clinic. The neighbor, Mrs. Law, has also assisted family. But the family, because of its continual moving, has not developed an adequate social support system.

  3. Dysfunctional adaptive tactics:

  Use of spousal withdrawal—both spouses do not communicate openly with each other; husband withdraws from family physically and through his drinking.

  Use of denial as to the family's real problems. They have seen their major family problem as John's "meddling mother." Use of *family myth* around this source of conflict was apparent. The family myth, more specifically, has been that "we are a happy family as long as John's mother stays away."

17

Cultural Differences among Families

LEARNING OBJECTIVES

Foundational Content

1. Explain why an understanding of a family's cultural background is crucial for family health practice.
2. Discuss several of the major problems which result when cultural insensitivity and ignorance exist on the part of the health professional.
3. Recall the salience and meaning of ethnicity for society, family, and the individual.
4. Discuss the importance of the cross-cultural approach to family health care.
5. Define these basic concepts: culture, ethnic groups, cultural pluralism, ethnic identity, stereotyping, acculturation, assimilation, cultural relativism, ethnocentrism, cultural imposition, cultural conflicts, cultural shock, indigenous health care system, and self-fulfilling prophecy.
6. Analyze both the negative and positive aspects of ethnic self-help.

The Chicano Family

7. Explain why the Chicano family has not integrated into the mainstream of American society to the extent that other ethnic groups have.
8. Discuss the four major family characteristics of the Chicano family: familism, male dominance, the ethnic of reciprocity among kin, and respect for the obedience to the older family members.
9. Explain the meaning and importance of *machismo* and *compadrazgo*.
10. Describe briefly the traditional role and power structure of the Chicano family.
11. Compare American core values with traditional Mexican-American values.
12. Identify the most important structural change occurring in Mexican-American families today.

13. Describe the basic differences in socialization patterns between American and traditional Mexican-American families.
14. Recognize the functions and primary role of the following folk healers: *yerbero, curandera(o), espiritualisto(a),* and *brujo(a).*
15. Recall several common Mexican-American folk illnesses.
16. Explain three health care practice implications based on Chicano culturally patterned beliefs and practices.

The Black Family

17. Point out some of the major problems (according to statistics) facing the black family today.
18. Compare the family roles and power structure of black middle-class, working-class, and lower-class families.
19. Broadly describe differences in socialization and marital stability among middle-, working- and lower-class black families.
20. Identify two traditional folk practitioners in the black communities in the past.
21. Recall two commonly seen tactics blacks utilize when coping with white health institutions.
22. Explain three health care practice implications based on black family beliefs and patterns.

Consideration of culture has been left to this a final chapter related to family theory and content for the purpose of emphasizing its vital, critical nature. Up to this point in the text, culture has been touched on as an important variable in assessment of both the structural and functional aspects of the family. In addition, Chapters 8 and 12 have covered the salient cultural aspects of acculturation and value orientations. Both of these aspects provide crucial background for practice, yet cultural factors cover much more than formation of one's values or assessment of the extent to which a family is acculturated. Because culture permeates and circumscribes our individual, familial, and social actions, its consequences are pervasive and its implications for practice broad in scope. This chapter can only hope to acquaint the reader with some of the rudimentary concepts and terms, cross-cultural barriers and problems, and assessment and practice implications. A discussion of the special problems or quandaries minority families face, as well as a description of families from America's two largest minorities or ethnic groups, is also included to show the significance of cultural variation in family life.

IMPORTANCE OF CULTURE FOR PRACTICE

To understand an ethnic group and to be able to work efficaciously with families from cultures different from one's own, one must be aware of that culture's unique, distinctive qualities and the variety of life styles, values, and structures found within that group. Hence the importance of culture lies in its vital character. Since cultural differences are often at the root of poor communication, interpersonal tensions, avoidance in working effectively with others, and poor assessment of health problems and their remedies, successful nursing care of clients of various ethnic backgrounds is dependent on the knowledge of and sensitivity to the clients' culture that nurses have.

In family counseling the importance of culture is paramount. Coddy points out that in family therapy the health professional and client must have interlocking cultural patterns. Without knowledge of the differences in cultural norms and patterns, behavior that differs from normative patterns is usually labeled as deviant, crazy, immoral, or illegal (depending on the type of prescribed behavior violated). In the absence of cultural data, it then becomes impossible for the health worker to recognize the possible cultural meaning of the client's behavior or actions. In addition, Coddy identifies four other important areas where cultural dissimilarity may permeate and disrupt counseling: (1) goal expectations; (2) establishment of rapport; (3) communication styles; and (4) acceptance of ideas.[1]

The importance of nurse–client cultural congruence is well documented. Several noted authors have pointed to the greater ease and efficacy when the client and the health professionals have similar ethnic and religious backgrounds. When similar frames of references exist in a relationship, the possibilities of greater freedom of expression, deeper identification, and increased empathy present themselves.[2] However, having a health worker and client of the same ethnic background is, in many cases, an ideal situation. In reality it is not often possible, and perhaps may not even be socially desirable. Otherwise, how are we to learn to live and relate well to one another?

The critical nature of language barriers also deserves mention. In some regions, where a majority or plurality of one's clients are from a different culture and speak a different language, learning the culture's language will not only result in dramatically improved communications, but also in a much greater understanding and appreciation of the culture. Padilla verifies this fact in his study of lower-class Mexican-Americans seen in therapy in a counseling center in East Los Angeles. He states that it has generally been assumed that lower-class persons have difficulty benefiting from psychotherapy because of their nonverbalness, inarticulateness, and lack of ability to think abstractly. Padilla reports, however, that in counseling Chicano clients, this generalization does not hold true when clients were given the opportunity and encouraged to communicate in Spanish, English, or a combination of both in order to enhance the meaningfulness of their communication. He concludes that, "It now seems clear that the Chicano poor are quite capable of verbally expressing themselves in the most intensive 'insight' therapy situation, if they are not forced to communicate in English, a language that may be partly or completely foreign to these individuals."[3]

CULTURAL-ETHNIC PLURALISM

Our country is truly a matrix of many ethnic groups or subcultures. Massive waves of immigration have continued to mold and revolutionize the character of the United States throughout the last two centuries. The myth of the American melting pot has been intellectually recognized, though its implications not eradicated. This myth encouraged all diverse ethnic groups immigrating to the United States to succeed in American society by becoming part of the one predominant group. Any differences were typically seen as deviant and inferior. Ethnic variation was perceived as an element of the lower social class and of recent immigrant groups. Moving up the social class ladder to success meant discarding one's ethnic traditions and values and assimilating into the mainstream of society.

The social protest of the 1960s brought about the harsh realization that the society had not, and did not wish to, move toward one homogeneous entity. The civil rights movement and the rise of black consciousness and identity set the model for all other ethnic groups. This model stressed a reaffirmation of cultural differences, a greater demand for equal treatment, and an acceptance of the value of ethnic or cultural diversity in society. This movement was quickly followed by similar demands for ethnic pluralism among white ethnic groups (Jewish, Irish, Italian, etc.), Asian-Americans, and Mexican-Americans.[4] Stemming from this push for cultural pluralism, American values have been changing, reflecting a greater tolerance for diversity (see Chap. 12).

Kobrin and Goldscheider, researchers of ethnicity, discuss the salience and meaning of ethnicity for society, family, and the individual:

> Ethnic pluralism is an integral feature of human societies and ethnicity continues to be an organic part of social and cultural changes. The major processes associated with industrialization and urbanization have not resulted in the disappearance of ethnic communities nor the eradication of ethnic differences in major social processes.... The conspicuousness of ethnic communities suggests that ethnic institutions and social networks even as they change remain major sources of group identification.[5]

The authors point out that with the recent reemergence of ethnicity, one's cultural heritage and ethnic identity has become an even more tangible and acceptable basis for group cohesion in America. One important reason for placing greater importance and recognition on ethnic or cultural roots is that ethnic identification provides for many persons and families an alternative link to the broader society, partially compensating for the cold, impersonal, and bureaucratic qualities of society today.[6] Moreover, ethnicity can be seen as enriching family life and strengthening its bonds of intergenerational continuity.

THE CROSS-CULTURAL APPROACH

The cross-cultural approach used in anthropology provides a broad comparative picture of human nature and human behavior.[7] This approach to nursing care is both a practical necessity and a social reality, due to the awareness of the pervasive part culture plays and also to recognition of the growing numbers of persons in the United States from different cultural backgrounds. As we become familiar with other cultures and learn to appreciate why certain values and norms are effective through time for those cultures, health workers, it is hoped, will become more sensitive and effective in providing family health care. Leininger asserts that it is not only sound for nursing to use a cross-cultural approach, it is mandatory: clients have a *right* to have their sociocultural backgrounds understood in the same way that they expect their physical and psychological needs to be recognized and understood.[8] Whereas health professionals have primarily emphasized physiological principles in their interpretation of individual health–illness phenomena, the cultural or the social level of analysis has been, until only recently, largely ignored.[9] Even now, as with the use of the family-centered approach, we pay lip service to assessing sociocultural factors and in practice carry on as usual.

BASIC CONCEPTS

As with other facets of social science, cultural anthropologists also have their own lexicon of terms and concepts which are of fundamental importance for the understanding of cross-cultural principles and processes.

Foremost among these concepts and terms is that of *culture*. Culture is usually viewed as a blueprint for man's way of living, thinking, behaving, and feeling. It circumscribes and guides the ways in which societies and ethnic groups solve their problems and derive meaning from their lives. From a systems perspective, culture is defined as systems of socially transmitted behavioral patterns that link human groups to their environmental settings, as well as systems of social change and organization which act to mediate societal adaptation.[10] It involves patterns of learned behavior and values which are transmitted from one generation to the next.

In other words, culture is a mold from which we all are cast. And it constrains and regulates our daily behavior, attitudes, and values in many latent and manifest ways. Since people rely on learned behavior or culture for survival, it is the prime source of our adaptability. Hence only through the understanding of culture can one hope to understand our humanity and our personal and social actions and needs.

Webster's Dictionary defines *ethnic* as an adjective related to people of a particular race or cultural group who are classified according to common traits and customs. In this chapter, ethnicity is used interchangeably with cultural group or subcultural group, even though ethnicity is defined more narrowly (in terms of a group of people) than culture is. Subcultures are groups within a society whose members have their own particular set of cultural values, beliefs, and practices, i.e., an ethnic group. Minority groups have sometimes objected to the term subculture, since some feel this term denotes "less than" or "under" the general culture.

Thus this term is used less frequently here, although it is in general usage in the social sciences.

Ethnic identity is another related term. This term refers to the way in which individuals classify themselves vis-à-vis other persons and the extent to which they associate or fail to associate themselves with persons of similar cultural backgrounds.

Just as there are enormous differences between cultures, there is also a great *variation within cultures*. Since nursing care is extended to individuals and families, it is of utmost importance to take into account the diversity among individuals within the various ethnic groups.[11] Yet the tendency is to simplify things by labeling people. Kay discusses the perennial problem of generalizing about a group of people in anthropologic-ethnographic descriptions:

> Most ethnographies, or accounts of the life style of people who participate in a specific culture, are like still photographs. They describe people staggered in time and space. We call such fixed images stereotypes. Model personalities are frozen in a changeless place, and subsequently are supposed to represent millions. But if we try to qualify groups by describing certain differences (e.g., 72 percent of *barrio* women make their own tortillas as compared with 12 percent who buy Rainbo bread), we end up by describing no one.[12]

Hence the knowledge that the father holds primary power in the Mexican-American home or that the Jewish mother is "the power behind the throne" in the Jewish culture provides data to look for when doing an assessment. However, these patterns need to be verified with the particular family the nurse is assessing.

Lack of recognition of individual differences or labeling is termed *stereotyping*. Cultural stereotyping involves the nonacceptance or disallowance of individual or group diversity; i.e., everyone from a particular culture is viewed as the same and perceived of as fixed in their characteristics. Although one needs to generalize about a culture in order to learn and teach others about it, health professionals must also realize that cultures change, as well as individuals within that culture, as a result of varying degrees of exposure to other cultures, of family differences, and of personal idiosyncrasies.

This exposure to another culture leads to a sociocultural process called *acculturation*. As one of the major causative factors of variation within an ethnic group, "acculturation comprises those gradual changes produced in a culture by the influence of another culture which results in an increased similarity of the two."[13] In the case of cultural groups immigrating to the United States, the influence is usually overwhelmingly one way, that is, the American culture exerts greater influence on the ethnic group to conform to its cultural patterns than vice versa. The resultant *assimilation* may proceed so far as to practically extinguish the ethnic culture (as occurred with the African culture during slavery) or factors may intervene to counterbalance the forces of assimilation and keep the two cultures isolated from one another. For example, language, religious, economic, and geographic barriers have kept Mexican-Americans and Native Americans fairly separate from American society, and the strong cultural traditions of the Jews have to a large extent curtailed their assimilation. Assimilation denotes the more complete and one-way process of one culture being absorbed into the other.

Kluckholm hypothesizes that the rate and degree of acculturation of any ethnic group into the dominant culture depends primarily on the degree of congruency between the group's own basic value orientations with those of the dominant (American) culture.[14] Also, certain groups within a particular ethnic subculture are more receptive to social and cultural change. For instance, urban residents, the more educated, occupationally successful, or higher socioeconomic groups are more likely to experience assimilatory changes. Hence socioeconomic and class factors are crucial elements to consider in learning about ethnicity.

Acculturation then implies that members of cultures other than the dominant culture of the society have internalized to a great extent the norms and values of the dominant culture and, moreover, that the wider society has been influenced to varying degrees by its exposure to each of the ethnic or subcultural groups within its boundaries.

Acculturation does not necessarily suggest the loss of ethnic identity—of a detaching of oneself from an ethnic community[15]—nor does it imply the loss of many of the customs related to that culture. Customs which continue, more or less unscathed, are those that are not stigmatizing or illegal, customs such as involving food, religion, music, and dance. In many instances these become the major tangible cultural difference, remnants of cultures quite different. Price states that sociocultural groups in America become transformed into ethnic subcultures. Although outright destruction never completely occurs, transformation (acculturation) begins immediately on participation in the American economic system—the adjustments necessitated in order to join the work force produce social change. As elements of the old and new culture intertwine, a unique subculture is formed.[16]

Our aim in working with clients from various cultural backgrounds is to eliminate our ethnocentric beliefs and substitute instead a relativistic cultural perspective. *Cultural relativism* refers to the perspective "holding that cultures are neither inferior nor superior to one another and that there is no single scale for measuring the value of a culture. Therefore, customs, beliefs, and practices must be judged or understood relative to the context in which they appear."[17] To do this, the health worker must be flexible enough to assume the cultural perspective of those with whom he or she works.[18]

Ethnocentrism implies the lack of cultural relativism. The tendency for health professionals to be ethnocentric is pervasive when working with families from different sociocultural backgrounds. From this springs the importance of studying families from other cultures—to counter the tendency to believe that the way "our" families operate is the way in which all (normal) families do and should operate.

A result of ethnocentrism is the problem of *cultural imposition.* Because health workers feel either consciously or unconsciously that their beliefs and practices are superior and proper, they use subtle and/or apparent ways to force their own values, beliefs, and practices on individuals from different cultural orientations.[19]

Cultural imposition may then lead to cultural conflicts—situations in which health professionals have covertly or overtly tried to impose their health practices on their clients and the clients have reacted negatively. As nurses we can think of many ways in which clients will "fight back," many times to their own detriment, because of the health system's lack of recognition of their culturally patterned beliefs and practices. The commonly seen reticence of Hispanic families to place one of their members in a hospital because of being forced to separate from the family member is a case in point. If family visiting and participation rights were relaxed to allow for a flexible consideration of client and family attitudes and patterns, both client and health care system would benefit.

To counter the frequently experienced problems of cultural imposition and cultural conflicts, Leininger suggests:

> The nurse must truly understand a culture before imposing any changes on the people. Sensitivity and foresight are essential to work in diverse cultural contexts.[20]

In order to provide *culturally sensitive* care, one must first be aware of the different nursing and health care patterns in one's own culture, followed by an understanding of the culture.[21]

Family health nurses and students commonly experience feelings of *cultural shock* when visiting with or interacting with families whose culture is (1) at great variance with their own, (2) one about which they are uninformed, and/or (3) one to which they have had little exposure. *Cultural shock* refers to a condition in which a person, in response to an environment which is so altered that meaningful objects and experiences have been replaced by those from a different culture, feels confused, immobilized, and "lost."[22] Feelings and sensations of discomfort are more pronounced or noticeable when visiting in the home, since the family's

differences are much more obvious, as well as the fact that health worker is in the client's "territory."

Life-style and value differences are not easy to deal with. Our own values and attitudes will greatly influence our perceptions and nursing assessments and interventions. Therefore, personal feelings, beliefs, and attitudes must be identified, discussed, and accepted before we can effectively help families seeking assistance.[23]

The last of the more general cultural concepts has to do more specifically with health care practices. Every culture has devised its own *indigenous health care system* as opposed to the Western *scientific or professional health care system.* This indigenous (or folk) health care system uses traditional folk care modalities. Practitioners of the indigenous system are often the first-line, primary care practitioners—the first healers to be consulted. As part of the cross-cultural approach proposed earlier, it is recommended that professional systems need to become more culturally attuned to these systems and to learn ways in which to work cooperatively with folk systems, rather than in opposition to them. Health professionals tend to down play the significance and value of folk health care and practices. These feelings are both inaccurate and detrimental, however, because much folk medicine is effective.[24]

In fact, in most cases the merits of any treatment depends on whether the sick client recovers or not, and indigenous health care does work in many instances. This is particularly true in illnesses where psychogenic factors are prominent, where effective treatment of the disease depends on a knowledge of the context of the person's cultural belief system—and who knows or appreciates this better than the folk practitioner?

MINORITY FAMILIES

Minority families are those families who are classified as belonging to ethnic or cultural groups other than white ethnic groups, such as the Irish, Poles, and Jews. More recently termed "ethnic people of color," this group comprised about 20 percent of our population in 1978. Minority families, then, in contrast to *all* ethnic families (both white and people of color), have certain common attributes and problems. One major thing they share is that while facing all of the same stressors experienced by all other families, they have the added burdens of the effects of discrimination.[25]

Cultural Variation or Deviance?

Families are not isolated groups which exist independently from the society of which they are a part or subsystem. Thus if a disproportionately large number of families of a particular minority or ethnic group are poor, unemployed, and "dysfunctional to the whole society," a comprehension of their status can be achieved only through an examination of the role played by the larger society. Eshleman notes that poverty, racism, and/or inferior schools may be due less to an inherent weakness within ethnic groups and families than to

1. social and cultural systems which place a higher value on moon walks, military strength, and corporate profit than on human needs;
2. religious institutions that stress a chosen ingroup as God's people to the exclusion of "nonbelievers" (i.e., anyone who is different);
3. educational systems that admit and serve those who pass "middle-class" exams, speak the "proper" language, and wear the "acceptable" hair and clothing styles, and, in general,
4. a society that in many ways places higher values on "things" and goods rather than on the needs and social conditions of people.[26]

If we live in a society in which minority families and their members are devalued and seen as inferior, this message and perception very effectively becomes the perception and beliefs of those people. It is a well-known tenet of social psychology that people develop their identities and perceptions of their worth in interactions with others. As the minority family and individual interacts in a white majority world that encourages feelings of inferiority and degrades self-esteem, the minority family and its members begin to believe what the outer world is saying about them. This trap is termed the *self-fulfilling prophecy*: people will conform to other's expectations and perceptions of them by internalizing their beliefs, even negative ones, and thus seem to fulfill the "prophecies" that were made about them.[27]

Problems within society set up conditions to which minority families and individuals must adapt. Some of these adaptations—such as going on welfare, dropping out of school, or formation of gangs—are viewed as "dysfunctional." The tendency becomes one of blaming the victim—the welfare mother, the unskilled, unemployed black male, the black family, the Chicano gangs—instead of looking more broadly at the problem. By seeing the ways in which the entire system is involved (the institutions of society and the individual's interactions within this larger environment), contextual solutions may be identified and the tendency to blame the already stigmatized individual or group will be curtailed.

Controversies about Minority Family Structures

One way in which social scientists have unwittingly stereotyped and stigmatized whole ethnic groups is by attempting to describe a particular cultural group in toto by data that is actually derived from, and so appropriate to, only *poor* segments of that group. In many of these instances, the particular segment of the ethnic group being described is not clearly identified, thereby giving readers an erroneous notion of what the cultural group is like as a whole.

Casavantes and others have asserted that this overgeneralization has certainly been true of social science studies of Mexican-Americans: "The net result of this extraordinary scientific oversight is the perpetuation of very damaging stereotypes of Mexican Americans."[28] Willie and Billingsley have pointed out the same criticism and conscientiously described life styles and values of the black family according to the family's social class position.[29, 30] Research has concentrated predominantly on the most oppressed families, the findings then being generalized to include all minority families in a process that perpetuates and reinforces biased attitudes. As part of this bias, the majority of stable ethnic families, and the processes by which they have become economically mobile, have largely been ignored.[31]

The importance of social class does not mean, however, that the middle class of a particular American ethnic group are like the white majority middle class. Although ethnic middle-class families are indeed closer to the dominant culture in life styles, values, beliefs, and so forth, they are still distinctive from the majority culture because of their ethnic identity and sense of peoplehood. Billingsley explains that families of the same social class but a different ethnic group show behavioral and value similarities, but not the same sense of historical identification of peoplehood. And conversely, those of the same ethnic group but of different social class manifest a sense of peoplehood, but not similar life styles.[32]

Ethnic Self-help

Social stresses, economic hardships, and discriminatory practices, with resultant feelings of social isolation from society, have forced minority families to rely more heavily on themselves for support and socialization. Rather than call on community agencies, reliance has been extended to a social network based on ethnicity. Many ethnic groups such as the Chinese-Americans and the Japanese-Americans have developed extensive community organizations that provide support and a multitude of services to families in need. The kin-help system is most apparent in the early phases of immigrant experience. Ethnic groups have clustered into areas where kin or other members of their culture already live. In these settings they have been able to provide support for each other until they were able to learn about the new environment, acquire a new language, and begin to be self-supporting.[33]

The kin-help system, where the ethic of mutual reciprocity of all helping each other exists, has been essential to minority groups for support in coping with a hostile or an impoverished environment. Yet, this ethic has some unintended, latent consequences also, since reciprocal responses tend to perpetuate the network. Upwardly mobile families in a Midwestern low-income black community were found to have heavy, unequal financial burdens and strains imposed by the heavy demands less fortunate kin made on them. The extensive kin-help system found there provided sustenance, but strong reciprocal obligations frequently threatened stable marriages and hindered the mobility of younger family members.[34]

ASSESSMENT PROCESS

As stated before, a cultural assessment of a client (individual and/or family) is an essential facet of assessment. Just as a family nurse would not intervene without an assessment of the biopsychosocial aspects of the family and its members, she or he should also not proceed until a cultural assessment has been completed.[35]

Developing skill in eliciting and recording cultural assessments of the client and the context in which the care is being given (the home, health care setting) is one significant strategy appropriate for nurses working in transcultural settings. As part of the broader assessment process, Armodt suggests three additional strategies:

1. becoming informed about the cultures of the persons with whom one interacts,
2. identifying alternative coping tactics to use when dealing with clients from a different culture, and
3. continuously reexamining problems and solutions related to sociocultural practices.[36]

Before community health nurses go into the community of a different culture, it is extremely important that they try to obtain the perceptions, views, values, and practices of people from the particular ethnic group in which they are working. "It is significant to remember that the ability to work with cultural groups is dependent upon the ability to understand the group in terms of their background as they view it and not in terms of our interpretations of their background."[37]

In this text, cultural assessment is integrated throughout the entire family assessment guidelines. For instance, within the identifying data section of the family health assessment guidelines, the family's religious and cultural orientation and the family's degree of acculturation (if the family's cultural background differs from the majority culture) is described. By completing the entire family health assessment, one should have culled comprehensive data on cultural influences pertaining to the family organization (role, power, values, and communication facets), child-rearing practices, affective responses, health care practices and beliefs, and coping strategies.

THE CHICANO FAMILY

The Hispanics

Mexican-Americans, or Chicanos, are the largest ethnic group within the larger Hispanic or Spanish-speaking populations within the United States. In 1978 it was reported that the Hispanic-American population was rapidly increasing and would soon become the largest minority group in the United States. According to the United States Census Bureau, in 1960 there were 3.1 million Hispanic-Americans; in 1970 there were 9.1 million Hispanic-Americans, and in 1978 there were 12 million Hispanic-Americans, with some sources estimating an additional 7.4 million illegal aliens of Hispanic background. As of October 1978, this would bring the total number of Hispanics in the United States to 19 million persons, representing about 9 percent of the total United States population. (In comparison, blacks comprise about 12 percent of the total population.)[38]

What specific factors are involved in the tremendous increase of the Hispanic population? The rate of natural increase (births over deaths) among Hispanics is 1.8 percent, one-third higher than that for blacks. Also, Hispanic immigration (legal and illegal) is running at the astonishing rate of an estimated one million persons per year. Extrapolating from these figures, Hispanics will outnumber blacks within the coming decade.

Whereas blacks are united by race and a common historic experience of slavery, Hispanic-Americans are united by two powerful forces: their language and their strong adherence to Roman Catholicism. Nevertheless, there are also many factors which make them into a diverse group. Hispanic-Americans may be Castilian Spanish, Cuban, Carribean Island black, Mexican, or Puerto Rican. Due to differences in social class and historical experience, and the lack of other roots in common, these groups cannot be considered a single, monolithic ethnic group. And because of this heterogeneity, only the Chicano—the largest single group of Hispanics—will be considered here. They comprise some 7.2 million people of Mexican origin and are concentrated primarily in the southwestern United States.[39]

The Chicano Interface with American Society

Just as slavery provides important keys to understanding the black family, the pattern of labor utilization of Mexicans and Mexican-Americans provides a significant path for understanding the growth and obstacles to growth of the Mexican-American subculture and its assimilation into the American cultural mainstream. Immigration has been closely tied to Southwestern labor needs. Until recently, job-starved Mexican nationals worked competitively and at lower wage scales than Mexican-Americans either by crossing the border daily, or coming over as *braceros*. (The bracero program, now defunct, permitted Mexican workers to work under contract to the United States when the supply of field workers in this country was evaluated as insufficient.)[40]

According to Queen and Haberstein, the Mexican-Americans, because of their proximity to Mexico, the fluidity of the border, and the exploitation of the Anglo-dominated agricultural system, have never been able to participate in the usual social processes used by European immigrants to become integrated into and socially mobile within the mainstream of American society.[41] Chicanos have been, and continue to be, isolated from wider society by religion, language, culture, and social class. Language has served a vital role in maintaining the culture: the Mexican-American family, more than other immigrant families, has continued to speak its native language—Spanish—in the home and community. Social class has also served to isolate Mexican-Americans from the mainstream of the American middle-class society. Quesada and Heller refer to this alienation as "structural," denoting by it that which results from class position within society where strong feelings of alienation are coupled with communication problems and enforcement of folk ways.[42]

Furthermore, the Anglos' oppressive and discriminatory practices and stereotypic view of the culture has created further problems of social integration. Adding to this situation is the view that many Mexican-Americans hold: that the *gringo* is someone from a world *alien* to their own way of life.[43]

Compounding the problem of incompatibility between the larger society and the Mexican-American culture is the ferment being generated by the drastic increases in the population of Spanish-speaking, mostly Mexican, immigrants in many of the areas in the Southwest. The vast influx of Hispanics in some states has been identified by Russell and Satterwhite as a prime source of conflict and dissension because of

the social, economic, political, law enforcement, educational, and health impact this rapid population influx has had.[44]

Variation in Acculturation

Martinez points out that one of the major problems in learning about the Chicano family from the literature is that most social scientists have limited their studies to the lower social class, albeit 60 to 70 percent of Mexican-American families are working, middle, or upper class.[45] Furthermore, individuals and families are in various stages of acculturation. At one extreme are those who have almost completely rejected Mexican family values, and at the other end of the continuum are those who continue to be fully immersed in their Mexican heritage and traditions.

The descriptions of the Chicano family that follow are culled from various classic and recent sources; however, the reader should continually keep in mind the possible bias of social class particularly. Moreover, family and health practices will focus on traditional patterns typical of the first-generation family.

Family Characteristics

Familism

Although there are differing perspectives of the Chicano family in the literature, total agreement is found concerning the existence and persistence of a strong familistic orientation whereby individual needs are subordinated to familial needs. This is termed *familism*. In fact, familism is identified as being the most significant characteristic of the Chicano.[46]

Within the culture, the family remains the single most important social unit. The theme of family honor and unity infuses Mexican-American society, irrespective of social class variation and geographic location. Mexican-Americans perceive of themselves first as family members, and secondly as individuals. Familism extends beyond the nuclear family to include relatives or the extended family on both the maternal and paternal sides. Even when the dominance of the male role is in the process of being weakened among families living in urbanized settings, the importance of familism persists. The family is not only the main source of one's identity, but is also the focus of obligations and the source of nurturance, assistance, and recognition for accomplishment.[47] Thus familial obligations, as defined by the patriarchal father and/or the family, take precedence over individual interests and needs. Individualism must accommodate to the collective needs of the family.

Traditional Family Roles

All of the literature about Chicano culture takes cognizance of male dominance in the home. The father is unquestionably the head of the family. Much has been written of the adult Mexican-American male. He is described as "hard, unyielding and strong," exemplifying the traits of *machismo*.[48] Family members must show respect for him or he will become angry and may give vent to his wrath by physically striking out. Paz, a noted Mexican author, has described the *macho* or masculine role as incorporating the following elements of arbitrary power: superiority, aggressiveness, insensitivity, and invulnerability.[49] Along with the Chicano male's authoritarian role, he is characterized as providing for his family in the best possible manner he can. Often Chicano men will work long hours or two jobs to support a large family. He prides himself in being the sole provider and being economically self-sufficient.

Within the family structure, the Chicano male is little affected by any incongruity between himself and his Anglo counterpart. He tends to see his role in the family as better than the gringo's role; after all, the Chicano male is in charge and has the power and authority to wield. Any ambivalence he experiences concerns his role as *macho*. "But within his culture, to question one's *machismo* is to question one's entire concept of himself as a man."[50] Therefore, strong defenses are created to forestall any questioning which might be so devastating to his very ego and identity.

The ideal mother is seen as a soft, nurturing, and self-sacrificing woman, with her place in the home and her responsibility to her husband and to her children. In fact, her status and roles are usually defined solely by her marriage and her children. She does not openly question her husband's decisions or actions.

The adult woman finds comfort and fulfillment in her maternal role, but many times feels ambivalence about her marital role. Queen and Haberstein attribute this in part to her prudish sexual orientation or socialization and her sexual ignorance.[51] Herrera and Wagner confirm that sex education and a more realistic, accurate understanding of sexual behavior is sorely needed among Chicanas.[52] Due to the Chicana's sexual inhibitions and beliefs, she typically feels she cannot trust herself in her sexual relations. Thus in her sexual relations with her husband, she makes no sexual overtures. Likewise, the husband finds it difficult to have sex with his virginal, good wife, and being culturally free to have extramarital affairs, he continues his sexual activity outside the home. In fact, among his friends, this is usually an important way to demonstrate his *machismo*. The unfortunate outcome is that the husband spends less time in the home and the marital relationship becomes more formal and distant.

The wife, in response to the emotional distance and her marital expectations, turns to her children and female kin for the meeting of her affective and companionship needs.[53]

The role of a Chicana mother and wife is not easy for some. Castro studied a group of Mexican-American women seen at a mental health clinic, and he concluded that the role of the mother within the Mexican-American culture is probably the most onerous and incongruous with the comparable roles of the wife and mother in the dominant culture. Castro's clients all had symptoms of depression and anxiety associated with the husband's *machismo* role, and they felt ambivalent about their role. On the one hand, they envied the *gringa's* power and freedom vis-à-vis her husband; but on the other hand, they socialized their children to show absolute respect and obedience toward their father. They complained of the burden of daily house cleaning and caring for children, but then expressed "great pride concerning their undying devotion to and sacrifice for their children."[54]

In poor families, children are expected to help with the running of the house—the girls with the household chores and child-care activities and the boys monetarily, by finding jobs outside of the home as soon as possible. Older siblings are respected by younger siblings and the female siblings are respectful of their brothers. Children usually confide in their mothers, rather than their aloof fathers. In all traditional families, children are expected to place familial duty before their personal ambitions.

Because of the contrasting expectations of men and women, the adolescent son is encouraged and given freedom to move about and gain experience in the world. Usually he joins youth groups that afford him the opportunity to demonstrate his *macho* among his peers. In contrast, the adolescent daughter's world is much more constricted—to the home and family—and is mother-centered.[55]

Family Power

A third characteristic of the Chicano family about which there is widespread concensus is the presence of "rigid, sex-age grading so that the older order the younger and the men order the women."[56]

One can easily surmise the power structure of the traditional Chicano family from the description of family member's roles. The father holds primary authority or legitimate power—a culturally determined power given to him by virtue of his sex and his status in the family. Both he and his family accept his right to exercise this power. This power is translated into *machismo* and authoritarianism. The male head directs activities, delegates responsibilities, arbitrates disputes, polices behavior, sanctions family members, and represents the family within the community and society.

The actual routine, everyday decisions are usually delegated to the wife or eldest female family member. The father remains distant from the household and child care, considering these to be mundane affairs, and is concerned primarily with being the family's provider. Mothers learn to manage everyday life by manipulating their dominant men to satisfy their needs as best as possible. Grandparents are an important source of warmth and support, and possess referent power in the family.[57]

Traditional Values and Value Conflicts

Traditional Mexican-American values are found among the unacculturated and the poor primarily. Moreover, social class status is a prime determinant of the viability of traditionalism.[58] Martinez asserts that the poor Chicano family shares many values with other poor families and that these values are actually not so different from those of the middle class. The main difference is in their realistic assessment as to whether they can achieve the same goals as the middle class of the dominant American culture. "This realistic assessment of their capabilities, instead of being received as a healthy and adaptive attitude, has been called fatalism, contentment with their lot, and lack of concern, all implying pathology, differentness, and wrongness. It is this sort of stereotyping that leads people in positions of dominance and control to expect the stereotyped behavior and to plan accordingly."[59]

Murillo and others have explained some of the most relevant differences in the values of the Mexican-American, irrespective of social class, and the American majority cultures. These are summarized in Table 17.1

TABLE 17.1
American and Traditional Mexican-American Value Differences

Area/Issue	American Central Value Orientation	Traditional Mexican-American Value Orientation
Family	Americans see themselves as individuals first and secondarily as members of families.	Chicanos see themselves as members of families first and as individuals second.
Self vs kin obligations	American culture stresses individuality and independence from family after a certain age. Self-reliance and autonomy are emphasized.	Chicanos believe in ethic of reciprocity within family and kinship group.
Respect and authority structures	Americans value democratic ideals and egalitarianism (to a much greater extent). The elderly do not receive great respect. The authority of the masculine role is gradually diminishing as a result of feminist struggles.	Value in male dominance and respect for and obedience to the elderly predominate. Authoritarianism is valued over democratic ideals.
Progress vs tradition	Americans value progress and change.	Mexican-Americans show more reverence and respect for tradition.
Work	Work and productivity are central, prominent values of the Anglo culture. Work often becomes a value in itself (more true in the past than today).	Work is seen as a necessity in order to live. Other life experiences—social and emotional experiences—are valued more than work.
Materialism	Materialism is another central American value. Possession of material goods is seen as a sign of success and becomes an end in itself. The cynosures of society are the businessman and financier.	Material objects are viewed as necessities and not as ends in themselves. Social status and prestige are more likely to be derived from an ability to experience things directly and/or through social and family relationships rather than through past successes and accumulation of wealth. Mexican-Americans generally have great reverence for philosophers, poets, musicians, and artists.
Time	"Time is money." Punctuality is equated with goodness and being responsible.	Time is a gift to be enjoyed. The concept of wasting time is not understood. Punctuality is not an important moral value.
Present vs future time orientation	Making plans for the future (planning) is highly valued as a means of getting ahead. Future-oriented.	Enjoyment of the present. Less concern for always living in the future. More present-oriented.

TABLE 17.1
American and Traditional Mexican-American Value Differences (cont.)

Area/Issue	American Central Value Orientation	Traditional Mexican-American Value Orientation
Interpersonal relationships	Americans value openness and directness in communications. (Americans are viewed as being blunt and succinct by Mexican-Americans.) Use of kidding to get messages across more indirectly is acceptable. In interpersonal conflict situations, Americans value "leveling," open dissent, and criticizing each other. Value rational expression of thoughts and not emotional expression as much.	Mexican-Americans value diplomacy and tactfulness, and show concern and respect for other's feelings and dignity. Their manner of expression is more elaborate and indirect. Mexican-Americans value agreement and courtesy, and are very sensitive to criticism regardless of manner presented. Value being expressive and showing feelings toward another person.
Environmental responses	Americans are less sensitive to the environment and its various forms of stimulation.	Mexican-Americans value greater sensory stimulation within their environments, using the full range of senses to experience their environment (vivid colors, expressive music and art, spicy foods).
Relationship to environment	Americans see themselves as mastering the environment.	Chicanos value living in harmony with the environment.
Education	Education highly valued as means to success and way to be productive. Correlated with work and productivity ethics.	Education is not valued highly, primarily because it has been so inaccessible and schools so culturally incongruent with the Mexican-American values. Also, many Chicanos are not in tune with the success and scientific values which are associated with education. They are not as competitive as Americans generally and education is not pursued with the aggressiveness needed to succeed.

Adapted primarily from: Murillo N: The Mexican American family. In Hernandez CA, Haug MJ, Wayner NN: Chicanos: Social and Psychological Perspectives. St. Louis, Mosby, 1971, pp 97–108

One of the serious problems which occurs as the Mexican-American family interfaces with the larger society is that value conflicts arise. Many of the primary values of the Mexican-American are incongruous with the core values of the American central value system. This naturally poses significant adaptation problems for Chicano families and individuals. When these children start school, they soon learn that they and their families are "out of synch" with the wider society. Castro, in a research study of mental health clinic clients of Mexican-American descent, in which the respective impacts on clients of the Mexican culture and the dominant culture were ascertained, concluded that "there is a definite correlation between the culture of the Mexican-American and his state of mental health." The mental health of these clients was negatively affected by the fact that their cultural values and patterns were at odds with the values and patterns of the dominant culture, and the language barrier and barriers between client and professional worker were both significant.[60]

Communication Patterns

Communication patterns in the family are quite congruent with the family's role, power, and value structure. Authoritarian lines of communication are present, with the male and older members of the household directing the women and children. There is much warmth and affection shown between mother and children when children are young. Respect is shown by children to parents and elders, and females show respect toward the males of the family.

The Spanish language, being more expressive and elaborate than English, shapes the cognitive structure of its speakers. Interpersonal relationships are noted for their tones of respect and hierarchical (dominant–submissive) relationships. As seen in the summary of values, Mexican-Americans value courtesy, respect, maintaining of one's dignity, diplomacy, tactfulness, expressiveness of feelings (emotionality), and agreement. Kidding and open confrontation are not sanctioned, since the need to show respect and to "save face" are important.

Recent Changes in Family Structure

Several authors have noted the influence which urbanization, social mobility, and acculturation have on the Mexican-American family. Additionally, the Chicano family is being subjected to many of the same societal changes that the Anglo family is facing. The most noteworthy and profound change revolves around the declining primary authority of the male and the greater egalitarianism of spousal roles. The husband's pervasive power has given rise to the wife's feeling a sense of injustice, particularly as she is exposed to American mores and values. Large families and the difficulties of finding employment with good wages also compromise the husband-father's ability to provide adequately for the family, which tends to diminish the base for his authority.

Many women, especially the younger ones, are challenging their traditional roles. In the urban areas, the *chicanitas* (adolescent girls) are venturing outside their homes to join social clubs and gangs. *Chicanas* are fighting for greater equality in the family and society. Given the increasing occupational opportunities for women and the wish for a higher standard of living, more and more Mexican-Americans are working. As a result, traditional male–female roles are changing among the younger and middle-class couples particularly, and the women of these groups are finding a greater flexibility and choice of options.[61] As with the Anglo families, when women take advantage of educational opportunities and find employment outside the home, their self-image and role expectations change drastically. This is beginning to effect revolutionary changes in the Mexican-American family. Hence the Chicano family will face substantial stress due to women's emancipation, generational conflicts, and the decline of the male's patriarchal authority.

Socialization

Traditionally, the raising of children is the mother's job; the father's role is to work and to form associations with his *compadres*. Marked gender differences in child rearing occur, as men and women are seen to live in different worlds.

Mexican-American babies are "wanted, cherished, pampered and thoroughly spoiled." They are regarded as *angelitos*, untouched by evil and sin. Parents and older siblings respond to them in very indulgent, affectionate ways.[62]

Gender awareness and differing socialization patterns for male and female children begin early. The son–father relationship becomes a formal, distant one as soon as the child is judged to be "responsible"; it is a relationship in which the son is continually attempting to meet the demands and the expectations of his father.

The mother tends to act as a buffer between the son and father, in order to soften the demands of father and to provide the nurturance the father does not give. The only time the father and son relate closely together is when they are performing some work together, which in agrarian settings can mean many hours together, but in urban settings does not allow much opportunity for relating closely.[63]

Father–daughter relationships are warmer and less distant, since the father does not have to act as a role model to his daughters. Mother–daughter relationships are very close during early childhood, with the same dominance patterns over daughters as fathers have over their sons. The mother gives more attention to her daughter than to her son, and as a result of this emotional intimacy, as well as a close working relationship revolving around household chores, a positive identification of daughter with the mother fully takes place.[64]

Kinship Patterns

The idealized family structure is the extended family. Kay reports that the stereotypical Mexican-American family is composed of a resilient grandmother, her son, his wife, and six children, with the brothers and sisters of both the wife and husband living nearby. Though still common, the extended family living under one roof is not found as frequently today as it was in the past—the more common family form is nuclear with extended family living close by.[65]

Children do not separate from their families of origin psychologically or socially. As children grow up and marry, their families become extensions of the original unit, even though they probably do not live within the same household. Mother's and father's kin are generally of equal importance, with special recognition given to mother's sisters. Both sets of grandparents are revered. First cousins are especially important colateral kin and are somewhat like sisters and brothers.[66] Most social relationships are still based on kinships, and relationships among the extended family are very close.

Godparents (*compadrazgo*) may hold an important place in the family. *Compadrazgo* refers to the ritual kinship pattern whereby a special linkage is established between two families or two persons by the baptismal ritual. *Compadres* provide coparenthood in time of need but also generate social and interpersonal cohesion, and godparents and godchildren are expected to visit each other and cultivate a close relationship.[67]

There is agreement among all authors on the clearly established patterns of reciprocal help and mutual aid existing between and among extended family members.[68] This system offers assistance and feelings of security. An example of reciprocity occurs when poor families become too large to support all their members and, as a result, some of the children are then raised by grandparents, uncles, or aunts.

The Health Care Function

Among Mexican-Americans the structure and values of the family are the most important influencing factors relative to understanding an individual's health attitudes and practices. One can also understand the shorter longevity and the higher mortality and morbidity rates of Chicanos when the high percentage of this group living at or below the proverty level is taken into account.[69]

Health Beliefs

Most of the Chicano health beliefs are based on assumptions and traditions which have evolved over centuries. In the blending of older European, Spanish-Catholic, and Indian traditions, three basic aspects of Chicano traditional folk health concepts and practices emerge. One aspect is concerned with the specific health beliefs and practices. A second consists of a set of ritualistic acts which are believed to improve health. And lastly, the use of folk practitioners or *curanderos* has evolved.[70]

Basic to Chicano health beliefs and practices are the health philosophies and ideologies of the culture that circumscribes these beliefs and practices. Dorsey and Jackson write that the basis for many health beliefs is the concept of equilibrium. Man is viewed holistically, as being in harmony and unity with his natural and supernatural environments. Health is a result of maintenance of this natural state of balance between man and the natural and supernatural worlds. Illness and disease stem from a loss in homeostasis or balance.

Preventive beliefs and rituals are exercised to promote this balance. Prayers, relics, faith, herbs, and spices are all used to ward off disease or to prevent complications of long-term illness. Two examples of the Chicano's concern with maintaining balance is in the consumption of hot and cold foods and pregnancy practices. Foods which are thought of as "hot" (heavy foods, meats, fatty or spicy foods) are eaten with "cold" foods (vegetables, ice cream), which are considered soothing and fresh to the body to achieve the necessary balance in the body. Since pregnancy is seen as a delicate time when imbalances occur easily which can cause great harm to the fetus, the practice of the mother's wearing keys on the night of the lunar eclipse is thought to be protective. Mothers are also urged to maintain good diets, exercise, and take herbs and teas recommended by the *yerbero* (herbalist) or health leader in the family, thus maintaining the delicate bal-

ance during the months of pregnancy.[71] Furthermore, disease may be inflicted on an individual as a form of punishment for wrongdoing.[72]

Some of the specific folk health beliefs, as expressed in form of folk illnesses, are the following. *Mal ojo,* literally translated "bad or evil eye," is believed to be a result of excessive admiration or desire on the part of another. *Mal de susto,* literally translated "illness from fright," is a syndrome believed to be the result of an emotionally traumatic experience. *Empacho* is believed to be caused by food clinging to the wall of the stomach in the form of a ball. *Caida de la mollera* (fallen fontanel) is the one illness that is felt to affect children only. *Mal puesto,* or sorcery, is considered to arise as a consequence of one of three kinds of social relationships: (1) a lover's quarrel, (2) unrequited love, or (3) as a reflection of invidiousness between individuals or nuclear families. Most folk illnesses are believed to be intimately related to faulty social relationships.[73, 74]

Castro reports that Chicano clients see mental illness as a "dreaded affliction," analogous to *mal de sangre* (venereal disease), or "bad blood." When a person acquires "bad blood" he or she loses the respect of friends and extended family and is viewed as no longer fit to have children or raise a family. The person is socially ostracized and believed to have offended God in some way or be under the influence of a "hex." The mentally ill person's nuclear family feels social disgrace, but continues to love and feel compassion for him or her, in spite of the belief that the individual will never be the same again. Thus for the Mexican-American, mental illness is perhaps one of the most difficult heath phenomena with which to cope or for which to seek professional help.[75]

Health Practices

Folk medicine does not treat symptoms of disease conditions alone. Folk medicine views the sick person as a whole psychobiocultural and spiritual being in relationship to the natural and supernatural environments. Whereas Western medicine focuses on epidemiology and pathophysiology, Chicano folk medicine focuses on holistically treating the person.

When an individual becomes ill, he or she usually consults the health expert in the family and tries to cure illness with self-care methods (prayers, diet, household remedies). If this does not relieve the symptoms, he or she usually consults the *yerbero,* and then the *curandero.* The types of healing or remedies prescribed are reflective of the healer's perceptions of etiology. All healing is geared toward restoring the necessary equilibrium or preventing disequilibrium. There are specific household remedies, such as those for being wet and chilled and those for menstruation. Spiritualistic practices are appropriate for helping persons suffering illness considered supernatural in origin. Prayers and ritualistic activities are performed by *espiritualistas*, family, and patient. Herbs are extensively used for treating a multitude of illnesses, some of which have been found scientifically to have great benefit.[76] Recent studies of Chicano folk health practices demonstrate that Mexican-Americans do not rely entirely on folk practices for cure, but consider them an important adjunct in expediting solutions to various health problems.[77]

Folk Healers

Margaret Clark, an anthropologist who conducted an extensive ethnographic study of the Mexican-Americans, explains why the Mexican-American people consider folk healers to be vital for meeting their health needs.

> Folk healers are not professionals in the sense that they have formal training in the art of medicine or earn their living by their practice; they are members of the community who are regarded as specialists because they have learned more of the popular medicinal lore of culture than have other barrio people; use language which patients understand and vocabulary familiar to patients; never dictate what must be done, advise the patient what she or he considers appropriate.[78]

There are several levels and types of folk practitioners in most Chicano communities, as described below.

Yerbero(a). The herbalist is an expert in the source, purposes, and derivatives of herbs and spices useful for cure and prevention of disease. As a grower and distributor of herbs, as well as a teacher about their uses, the *yerbero(a)*'s position in the community is one of respect and esteem. Patients will often try family remedies first, herbs from the *yerbero* second, and thirdly visit the *curandero* or physician separately or cojointly.[79]

Curandero(a). The *curandero(a)* is the most respected and specialized healer in the Chicano community. The following characteristics of *curanderismo* have been noted: (1) *curanderos* are chosen through divine calling and live in the community; (2) they usually have their practice in their home and their reputation is established from their rate of success; (3) if respectable, they will not try to cure someone who is incurable, critically ill, or "hexed" (under the influence of a witch or magic); (4) most prescribe prayers, teas, poultices, and herbs; and (5) they do not charge fees, but do accept donations from families.[80, 81]

Espiritualisto(a). This person is a spiritualist who has the ability to analyze dreams, fears, foretell the future, and treat some supernatural and magical diseases (those caused by *brujos*).

Brujo(a). The *brujo(a)* is skilled in the use of magic and witchcraft and can cast spells or hexes on individuals, as well as remove those cast by other magicians. They are honored out of fear rather than admiration.[82]

Attitudes toward Western Health Care

Mexican-Americans generally tend to dread illness and hospitalization more than Anglos do. Perhaps this is due to higher mortality rates or the poorer health the Chicanos experience. Certainly the huge medical expenses which the family cannot afford and the estrangement Chicanos often feel when dealing with the health care system contribute to their apprehension of being sick, injured, or hospitalized.[83]

Many authors have mentioned that Chicano feelings about health providers and the "scientific" or Western health care system are usually negative. There are several reasons for this.

1. Health providers use their own medical jargon which is not comprehensible to Chicano clients.
2. Fee-for-service arrangements between doctors and clients results in feelings of stiffness and mistrust.
3. The Chicano feels alienated and lacks confidence in health providers for their ignorance and arrogance regarding their own traditional beliefs and practices.[84, 85]
4. Chicanos generally object to authoritarian, objective attitudes of physicians and nurses (clinical, cold approaches) and the concept of efficiency involving a time orientation valuing speed and resulting in not getting to know the patient.

Although there is an increasing reliance on physicians and "scientific health care," especially among second- and third-generation Chicanos, significant barriers to utilization still exist. For example, when the Mexican-American is in need of support, nurturance, and assistance, he or she is expected to turn to his or her family first in order to have these needs met. Only when familial resources have been exhausted or under unusual circumstances is it acceptable for the Chicano to seek outside help, and then this is seen to compromise one's sense of pride and dignity. This cultural fact is often cited as a reason why it is so difficult for Chicano families and individuals to seek professional help soon enough for their problems.[86]

The use of hospitalization for the Mexican-American should be considered seriously by health professionals. Integration into Mexican-American culture and the social structure runs counter to the acceptance of health care which involves separation of a patient from the support of family and kin group. This separation is exceedingly difficult for Mexican-American, since the culture and family build into the modal personality a high degree of psychological dependency.[87]

Practice Implications

Several practice implications, based on Chicano culturally patterned beliefs and practices, suggest themselves as germane for family health workers.

1. Health workers should not expect a Chicano client to make a medical decision until he or she has a chance to consult with family members. Group responsibility should be recognized. Family health professionals should make an effort to consult with those of the patient's family who have real authority in the family group. Also, including an older person, such as the grandmother, in a family discussion is helpful, since she or he could be a powerful influencer of medical decisions.
2. It is best to encourage the whole family or the extended family to adopt a new health program—such as dietary regimens or immunization—rather than encouraging a sole individual to go it alone. Persons may be more influenced by what other significant family members will say than what the physician will think.
3. It is well to remember that other family problems may supersede the resolution of health problems. Helping a family tackle their other health-related problems first may leave the way open for the family to engage in solving their primary health concerns.
4. Interactions with Chicanos need to be friendly and warm, with sensitivity shown toward the client's feelings.[88] Since the Chicano tends to look on the health professional as an authority, a structured instructive approach is usually expected and responded to favorably.[89]

THE BLACK FAMILY

Historical Background

The development of the contemporary black family is overshadowed by the disastrous legacy of slavery. During the era of slavery, the black family existed only by the consent of the slave owner for the purposes of perpetuating the system and improving his economic status. The black family was not autonomous or self-sufficient. Slaves were able to construct a partial family unit, when it suited the needs of the slave owners. These units often were mother-centered, with the mother–child relationship primary and the husband–wife and father–child relationships tenuous.[90]

The matrifocal family, which had its inception during slavery, does not exist within the black families to any great extent in the rural areas today. Blacks in rural areas have been able to maintain two-parent nuclear families almost as well as similarly situated whites. In agrarian regions, men and women by necessity must function together. In the rural setting, the man has important functions, and it is difficult for women to get along on the farm by themselves. It is the migration to cities where the black family has disproportionately been headed by women. Here women can earn wages just like a man, and in many cases more easily, because of the large number of domestic jobs available. It is also easier for a mother to receive welfare payments, since she is the bearer and rearer of the dependent children.[91]

The black family has adapted to the larger society of which it is a part in various ways, with the common experience of racial discrimination and economic adversity playing the most significant roles. The various structures and functions of black families have resulted largely as adaptive reactions to varying socioeconomic conditions and stressors which threaten their survival.[92]

Status of the Black Family Today

In 1965, Daniel P. Moynihan, who was then Assistant Secretary of Labor, wrote a report indicting the black family for "the tangle of pathology" and deterioration of Negro society.[93] He concluded that black families were falling apart, basing his conclusions on a myriad of statistical data showing such phenomena as numbers of absent fathers, children on welfare, and juvenile delinquency.

One of the significant points of clarification to come from the ensuing debate about the status of the black family was that the issues concerning the black family were issues concerning "the black lower-class family." Notwithstanding the recognition that racism exists against all blacks, the black middle-class family is similar to its white counterpart and is thus accepted and integrated into society.

The major issue is whether events that take place inside of the family are to any extent attributable to the family itself, or whether these events are to be understood only as the result of poverty, discrimination, and exploitation. Moynihan pointed out that the societal treatment of blacks was ultimately to blame, but that the black family itself, as a result of its weakening, possessed characteristics which were inimical to its welfare, as well as to the welfare of its family members and the black community. He identified the black family's matriarchal structure as a key contribution to the deterioration of the black family. Billingsley and others disagreed. They see the black family as a resilient and adaptive system.[94] They maintain that black families survived their long journey from Africa to urban America by developing characteristic strength— chiefly a sense of extended family that provides support and nurture during crisis or parental absence.[95] Willie emphasizes that "the black family, in spite of generations of family break-up due to slavery and other socioeconomic and discriminatory pressures, has not only survived, but in many cases, has grown stronger over the years."[96]

The black family, regardless of social class status, has been repeatedly termed a matriarchal structure, forced into this family form because of the separation of husband and wife during slavery and more recently due to ecnomic realities and welfare restrictions. But according to Billingsley and Willie, this assertion does not properly account for the total range of black families in our society. First, 80 to 90 percent of adult black men work to support their families. Although still below the proportion of two-parent white families, 60 to 70 percent of black families are two-parent families. Willie concludes as follows:

> Most of the family instability among blacks is more a function of contemporary economic circumstances and racial discrimination than of historical circumstances such as slavery. An indirect [inverse] association, we know exists between family income and family instability: As the family income decreases, the proportion of families headed by one parent increases.[97]

Although notable gains have been made by middle-class black families in the last 10 to 15 years, the preponderance of black working-class and lower-class families are in a poorer position economically and structurally today. More black children are born out of wedlock (most to girls in their teens), more black heads of households are unemployed, the number of female-headed households has risen steadily to 37 percent of all black households, and the percentage of black children on welfare rose from 14 percent in 1961 to 38 percent in 1977.[98] As the American economy contracts, the lower class is the hardest hit, and this fact, together with lack of effective government action, has further compounded the problem.

Family Form and Kinship System

Although the modal black family is nuclear (either single- or two-parent), one of the distinctive character-

istics of black families is the fact that their households have a much higher proportion of extended family members living with them than do white families. Working-class and middle-class black families are likely to have an older relative living in the home providing child care while both spouses work. In the poorer family, the more common pattern is of an older female relative bringing under her wing a younger woman and her children. Three-generation households such as the one just mentioned exist only when there is no husband present. Almost all married couples have their own apartment or home.

Strong kinship bonds are evidenced by the high frequency with which the black families take relatives (especially children under 18) into their households. Black families have developed their own network for the informal adoption of children. Babies born out of wedlock are routinely kept in the home: in 1978 fully 90 percent of such black children were reared by parents or relatives, whereas in white families only 33 percent of illegitimate children were kept in the home. Financial resources, food, and child care are extensively shared among the extended family, to the point of informally adopting children for long periods of time. This constitutes a tremendous self-help effort among families who are already economically strained. Robert Hill, of the National Urban League, asserts that "the extended family is still one of the most viable institutions for the survival and advancement of black people today."[99]

Concerning living patterns, young black couples prefer to live near their families of origin. It is common practice for long-time friends and neighbors to be brought into the family circle, as well as those persons who have expressed some interest in the family, including the beautician, barber, physician, and dentist.[100]

To cope with the enormous sociocultural stresses of daily life, the black family has adapted by developing a variety of family structures, including the patriarchal, egalitarian, and matriarchal forms. The differences in family structure and function can best be understood when one looks at the social class differences. Eshleman and Billingsley both state that the most important variable in understanding the life style of black families is social class.[101, 102] Nevertheless, it must be restated that black–white family differences are not reducible to simple social class distinctions, since the black and white middle-class families lack the common identity created by "a sense of peoplehood" (common ethnic identity). Even though lower-class and upper-class black families exhibit dramatic differences in life styles, they still share a common experience and ethnic identity that makes them feel as "one people," as well as distinct from white families, regardless of their social class similarity.

Since social class is the major determinant of family

patterns among black families, the family descriptions that follow are organized by class strata. Upper-class black families are not included here, since there was insufficient data to make a discussion of this class of family worthwhile.

The Black Middle-Class Family

Black middle-class families comprise 25 percent of all black families and tend to be nuclear in form, generally consisting of husband, wife, and two to three children. Both parents usually work. The wife is often a professional, while the husband may or may not be. (If not a professional, he may have a clerical job or be a skilled worker.) Both parents usually make about equal income and are frequently employed in the public sector; one or both parents are college graduates, and they plan a college education for their children.

Because of their dual employment, cooperative work and team effort of husband and wife are needed. Thus many family tasks such as cooking, cleaning, and shopping are shared, and there is extensive adaptability or flexibility of roles. "Probably the best example of the liberated wife in American society is found in the black middle-class family. Spouses are partners out of economic necessity and have an equalitarian pattern of interaction."[103] Equalitarian patterns include the sharing of decison making by spouses. From this arrangement of power and roles, one can infer that communication patterns are a two-way process and democratic in nature.

The middle-class black family's value system and, consequently, its socialization patterns are largely congruent with those of the dominant culture. For instance, these families have a strong work orientation, a strong achievement orientation, and highly value self-reliance and education.

Religion, however, generally has a higher priority for the black middle-class than for WASP families. Parents tend to be active participants in church affairs, the church serving not only important emotional-spiritual needs, but also as a central institution for black social life.[104] Additionally, grandparents, older siblings, or extended family members usually play a more active role in the socialization process than in similar white families.

The Black Working-Class Family

Working-class black families tend to be nuclear households, but usually have more children (four or more) than do the middle-class families. There is also a greater likelihood that a relative or boarder may be part of the household. Again, both parents generally hold jobs. Men tend to work in semiskilled factory, restaurant, or janitorial positions and women are frequently employed at a similar level in community in-

stitutions. The parents have often not completed high school, but they desire more education for their own children, and encourage the more motivated children to go to college. Couples usually marry early and begin a family very soon after marriage.

The relationship between husband and wife usually takes on an egalitarian character, since cooperation for getting by and survival is a necessity. Nevertheless, husbands and wives usually have traditionally assigned roles, except for the shared provider role, although these may change in time of crisis. Additionally, there is a tendency toward some flexibility concerning child-care tasks based on the sex of the child. Lastly, the mother also takes on the social liaison role, primarily with the school and the church.

Power is also egalitarian, although perhaps not as shared as in the black middle-class family. Because the mates carry out traditional family roles, women generally have more economic control in matters pertaining to the home and children.

Respectability is important among black working-class families, with the ownership of one's own home and the good character of one's children being important symbols of the attainment of this value. Of a great significance is one's family. The size of the family may be a source of pride for the parents, as the bearing and rearing of children is considered to be an important responsibility. Working-class parents often make great personal sacrifices for their families, and kinship relationships are strong.[105]

Again, religion and the church play a central role in the lives of these families. And the church is often second only to the home as the emotional center of black life.[106]

In regard to child rearing, parents raise their children to assure that they receive the skills and attitudes necessary to survive in the world as the parents perceive it. Thus respectfulness, obedience, conformity to rules, and being "good" are stressed. During childhood, children are assigned household chores as part of their family responsibility and are encouraged to seek away-from-home jobs for pay when old enough.

Fulfilling the affective functions in the family poses difficulties because of the long hours both parents usually work to provide the necessities of life. Most black working-class families have to give up doing things together as a whole family. Many husbands hold down two jobs, and it is not uncommon for spouses to work different shifts to cover child-care responsibilities. Free time is at a premium, but in spite of this, marriage and constancy of family residence are maintained in most families.[107]

The Black Lower-Class Family

The black lower-class family comprises about 40 percent of all black families, a proportion twice that for the white lower class. A chief cause continues to be racial discrimination and economic adversity. About three-fourths of these are working poor; the other one-fourth constitute the underclass described in Chapter 12. Most married couples have their own households. Poorer black households are much more likely to be single-parent families. It is common to find extended families also, consisting of the grandmother and the mother and her children when no husband is present. Moreover, lower-class black families generally have more children than either the poor white family or the working- or middle-class black family.

In the lower class, desertion and divorce are chief causes for family disruption, although single-parent families are usually not entirely devoid of a male presence. Often the mother will have a boyfriend who visits frequently and acts as companion to the family. If a husband-father is present, he is often unemployed, with the mother on welfare or working in an unskilled job. Even when either spouse is working, the possibility of unemployment is a continual threat.

The primary feature of the lower-class black family is its low-income status. Due to the family's impoverished state, they are coerced into making various adaptations, some of which are heavily criticized by the wider society. These adaptations include multigenerational living arrangements and taking in boarders or foster children for pay. Adult heterosexual relationships may involve both marital and parental responsibilities in the absence of marriage. Poor households sometimes forgo conventional morality in order to provide an expedient arrangement for earning sufficient money to live on. "The struggle among poor families is a struggle for existence."[108] Movement and instability are great in areas of jobs, residence, and relationships.

Adolescent girls and boys have sexual experiences at an early age and tend to get married earlier than their counterparts in the working and middle classes. Premarital pregnancy, though not condoned, is accepted by the family after the fact, as is the belief that, though it may be desirable, it is not necessary to have a man around the house in order to have and raise a family. Most poor black men and women do marry and stay together for various periods of time. Marriage is looked upon ambivalently and in many cases negatively by both sexes, because of the stresses and strains associated with family life.[109] This ambivalence and negativity has a reality base. Much greater marital instability exists generally due to economics (unemployment), and, in addition, affectional problems (extramarital relationships) are commonplace.[110]

The husband–wife relationship in both the black and white lower classes is characterized by a high degree of conjugal role segregation. There are few shared roles, and the wife and husband pursue separate recreational and outside interests. The husband is expected to be the provider—to bring home the paycheck. Even though he is the titular head, he plays a minimal role in family life. The wife is expected to care for the children and home and to make the husband feel welcome and comfortable when he is at home.

These families are matrifocal in the sense that the wife makes most of the necessary decisions and has the greatest sense of responsibility for the family. There is intense loyalty between mothers and grandmothers and their children/grandchildren. Mothers extend every effort to assist their children, even into adulthood; and the grandparents often take on the child-care role and act as prime socializers. Strong loyalty and reciprocity also exists among siblings. The problem here is that when one is in need, all of the siblings are struggling too. Nevertheless, they share their already overcrowded living quarters and often give whatever assistance they can.

The family's values are distinct and incongruent with the wider society's values, thus helping to create the malintegration of this group within and the stigmatization by society of the black lower class. A few selected values will be explained. Fatalism is a common value and one associated with poverty. Black lower-class families learn to hope for little and expect even less. Men and women get sexually involved, but are afraid to trust and commit themselves to each other due to their experience of repeated disappointments. Dependency, rather than self-sufficiency, is an orientation—not really valued, but accepted as a reality and a way to "get by," e.g., it is all right to lean on extended family and society (receive welfare). The lack of the achievement and work ethic is apparent, as is the lack of the value on education and future planning. It must be remembered that family values are reality-based—a reflection of what families can aspire to and expect in life.

Irrespective of social class, kinspeople (grandmothers, aunts, cousins, older siblings) play a more active role in the socialization of black children than is true of white families. In three-generation maternal households, it is the grandmother who is expected to stay at home with the young children (infants and preschoolers), since the mother has the right to continue outside activities.

Writes Rainwater of the black lower-class family, there is little sense of the awesome responsibility of caring for children that the middle-class parent experiences. Although the confinement of being home with infants and preschoolers is also difficult for mothers and grandmothers, there is not the deep involvement and constant solicitousness that is seen when observing working- and middle-class mothers from various ethnic backgrounds care for their infants. The babies' needs are attended to on a "catch-as-catch-can" basis.

In single-parent poor homes the maternal household is generally run with a loose organization. Children learn at an early age to fend for themselves, especially if the family is large, with school-agers beginning to shop, cook, go to bed and school on their own, and watch after themselves when mother is gone. The lower-class, three-generation maternal homes are busy and open to the world. Kin and friends come and go at all times of the day and evening on an unplanned basis. This openness of the home is a reflection of the mother's sense of impotence in facing the street system. Although the mother often tries to keep children away from the street when they are young, as they grow older it becomes increasingly futile, and she finally gives up, disengages, and lets the children have their freedom.[111]

The Health Care Function

A brief review of historical black health practice is instructive for a comprehension of the present-day situation. After slavery and during the reconstruction period in the South, a rise in the use of folk remedies and the midwife or "granny" occurred. As late as 1962 the black midwife was still delivering 42 percent of black babies in the state of Mississippi.[112] The use of the conjure doctor, voodoo or hoodoo man, or witch doctor—a practice brought from West Africa—also continued throughout the post-emancipation period. Certain diseases were thought to be caused by God or the supernatural, one effect of which was to lead to the fatalism felt by many rural blacks.

The use of conjure doctors, magical thought patterns, folk practices, and feelings of fatalism are all health attitudes which migrated north with the poor black families. In some black ghettos today, lower-class black families continue to use herb doctors, spiritualists, and faith healers, but in most black communities their use is minimal.[113]

For the poor black family today, professional health care is generally available through the public sector and the small percentage of private physicians who accept Medicaid and/or Medicare or charge affordable fees. The percentage of black physicians and health care professionals is still substantially below the proportion of the black population as a whole. Furthermore, health care agencies to the black poor represent an alien world of the middle-class and white society.

Since many blacks live in urban ghettos, slums, rural areas, and overcrowded surroundings, the health of these individuals is adversely affected. As explained before, the positive correlation between poor general health status and unsanitary, overcrowded, and poor environments has been clearly demonstrated.[114]

Folk medicine has remained important in the urban ghettos and in the rural South. Low-income blacks commonly make use of patent medi... remedies, secure medical advice from f... reluctant to seek professional health care... poor black person will endure blatant sympt... health such as unexplained weight loss, a... pain, and frequent breathlessness without se... care. In other words, for families whose socioecon... status is low and/or who feel socially and cultura... alienated from available health care, the period of delay is longer. These families will generally exhaust all the home remedies known to kin, friends, and folk practitioners before feeling forced to turn to establishment health care facilities for help.

Bullough and Bullough explain that home remedies may have their origins in magical beliefs or have a logical, empirical basis. Two of the more common purely magical actions are putting a knife under the bed of a woman in labor to cut the pain and wearing amulets or charms to ward off disease. Empirical modalities include massage, heat and tub baths for rheumatoid arthritis, and the application of poultices and the use of herb teas for colds. Older women are the common repository of these folk remedies in today's black families.

As medical care has become more accessible to black Americans, the use of folk medicine and practitioners has declined considerably. Particularly among the working and the middle classes, only isolated home remedies remain as reminders of the days of "grannies," conjure doctors, and folk health practices.[115]

In the same way as Chicanos, black persons often feel strange or unwelcome in white health facilities. How do blacks cope with white medical institutions? The Harrisons write that black clients often go through a process of *testing* the agency to diagnose the degree of racism existing in a new situation. In making a preliminary analysis, they may come into a clinic waiting room, sit, stand, or observe for a while without registering to see what is going on, or they may send an older child to the clinic to report back his or her impressions. If testing results in unsatisfactory opinions, *avoidance* may result, which constitutes a second mode of coping. A third mode of adapting is to *demand* services or a voice in decision making. Increasing demands for control, either at the agency level or personal level, have been heard since the civil rights movement and must be generally considered as a positive move to increase the black consumer's health-seeking behaviors.[116]

Practice Implications

The following practice implications based on the characteristics of the black family are suggested in order to provide more culturally sensitive care.

nded family is usually intact and ubstantial amount of direct assis- upport, this family resource should be ed when working with families. For the or disabled person, help from extended nily is often an invaluable asset that makes the ifference between the client having to be placed in a nursing home or being cared for in the home. In working with a family with young children, the use of the extended family support system is also a central family strength and, as such, should be capitalized on in counseling families.

2. The importance of the role of the older woman or grandmother should be recognized in working with black families. As mentioned, she is usually the repository of both care-child expertise and health remedies. She can serve as both a critical asset and also as a stumbling block if her central role in health matters is not appraised and if she is not brought into important family health decision making.

3. In recognition of the powerful influence the fam-

ily social network exerts on personal behavior, the whole family should be encouraged to adopt a new health promotion program, if appropriate, rather than only a family member.

4. Poor families, from any cultural group, have survival needs which often supercede the resolution of health problems. Family health workers need to recognize that their role will need to be enlarged in order to assist families with their problems of greater priority. Only after these more pressing problems are resolved can any real energy be given to health needs. Improvement in educational, environmental, social service, and employment opportunities for the poor black families are crucial in elevating their health status.

5. Health professionals must be aware of the discomfort and alienation poor black families feel toward white health facilities. Interactions need to be warm, sensitive, and respectful of clients' needs, beliefs, and feelings.

REFERENCES

1. Coddy B: The therapist was a gringa. In Smoyak S (ed): The Psychiatric Nurse as a Family Therapist. New York, Wiley, 1975, pp 39, 44
2. *Ibid.*, p 40
3. Padilla ER: The relationship between psychology and Chicanos: Failures and possibilities. In Hernandez CA, Haug MJ, Wagner NN (eds): Chicanos—Social and Psychological Perspectives, 2nd ed. St. Louis, Mosby, 1976, p 286
4. McAdoo HP: Minority families. In Stevens JH, Mathews M (eds): Mother/Child; Father/Child Relationships. Washington DC, The National Association of the Education of Young Children, 1978, pp 178–179
5. Kobrin FE, Goldscheider C: The Ethnic Factor in Family Structure and Mobility. Cambridge, Mass, Ballinger, 1978, p 1
6. *Ibid.*, p 4
7. Leininger M: Nursing and Anthropology: Two Worlds to Blend. New York, Wiley, 1970
8. Leininger M, *op. cit.*
9. Aamodt AM: Culture. In Clark AL (ed): Culture, Childbearing and Health Professionals. Philadelphia, Davis, 1978, p 7
10. Leininger M: Transcultural Health Care Issues and Conditions. Philadelphia, Davis, 1976, pp 3–22
11. Koshi PT: Cultural diversity in the nursing curricula. J Nurs Educat 15:14, 1976
12. Kay MA: The Mexican American. In Clark AL (ed): Culture, Childbearing and Health Professionals. Philadelphia, Davis, 1978, p 89
13. Kroeber AL: Anthropology. New York, Harcourt, Brace, 1948, p 425
14. Kluckholm FR: Dominant and variant value orientations. In Brink P (ed): Transcultural Nursing. Englewood Cliffs, NJ, Prentice-Hall, 1976, p 77

15. Kobrin, Goldscheider, *op. cit.*, pp 2, 4
16. Price JA: North American Indian families. In Mindel CH, Haberstein R (eds): Families in America: Patterns and Variations. New York, Elsevier, 1976
17. Aamodt, *op. cit.*, p 9
18. Coddy, *op. cit.*, p 44
19. Leininger M: Transcultural nursing: a promising subfield of study for nurses. In Reinhardt, Quinn, *op. cit.*, p 7.
20. *Ibid.*, p 40
21. *Ibid.*, pp 42–43
22. Aamodt, *op. cit.*, pp 9–10
23. Clemen S: Concepts of culture and value clarification. In Clemen S, Gregerson M (eds): Family and Community Health Nursing: A Workbook. Ann Arbor, Mich, The University of Michigan Media Library, 1977, p 194
24. Leininger, *op. cit.*, p 48
25. McAdoo, *op. cit.*, p 178
26. Eshleman JR: The Family: An Introduction. Boston, Allyn & Bacon, 1974, p 203
27. *Ibid.*, p 219
28. Casavantes E: Pride and prejudice: A Mexican American dilemma. Civil Rights Digest 3:22, Winter 1970
29. Billingsley A: Black Families in White America. Englewood Cliffs, NJ, Prentice-Hall, 1968
30. Willie CV: A New Look at Black Families. Bayside, NY, General Hall, Inc., 1976
31. McAdoo, *op. cit.*, p 189
32. Billingsley, *op. cit.*, p 10
33. McAdoo, *op. cit.*, pp 178, 180
34. McAdoo, *op. cit.*, p 191
35. Leininger, *op. cit.*, p 43
36. Aamodt, *op. cit.*, p 15
37. Clemen, *op. cit.*, p 192

38. Russell G, Satterwhite B: It's your turn in the sun. Time 112:48, October 16, 1978
39. *Ibid.*
40. Queen SA, Haberstein RW: The Family in Various Cultures. Philadelphia, Lippincott, 1974, pp 423–424
41. *Ibid.*, pp 424–425
42. Quesada GM, Heller PL: Sociocultural barriers to medical care among Mexican Americans in Texas. Med Care 15(5):97, 1977 (supplement)
43. Castro EM: The Mexican American: How his culture affects his mental health. In Martinez RA (ed): Hispanic Culture and Health Care. St. Louis, Mosby, 1978, pp 19–32
44. Russell, Satterwhite, *op. cit.*
45. Martinez RA (ed): Hispanic Culture and Health Care. St. Louis, Mosby, 1978, p 1
46. Miranda A: The Chicano family: A reanalysis of conflicting views. J Marriage Family 6:(1):751, November 1977
47. Queen, Haberstein, *op. cit.*, p 427
48. Castro, *op. cit.*
49. Paz O: The sons of La Malenche. In Duran LI, Bernard HR (eds): Introduction to Chicano Studies. New York, Macmillan, 1973, p 24
50. Castro, *op. cit.*, p 24
51. Queen, Haberstein, *op. cit.*, p 435
52. Herrera T, Wagner NN: Behavioral approaches to delivering health services in a Chicano community. In Reinhardt, Quinn, *op. cit.*, pp 73–74
53. Queen, Haberstein, *op. cit.*, p 435
54. Castro, *op. cit.*, p 23
55. Queen, Haberstein, *op. cit.*, pp 425–430
56. Miranda, *op. cit.*, p 747
57. *Ibid.*, p 753
58. Moore JW: Mexican Americans. Englewood Cliffs, NJ, Prentice-Hall, 1970, p 131
59. Martinez C: Community mental health and the Chicano movement. In Hernandez CA, Haug MJ, Wagner NN (eds): Chicanos—Social and Psychological Perspectives, 2nd ed. St. Louis, Mosby, 1976, p 293
60. Castro, *op. cit.*, pp 19–32
61. Miranda, *op. cit.*, p 759
62. Queen, Haberstein, *op. cit.*, p 431
63. Philippus MJ: Successful and unsuccessful approaches to mental health services for an urban Hispanic American population. Am Public Health 61:(4):825, 1971
64. Queen, Haberstein, *op. cit.*, p 432
65. Kay, *op. cit.*, p 93
66. Queen, Haberstein, *op. cit.*, p 429
67. *Ibid.*, pp 435–437
68. Miranda, *op. cit.*, p 751
69. Moustafa AT, Weiss G: Mexican American Study Project, Advance Report II. Los Angeles, UCLA School of Public Health, 1968, p 1
70. Gonzales E: The role of Chicano folk beliefs and practices in mental health. In Hernandez CA, Haug MJ, Wagner NN (eds): Chicanos—Social and Psychological Perspectives, 2nd ed. St. Louis, Mosby, 1976, p 265
71. Dorsey RR, Jackson HQ: Cultural health traditions: The Latino/Chicano perspective. In Branch M (ed): Providing Safe Care to Ethnic People of Color. New York, Appleton, 1976, pp 54–55
72. Clark M: Health in the Mexican American Culture: A community study. Berkeley, University of California Press, 1970, pp 162–217
73. Herrera, Wagner, *op. cit.*, p 70
74. Prattes O: Beliefs of the Mexican American family. In Hymovich D, Barnard MV (eds): Family Health Care. New York, McGraw-Hill, 1973, pp 131–136
75. Castro, *op. cit.*, pp 26–31
76. Dorsey, Jackson, *op. cit.*, pp 60–73
77. Herrera, Wagner, *op. cit.*, p 70
78. Clark, *op. cit.*, p 207
79. Dorsey, Jackson, *op. cit.*, pp 58–59, 70
80. *Ibid.*, pp 59, 69–70
81. Prattes, *op. cit.*, pp 130–131
82. Dorsey, Jackson, *op. cit.*, p 59
83. Herrera, Wagner, *op. cit.*, pp 75–76
84. *Ibid.*, p 76
85. Farge EJ: La Vida Chicano: Health Care Attitudes and Behaviors of Houston Chicanos. San Francisco, R & E Research Associates, 1975, p 19
86. Martinez, *op. cit.*, p 1
87. Nall FC, Speilberg JS: Social and cultural factors in the responses of Mexican Americans to medical treatment. In Martinez, *op. cit.*, p 63
88. Clark, *op. cit.*, pp 231–232
89. Nall, Speilberg, *op. cit.*, pp 63–64
90. Rainwater L: Crucible of identity: The Negro lower-class family. In Bracey JH, Meier A, Rudwick E (eds): Black Matriarchy: Myth or Reality? Belmont, Calif, Wadsworth, 1971, p 81
91. *Ibid.*, pp 81–82
92. Billingsley, *op. cit.*
93. Moynihan DP: The Negro Family: A Case for National Action. Washington DC, Government Printing Office, 1965
94. Billingsley, *op. cit.*
95. Williams DA, Lord M: Blacks: Fresh trials. Newsweek, May 15, 1978, p 77
96. Willie, *op. cit.*, p 1
97. *Ibid.*, pp 3–4
98. Williams, Lord, *op. cit.*, p 77
99. *Ibid.*
100. Carrington BW: The Afro-American. In Clark AL (ed): Culture, Childbearing and Health Professionals. Philadelphia, Davis, 1978, p 37
101. Eshleman, *op. cit.*
102. Billingsley, *op. cit.*
103. Willie, *op. cit.*, p 20
104. *Ibid.*, pp 19, 22–23
105. *Ibid.*, pp 12–15
106. Fellows DK: A Mosaic of America's Ethnic Minorities. New York, Wiley, 1972, p 29
107. Willie, *op. cit.*, pp 59–62
108. *Ibid.*, pp 95–98
109. Rainwater, *op. cit.*, p 89
110. *Ibid.*, pp 90–94
111. *Ibid.*, pp 95–96
112. Harrison IE, Harrison DS: The black family experience and health behavior. In Crawford C (ed): Health and the Family. New York, Macmillan, 1971, pp 178–183
113. *Ibid.*, p 184
114. Stokes LG: Delivering health services in a black community. In Reinhardt, *op. cit.*, p 53
115. Bullough B, Bullough VL: Poverty, Ethnic Identity, and Health Care. New York, Appleton, 1972, pp 53–54
116. Harrison, Harrison, *op. cit.*, pp 193–196

STUDY QUESTIONS

1. Give a brief answer to the question of why it is essential to understand a family's cultural background when providing family health care.

Choose the correct answers to the following questions.

2. One of the assumptions made in dealing with families from different cultures is that we become less judgmental of other people's behavior as we attempt to:
   a. Give up our values and learn to accept people as they are.
   b. Recognize the origins of our own values and understand why we hold them.
   c. Work purposefully to overlook other person's values that are contrary to our own.
   d. Gradually work to change other's values when we consider them detrimental to their well-being.

3. Cultural ignorance and insensitivity lead to the following problems (choose the correct answers):
   a. Poor communication.
   b. Interpersonal tensions.
   c. Stigmatization.
   d. Inadequate assessments.
   e. Professional objectivity.

4. Ethnicity is an important resource for individuals and families because:
   a. It guides them in occupational choices.
   b. It compensates for the cold impersonality of modern society.
   c. Its traditions enrich family life and strengthen its continuity.
   d. It facilitates upward mobility.

5. The cross-cultural approach is relevant for family health care because it (select the *one* best answer):
   a. Provides information about different cultures.
   b. Takes on a cultural-equivalent perspective.
   c. Provides a broad comparative picture of individual and group behavior.
   d. Assumes a cultural deviant perspective in assessment.

6. Ethnic self-help measures have historically been most positive, since immigrants and peoples of the same ethnic background have desperately needed each other to survive and adjust to American society. Yet, self-help among kin can have drawbacks also. What is the primary drawback?

7. Several important factors have adversely influenced the Chicano family's integration into American society, even though some of these same factors may be "positive" for the family. Give three of these factors.

Are the following statements True *or* False?

8. Familism refers to the Mexican-American's propensity to marry early and have a family.

9. In the Chicano family the male and older person have both traditionally held positions of power and respect.

10. The ethic of reciprocity involves mutual sharing of resources and provision of assistance to those in need.

11. Match the proper definition with the corresponding concept.

Concept	*Definition*
1. Cultural conflict	a. Blueprint for man's way of living.
2. Acculturation	b. People of a particular cultural group.
3. Assimilation	c. Nonacceptance of diversity within cultural group.
4. Ethnic identity	d. Gradual changes created as one culture is influenced by another.
5. Ethnocentrism	e. The way individuals see themselves as to their cultural association.
6. Stereotyping	f. Denotes the more complete one-way process of acculturation.
7. Cultural relativism	g. Culture is viewed nonjudgmentally and understood within its own context.
8. Cultural pluralism	h. Lack of cultural relativity (seeing one's own culture as superior to others).
9. Cultural imposition	i. Local professional health care system.
10. Culture shock	j. Lay health care system.
11. Indigenous health care system	k. Primary tactic used in cultural anthropology to analyze cultures.
12. Self-fulfilling prophecy	l. Discomfort and confusion created by experiencing cultural differences.
13. Culture	m. Ethnic diversity.
14. Ethnic group	n. Forcing one's values and practices on another person because of ethnocentricity.
	o. A degraded person's tendency to conform to the beliefs and expectations others have about him.
	p. Negative responses of clients to culturally unacceptable practices of health agencies and health workers.

12. Machismo refers to (select all appropriate answers):
    a. A cluster of traits traditionally characteristic of the Mexican-American male.
    b. Masculine role incorporating elements of aggressiveness and power.

    c. Feminine attitudes of softness and respect.

    d. None of the above.

13. The institution of *compadrazzo* among Mexican-American families can be described as:

    a. Kinship patterns linking maternal and paternal sides of family together.

    b. The institution of godparenthood.

    c. A special linkage between two families established by the baptismal ritual.

    d. An institution which is declining in importance today as a result of acculturation pressures.

14. Match the appropriate family roles and power attributes with the family member most frequently associated with these roles and power characteristics in the traditional Chicano family (family members may have multiple attributes).

Family Members	*Role/Power Attributes*
1. Father-husband	a. Submissive, dependent role.
2. Mother-wife	b. Accorded respect in home by virtue of age and/or sex.
3. Daughter	c. Holder of legitimate power (primary authority).
4. Adolescent son	d. Holder of referent power.
5. Grandparent	e. Demonstrate *machismo*.
	f. Role most incongruent vis-à-vis dominant culture's corresponding family role.
	g. Acts as confidante to children.
	h. Stands aloof in child rearing.

15. For each of the following American central values, explain what the corresponding traditional Mexican-American value is.

Area	American Core Value	Traditional Chicano Value
Family	Americans see themselves as an individual first, a family member second.	
Work	Productivity and work are central and prominent values. Work often becomes an end rather than a means to an end.	
Materialism	Possession of material goods is a symbol of success. The greater the accumulation of goods, the greater the prestige.	
Time and punctuality	"Time is money." Punctuality is a moral value equated with being responsible.	
Interpersonal relationships	Americans value openness and directness in communication, as well as rationality vs emotional expressiveness.	

Are the following statements True *or* False?

16. The most profound structural change occurring in the Chicano family today is the resurgence of the value of familism.

17. Marked gender differences in socialization occur in the traditional Chicano family.

18. Democratic ideals and verbal facility is taught at a young age in the Chicano family.

19. In the traditional Chicano family, the father plays a continuining close role of companion to his sons.

20. In the traditional Chicano family, the mother tends to act as a buffer between father and son to soften the paternal demands on the son.

21. Match the description of the folk healer with the type of folk healer.

    1. *Yerbero*
    2. Conjure doctor
    3. "Granny"
    4. *Espiritualisto(a)*
    5. *Brujo(a)*
    6. *Curandero(a)*

    a. Herbalist
    b. Deals with supernatural illnesses.
    c. Practices witchcraft or magic.
    d. Black family's herbalist and midwife.
    e. Healer of folk illnesses in the Chicano community.

22. Fill in the name of each of the following common Mexican folk illnesses from this list of possibilities (mental illness, *empacho, susto, mal ojo, mal puesto, caida de la mollera*).
    a. "Bad eye," resulting from excessive admiration or desire on the part of another.
    b. Analogous to *mal de sangre*, placed by God or *brujo* as hex or punishment on the patient.
    c. Affliction caused by food adhering to the stomach wall in the form of a ball.
    d. Fallen fontanels (in infants).
    e. Sorcery.
    f. Illness caused by fright or emotionally traumatizing experience.

23. Based on what is known of black and Chicano families, and of families in general, identify which of the following practice suggestions would be most appropriate for which group (black family, B; Chicano family, C; and all families, A).

    a. Separation of patient from family member should be considered very carefully.
    b. Client should not be expected to make a health decision until he or she has had a chance to consult with his or her family.
    c. It is best to attempt to have the whole family adopt health promotion or maintenance program.
    d. Other family problems may take precedence over health problems, and

thus, the health worker may have to help family with their other problems in order for them to be able to resolve their health needs.

e. Families need to be spoken to in terms and concepts they understand and suggestions need to appeal to their basic values.

f. An authoritative approach, whereby the health professional conveys expertise and confidence in his/her ability to "heal" is expected.

24. Which of the following are some of the frequent effects on the black family of slavery, racism, and economic disadvantages (mark true or false after each statement).

a. The black male's self-esteem has been lowered.

b. The wife became submissive to her husband and his primary authority.

c. The self-fulfilling prophecy often occurs in the areas of education and employment.

d. Health-seeking behaviors are attenuated.

e. A mother-centered family became a practical necessity.

f. Traditional husband–wife family roles became rigidly defined.

25. When one examines recent family and economic statistics related to the black family, which of the following problems appear to be important? (Select all appropriate answers.)

a. Economic.

b. Parenting and child care.

c. Family planning.

d. Employment.

26. Match the following structural and functional attributes with the black family according to social class.

Structural-Functional Attribute	*Class*
a. Respectability is an important value.	1. Middle class
b. Both parents are college-educated and work.	2. Working class
c. Role sharing between husband and wife occurs extensively.	3. Lower class
d. More likely to be single-parent families and/or matrifocal.	4. Underclass
e. A strong achievement orientation is present.	
f. Has the largest family and largest number of relatives living in same household.	
g. Church is a central value and institution.	
h. More traditional family roles are present.	
i. Egalitarian-autonomic power pattern exists.	
j. Values most incongruent with wider society.	

27. Black clients have been described as coping with white health care agencies by first carefully evaluating them as to their possible racism or degree of prejudice. Which of the following ways do they employ?
   a. Testing.
   b. Creating conflicts and openly becoming argumentative.
   c. Avoidance of agencies perceived as prejudicial.
   d. Demanding more of a say in their own care.

STUDY ANSWERS

1. Gaining an understanding of the cultural background of a family is essential to family health care, since without this knowledge, family values and behavior cannot be understood nor accurately interpreted. Culture permeates and circumscribes familial actions. In the absence of being able to assess accurately, the health professional is then not in a position to work with the family to assist them in resolving their health problems.

2. b

3. all but e

4. b and c

5. c

6. Self-help, among kin particularly, creates a leveling effect in some families. Among poor families and communities, the ethic of reciprocity has tended to keep the upwardly mobile families down, since they are continually being asked to help the less fortunate members of their extended families. Under these situations the motivated, more successful families experience unequal kinship burdens. This may breed discontent and animosity between families.

7. List any three:
   a. Language differences.
   b. Religious differences.
   c. Social class differences (large numbers of peasant agricultural workers and laborers migrated).
   d. American discriminatory and segregation practices.
   e. Mexican-American closeness with Mexico, so that Chicanos could cross back and forth frequently. This consequently strengthened their ties to Mexico and reduced their need to become involved with some of the institutions within the United States.

8. False

9. True

10. True

11. 1. p 6. c 11. j
    2. d 7. g 12. o
    3. f 8. m 13. a
    4. e 9. n 14. b
    5. h 10. 1

12. a and b

13. b, c, and d

14. 1. b, c, e, and h
    2. a, b, d, f, and g
    3. a
    4. b and e
    5. b and d

15.

Area	Traditional Chicano Values
Family	Chicanos see themselves as members of families first, as individuals second.
Work	Work is seen as a means, i.e., as a necessity in order to live. Other life experiences (social and emotional experiences) are valued more than work.
Materialism	Possession of goods and objects are necessary for living, not ends in themselves. Status and prestige more likely derived from ability to intellectually and emotionally experience things. Social relationships and family more important than accumulation of wealth.
Time and punctuality	Time is to be enjoyed. Punctuality does not have the moral overtones it does in American society.
Interpersonal relationships	Mexican-Americans value use of diplomacy and tactfulness. They are concerned about showing respect and are more elaborate, indirect, and emotionally expressive in their communications.

16. False

17. True

18. False

19. False

20. True

21. 1. a
    2. c
    3. d
    4. b
    5. c
    6. e

22. a. *Mal ojo*
    b. Mental illness
    c. *Empacho*
    d. *Caida de la mollera*
    e. *Mal puesto*
    f. *Susto*

23. a. C
    b. C
    c. A
    d. A
    e. A
    f. C

24. a. True
    b. False
    c. True
    d. True
    e. True
    f. False

25. All (a–d)

26. a. 2
    b. 1
    c. 1
    d. 4
    e. 1
    f. 3
    g. 1, 2, and 3
    h. 2 and 3
    i. 2
    j. 4

27. a, c, and d

APPENDIX A

Guidelines for Family Assessment

The following guidelines represent a collation and abbreviation of the assessment questions which appear at the end of each of the chapters in Part II of the text, beginning with the assessment of identifying and environmental data, continuing through the assessment of structural and functional dimensions, and concluding with an assessment of cultural differences in families. After each broad heading, a footnote alerts the reader as to where the related family theory and further discussion of assessment areas may be found.

IDENTIFYING DATA

Foundational data which describe the family in basic terms is included in this section.

1. **Family Name**[1]
2. **Address and Phone**[1]
3. **Family Composition:**[1] In Table A.1, after the adult family members, record oldest child first, followed by each succeeding child in order of birth. Include any other related or nonrelated members of household next. If there are extended family members or friends who act as family members, although not living in household, include them also at end of listing. The relationship of each family member to each other, as well as birthdate, birthplace, occupation, and education, should be specified.
4. **Type of Family Form**[1]
5. **Cultural (Ethnic) and Religious Orientation**[2] (including extent of acculturation). In describing this, use the following criteria as guideposts for determining family's cultural and religious orientation.
   5.1 Family's stated ethnicity and religious preference?
   5.2 The family's social network (from the same ethnic group)?
   5.3 Family residence (part of an ethnically homogeneous neighborhood)?
   5.4 Religious, social, cultural, recreational and/or educational activities (are they within the family's cultural group)?
   5.5 Dietary habits and dress (traditional or Westernized)?
   5.6 Presence of traditional or "modern" family roles and power structure?
   5.7 Home decor (signs of cultural influences)?
   5.8 Language(s) spoken in home?
   5.9 The portion(s) of the community the family frequents—the family's territorial complex (is it within the ethnic community primarily)?

TABLE A.1
Family Composition Form

Name (Last, First)	Sex	Relationship	Date/Place Of Birth	Occupation	Education
1. (father)					
2. (mother)					
3. (oldest child)					
4.					
5.					
6.					
7.					
8.					

5.10 The family's use of health care services and practitioners. Does family visit folk practitioners, engage in traditional folk health practices, or have traditional indigenous health beliefs?

5.11 Length of time family has lived in the United States (what generation are family members, relative to their immigration status)?

5.12 How actively involved is the family in a particular church, temple, or other religious organization?

5.13 What religious practices does the family engage in?

5.14 What religiously based beliefs or values appear central in the family's life?

6. **Social Class Status**[3] (based on occupation, education, and income):
   Economic Status
   Who is (are) the breadwinner(s) in the family?
   Does the family receive any supplementary funds or assistance? If so, from where?
   Does family consider their income to be adequate?

7. **Social Class Mobility**[4]

8. **Developmental History of Family (optional)**[5]
   8.1 Family's present developmental stage.
   8.2 Family's history (from inception through present-day).
   8.3 Family's developmental (addition of new baby, retirement) and unique health concerns and experiences (divorce, death, illnesses, unemployment) during the family's existence as a unit.
   8.4 Both parents' families of origin (present and past relationships; what life in family of origin was like).

9. **Family's Recreational or Leisure-Time Activities**[6]
   Suggested assessment areas pertaining to the family recreational or leisure-time activities include:
   9.1 Identifying the family's activities—what types and how often do these activities occur?
   9.2 Listing the leisure-time activities of family subsystems (spouse subsystem; parent–child subsystems; and sibling subsystems).

ENVIRONMENTAL DATA

Environmental data covers the family's universe—from consideration of the smallest area such as aspects of home to the larger community in which the family resides.

10. **Characteristics of Home**[6]
    10.1 Describe the dwelling type (home, apartment, rooming house, etc.). Does family own or rent their home?
    10.2 Describe the home's condition (both the interior and exterior of house). House interior would include number of rooms and types of rooms (living room, bedrooms, etc.), their use and how they are furnished. What is condition and adequacy of furniture? Is there adequate heating, ventilation, and lighting (artificial and daylight)? Are the floors, stairs, railings, and other structures in adequate condition?
    10.3 In kitchen, observe water supply, sanitation, and the adequacy of refrigeration.
    10.4 In bathrooms, observe sanitation, water supply, toilet facilities, presence of towels and soap.
    10.5 Assess the sleeping arrangements in the house. Are they adequate for family members, considering their age, relationships, and their special needs?
    10.6 Observe for vermin (interior especially).
    10.7 Assess family's subjective feelings about home. Does the family consider its home adequate for its needs?
    10.8 Identify the family's territorial unit.
    10.9 Evaluate the privacy arrangements and how the family feels about the adequacy of their privacy.
    10.10 Evaluate the home's presence or absence of safety hazards.

11. **Characteristics of Neighborhood and Larger Community**[6]
    11.1 What are the physical characteristics of the immediate neighborhood and the larger community?
    Types of dwellings (residential, industrial, combined residential and small industry, agrarian).
    Condition of the dwellings and streets (well kept up, deteriorating, dilapidated, being revitalized).
    Sanitation of streets, home (cleanliness, trash and garbage collected, etc.).
    Incidence of crime in neighborhood (safety problems).
    Presence and types of industry in neighborhood (air, noise pollution problems).

11.2 What are the demographic characteristics of the neighborhood and community?
Social class and ethnic characteristics of residents.
Occupations and interests of families.
Density of population.

11.3 What health and other basic services and facilities are available in the neighborhood and community?
Marketing (food, clothing, drug store, etc.)
Health agencies.
Social service agencies (welfare, counseling, employment).
Family's church or temple.

11.4 How accessible are the neighborhood and community schools and what is their condition? Are there busing and integration problems which affect the family?

11.5 Recreational.

11.6 Availability of public transportation. How accessible (in terms of distance, suitability, hours, etc.) are these services and facilities to family?

11.7 What is the incidence of crime in the neighborhood and community? Are there serious safety problems?

12. **Family's Geographic Mobility**[6]
12.1 How long has the family lived in the area?
12.2 What is their history of geographic mobility?
12.3 From where did they move or migrate?

13. **Family's Associations and Transactions with Community**[6]
13.1 *Who* in family uses *what* community services or is known to what agencies?
13.2 How frequently or to what extent do they use these services or facilities?
13.3 What is the family's territorial cluster and complex?
13.4 Is the family aware of community services relevant to their needs, such as transportation?
13.5 How does family feel about groups or persons from whom it receives assistance or with whom it relates?
13.6 How does the family view community?

14. **Family's Social Support System or Network:**[7] Who helps family in time of need for assistance, counseling, family activities (babysitting, transportation, etc.)?
14.1 *Informal:* Family's ties with friends, neighbors, relatives (kin), social groups, employers, employees. Who are they and what is the nature of their relationship?
14.2 *Formal:* Family's relationships with helping persons from health and health-related agencies.

FAMILY STRUCTURE

15. *Role Structure*[8]
Formal Role Structure
15.1 What formal positions and roles do each of the family members fulfill?
15.2 Are these roles acceptable and consistent with family's expectations? In other words, does role strain or role conflict exist?

15.3 How competently do members perform their respective roles?
15.4 Is there flexibility in roles when needed?
Informal Role Structure
15.5 What informal or covert roles exist in family? Who plays them and how frequently or consistently are they enacted? Are members of the family covertly playing roles different from those which their position in the family demands that they play?
15.6 What purpose does the presence of the identified covert or informal role(s) serve?
Analysis of Role Models
15.7 Who were (or are) the models that influenced a family member(s) in his or her early life, who gave him or her the feelings and values about growth, new experiences, roles, communication techniques, etc.?
15.8 Who specifically acted as role model for the mates in their roles as parents, and as marital partners, and what were they like?

16. **Power Structure**[9]
Decision Making
16.1 Who makes what decisions?
16.2 And how important are these decisions or issues to the family?
More specific questions might include:
Who budgets, pays bills, decides how money is to be spent?
Who decides on how to spend an evening or what friends or relatives to visit?
Who decides on changes in jobs or residence?
Who disciplines and decides on child's activities?
Decision-Making Process
16.3 What specific techniques are utilized for making decisions in the family and to what extent are these utilized (e.g., consensus; accommodation–bargaining; compromising or coercion; de facto)? In other words, *how* family makes its decisions.
Bases for or Sources of Power: The various sources of power are authority (legitimate power) and a variation of it, "helpless" power; referent power; expert power or resources power; reward power; coercive power; and informational power (direct and indirect).
16.4 On what bases did (the family member) make his or her decision?
Variables Affecting Family Power
16.5 Recognizing the existence of any of the following variables will help the assessor interpret family behavior from which family power can be assessed.
Family communication network.
Control for implementation of decisions.
Interpersonal resources.
Formation of coalitions.
Social class and life cycle differences.
Overall Family Power
16.6 From your assessment of all the above broad areas, are you able to deduce whether the family power can be characterized as dominated by wife or husband, child, grandmother, etc.; egalitarian–syncretic or autonomic; leaderless or chaotic? The family power continuum can be used for a visual presentation of your analysis.

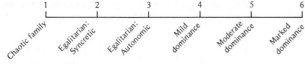

Family Power Continuum: If dominance is found, who is the dominant one?

16.7 To determine the overall power pattern, asking a broad, open-ended question is often illuminating (asking both spouses and children if feasible), examples of which are given below.

Who usually has "last say" about important issues?

Who is really in charge and why (getting at bases for power)?

Who runs the family?

Who wins the important arguments or issues?

Who usually wins out if there is a disagreement?

Who gets his or her way when they disagree?

Are family members satisfied with how decisions are made and with who makes them (i.e., the present power structure)?

17. **Communication Patterns**[10]

17.1 In observing the family as a whole and/or the family's set of relationships, how extensively are functional and dysfunctional communication used? Give examples of recurring patterns.

Are the majority of messages of family members congruent in content and instruction? (Include observations of nonverbal messages.) If not, who manifests incongruency?

How firmly and clearly do the members state their needs and feelings?

To what extent do members use clarification and qualification in interaction?

Do members elicit and respond favorably to feedback or do they generally discourage feedback and exploration of an issue?

How well do members listen and attend when communicating?

Do members seek validation from one another?

To what degree do members use assumptions and judgmental statements in interaction?

Do members interact in an offensive manner to messages?

How frequently is disqualification utilized?

17.2 How are emotional (affective) messages conveyed in the family and within the family subsystems? How frequently are these emotional messages conveyed?

What types of emotions are transmitted within the family subsystems? Are negative, positive, or both types of emotions transmitted?

17.3 What is the frequency and quality of communication within the communication network and familial sets of relationships?

Who talks to whom and in what usual manner?

What is the usual pattern of transmitting important messages? Does an intermediary exist?

Are messages sent that are appropriate to the developmental age of the members?

17.4 What areas are closed off to discussion that are important issues to the family's wellness or adequate functioning?

17.5 What are the internal (familial) and external (environmental, socioeconomic, and cultural) influences impinging on the processes and communication patterns?

18. **Family Values**[11]

18.1 Use of "compare and contrast" method suggested (with values of either dominant culture, family's reference group—ethnic group with whom they identify—or both).

American Core Values	Family's Values
Productivity	
Work ethic	
Materialism	
Individualism	
Education	
Consumption ethic	
Progress and mastery over environment	
Future time orientation	
Efficiency, orderliness, practicality	
Rationality	
Cleanliness	
Democracy, equality, and freedom	
Voluntarism	
"Doing orientation"	
Health	

18.2 How important are these identified values to the family?

18.3 Are these values consciously or unconsciously held?

18.4 Are there any value conflicts evident within the family itself?

18.5 How do these family values affect the health status of the family?

FAMILY FUNCTIONS

19. **Affective Function**[12]

Family Need–Response Patterns

19.1 Do family members perceive of the needs of the other individuals in the family?

Are parents (spouses) able to describe their children's and mate's needs and concerns?

How sensitive are family members in picking up cues regarding other's feelings and needs?

Do the family members each have someone they can go to within the family to unburden themselves to, i.e., a confidant?

19.2 Are each member's needs, interests, differentness respected by the other family members?

Does a mutual respect balance exist (do they show mutual respect toward each other)?

How sensitive is the family to each individual's actions and concerns?

19.3 Are the recognized needs of the family members being met by the family, and if so, to what extent? For questions 19.1, 19.2, and 19.3, it is suggested that a list of the family members be included with their needs identified (as perceived by family members) and the extent to which these needs are being met.

Mutual Nurturance, Closeness, and Identification

19.4 To what extent do family members provide mutual nurturance to each other?

How supportive of each other are they?

19.5 Is a sense of closeness and intimacy present among the sets of relationships within the family?

How well do family members get along with each other?

Do they show affection toward each other?

19.6 Does mutual identification, bonding, or attachment appear to be present? (Empathetic statements, concerns about other's feelings, experiences, and hardships are all indicative.)

Separateness and Connectedness

19.7 How does the family deal with the issues of separateness and connectedness?

How does the family help its members want to be together and maintain cohesiveness (connectedness)?

Are opportunities for developing separateness stressed adequately and are they appropriate for the age and needs of each of the family members?

20. **Socialization Function**[13]

20.1 Assess family's child-rearing practices in the following areas.

Discipline

Reward

Punishment

Autonomy and dependency

Giving and receiving of love

Training for age-appropriate behavior (social, physical, emotional, language, and intellectual development).

20.2 How adaptive are the family's child-rearing practices for their particular situation?

20.3 Who assumes responsibility for the child-care role or socialization function? Is this function shared? If so, how is this managed?

20.4 How are the children regarded in this family? What cultural beliefs are operating in their child rearing?

21. **Health Care Function**[14]

21.1 Family's definition of health/illness and their level of knowledge:

How does the family decide on who is sick or ill? What clues give them this impression, and who decides?

Does the family have pertinent information about health promotion, disease, treatment, and hazards?

Can the family observe and report significant symptoms and changes?

What serious health problems does family perceive family members to be susceptible or vulnerable to and what are family members' beliefs about the effectiveness and appropriateness of health actions to resolve these problems?

21.2 Family dietary practices:

Adequacy of the family diet (a 24-hour food history record of family eating patterns is recommended).

Function of mealtimes and family's attitude toward food and mealtimes. Does the family eat together? Is mealtime a pleasurable experience? Is food used as a reward or punishment?

Shopping (and its planning) practices.

Budgeting limitations (use of food stamps).

Adequacy of storage and refrigeration. Ways food is prepared.

Who is responsible for the planning, shopping, and preparation of meals?

21.3 Sleeping and resting practices:

What are the usual sleeping habits of the family? Are they suitable according to age and health status?

Are regular hours established for sleeping? Who decides when children go to sleep?

Where do family members sleep?

Do any family members take naps or have other regular means of resting or relaxing?

21.4 Exercise and recreation. This is duplicative of identifying data except for the following:

Does family believe regular exercise and physical fitness are necessary for good health?

Types of daily activities where exercise is involved (individual's work).

21.5 Family's drug habits:

Family members' use of alcohol, tobacco, coffee, cola, and tea (caffeine and theobromine are stimulants).

Is the use of tobacco or alcohol by a family member perceived as a problem by that person or another family member?

Does the use of alcohol interfere with their capacity to carry out their usual activities? How long has family member been using alcohol?

Family's use of over-the-counter and prescription drugs.

Does family "save" drugs over long periods of time and reuse them?

Are drugs properly labeled and in safe place, away from children?

21.6 Family's role in self-care practices:

Who is (are) health leader(s) in the family? Who makes the health decisions in the family?

How competent is family in self-care relative to recognition of signs and symptoms of common illnesses, diagnosis, and home treatment of common, simple health problems?

21.7 Environmental practices:

Family's exposure to air, noise pollution.

Family's hygiene, cleanliness practices.

21.8 Medically based preventive measures:

Periodic physical examinations appropriate for age, sex, and health status.

Family's feelings about having physical when well?

Eye and hearing examinations.

Immunization status.

21.9 Dental health practices:

Nutritional habits—amounts and types of starches and sugars consumed by family.

Brushing of teeth after meals.

Use of topical fluoride, fluoride tablets, or rinses if water supply not fluoridated.

Regular dental checkups, cleaning, and repair.

21.10 Family medical history. (Question regarding overall health of parents' parents and siblings and if specific diseases have been present.)

Identification of past and present environmentally related diseases of the family of orientation of parents (and parents' siblings).

Psychosocial problems: mental illness and obesity.

Infectious diseases: typhoid fever, tuberculosis, venereal disease, hepatitis, diarrheas, and skin diseases.

Identification of past and present genetically related diseases of family of orientation of parents (and parents' siblings).

Epilepsy, diabetes, cystic fibrosis, mental retardation, sickle-cell anemia, kidney disease, hypertension, heart disease, cancer, leukemia, vision and hearing defects, hemophilia, allergies, including asthma.

21.11 Health services received:

What physician and/or health agency(ies) does the family receive care from?

Does this source (physician, etc.) see all members of the family and take care of all their health needs?

21.12 Feelings and perceptions regarding health services:

What are the family's feelings and perceptions regarding the health services they receive?

Is the family comfortable and satisfied with the care they receive and their relationships with the physician(s), family health nurse, school nurse, and/or the other health providers they are currently seeing?

Do they have confidence in their doctor, nurse(s), social worker, etc.?

How do they perceive the role of the various health providers?

If you are the community health nurse visiting the home, what does the family see your role as being?

What has been the family's past experience with the community health nurse?

21.13 Emergency health services:

Does the agency or physician the family receives care from have an emergency service?

Are medical services by current health providers available if an emergency occurs?

If emergency services are not available, does the family know where the closest available (according to their eligibility) emergency services are for both the children and the adult members of the family?

Does the family know how to call for an ambulance and paramedic services?

Does family have an emergency health plan?

21.14 Dental health services:

What dental health services are/have been received by members of the family?

21.15 Source of payment:

How does the family pay for services it receives or might receive?

Does the family have a private health insurance plan, Medicare, or Medicaid; or must the family pay for services in full or partially?

Does the family receive any free services (or know about them)?

What effect does the cost of health care have on the utilization of health services?

If the family has health insurance (either private, Medicare, or Medicaid), is the family informed about what services are covered, such as preventive services, special medical equipment, home visits, etc.?

21.16 Logistics of receiving care:

What is the distance of the health care facility(ies) from the family's home?

What modes of transportation does the family use to get there?

If the family must depend on public transportation, what problems exist regarding hours of service and travel time to the health facility?

22. **Family Coping Function**[15]

22.1 What stressors (both long- and short-term and socioeconomic and environmental) are impinging on the family? (Refer to Holmes and Rahe's Social Readjustment Scale.)

Are you able to estimate the duration and strength of the family's stressors?

What strengths counterbalance these stressors?

22.2 Is the family able to make decisions (adapt) based on a realistic and objective appraisal of the situation?

22.3 How does the family react to stressful situations (what functional strategies are used)?

What are the coping resources of the family?

What coping strategies does the family use, or has it used, to deal with what types of problems?

What are the family's inner resources?

Family group reliance via greater control.

Use of humor.

Sharing of feelings, thoughts, and activities.

Development of strong subsystems and family members.

What are family members' problem-solving abilities?

Are they able to articulate their needs and concerns?

Can they outline ways of satisfying these needs, arrive at solutions, and implement and evaluate them?

Controlling the meaning of the problem.

What are the family's external resources?
Use of knowledge.
Increased linkages with the broader community (general external involvement)?
Social support systems.
Informal and formal.
In what problem areas or situations has the family, in its dealings over time, achieved mastery?
Is the family able to meet the usual stresses and strains of daily family life?

25.4 How does family react to stressful situations (dysfunctional strategies)?
What dysfunctional adaptive strategies has the family used or is the family using?

If there are signs of any of the following dysfunctionalities, record their presence and how extensively used:
Spousal violence
Child abuse
Scapegoating
Use of threat
Child neglect
Triangling
Family myth
Pseudomutuality
Authoritarianism (submission to marked dominance).

FOOTNOTES

1. Chapter 8.
2. Chapters 8 and 17.
3. Chapters 8 and 19 (primarily).
4. Chapter 8.
5. Chapters 8 and 5.
6. Chapter 8.
7. Chapters 8 and 16 (primarily).
8. Chapter 9.
9. Chapter 10.
10. Chapter 11.
11. Chapter 12.
12. Chapter 13.
13. Chapter 14.
14. Chapter 15.
15. Chapter 16.

The O'Shea family was referred to the community health nurse, Ms. Bell, by the county hospital's maternity service for the following reasons. "Mrs. O'Shea has expressed the desire to learn about family planning. She also needs referral for post partum and well-baby care." These bits of information were also on the referral: Mary—age 35; gravida VII, para V, abortions II. Delivered newborn son, Daniel—born 11/3 (5 days ago); birth weight—7 lbs., 2 oz.; length—19 in.; hypertension during pregnancy; normal labor and delivery; mother's post partum status and stay normal.

FIRST HOME VISIT

During Ms. Bell's first home visit, the father and two oldest children were at work and school, respectively. From her conversation with Mary O'Shea and her observations of the home and family members, the following family data was extracted from nurse's tape recordings. Family: Patrick, father—age 43; Mary, mother—age 35 (looks older, tired and slightly overweight); Joseph, son—age 6; Maureen, daughter—age 5; Betty, daughter—age 4; Richard, son—age 3; and Daniel, son—age 1 week. Pat works as a butcher in his father's small grocery store located in same neighborhood a mile away from home.

The family lives in an older (50 years or more) wooden, three-bedroom house in the Maplewood district—an Irish neighborhood—located five miles from a New England city with a population of 300,000. The immediate neighborhood is ethnically and socially homogeneous (working class) and residential, although located very near to a heavily industrialized factory district.

The family's home is rented from a cousin for $250 per month and is sparsely furnished, with a minimum of furniture in each room. The kitchen is clean, containing a small functioning refrigerator and stove. There is one bathroom with toilet and bathtub, and two dirty towels hung from hook on the wall. The parents have their own room, which they presently share with the newborn (who has a new bassinet the women's group at the parish donated). The girls, Maureen and Betty, have their own bedroom with a double bed, while the boys share the other bedroom, having twin beds and a small chest of drawers. A few area carpets are noted, but no pictures, books, art/craft objects, house plants, or other decorations—with the exception of several Catholic religious objects in parent's room, dining room, and living room. Curtains matching the tablecloth hung in the dining room, a wedding gift from Mary's mother to them when they were married. A color television set was the centerpiece of the living room. The mother said the home was adequate for their needs, although it was getting smaller with the arrival of another baby.

The outside of the house needed painting but was not cluttered and in fair repair. It was noted, however, that the stairs leading up to the front porch were loose, and there was no railing or lighting.

Mrs. O'Shea was quite talkative and responsive to questions. Ms. Bell felt that Mary did not have many visitors or adults to talk to. When Ms. Bell explained that she had come because of a referral from the county hospital where Mrs. O'Shea had delivered her last baby, Mary was quite pleased that nurse had been contacted to visit her.

Nurse: How are you managing since you have been home from the hospital with your new baby?

Mary: Not too bad, but it sure is harder with five than with four kiddies and being older doesn't help. I just don't have the energy to get up at night and feed Daniel.

Nurse: Do you have any help?

Mary: My mother came over the first day I was home and Pat's mother came over two days ago. They helped by cooking and cleaning up the house a little, and lookin' after the children. I also have a sister nearby who goes shopping for me.

Nurse: What about your husband? Does he help?

Mary: I wish! He thinks this is all women's work and that if I need help my sister or mother can come in. He does help with putting the younger children to bed when I ask him. Men sure have an easy time of it. The responsibility really falls on my shoulders. Pat tries to help every once in a while, but then he gets distracted by his football games, or TV, or running down to the tavern for a beer.

Nurse: Is this the way it's been with the other children too—you handling practically everything?

Mary: Yes, I'll just have to "offer it up."

Nurse: You sound pretty resigned to all your work?

Mary: I am!

Nurse: Have you found ways to save your energies?

Mary: Mainly it's a question of sleeping when the baby does, letting the other kids watch TV, and not worrying about the house cleaning.

Nurse: Sounds like a good list of priorities. Your health, children, and baby are certainly more important than housework. Is there anything which is important and needs doing that you can't handle?

Mary: Nothing immediately—my family lives here and they help—but I am concerned about getting pregnant again and having more children. I didn't think I would have the need to ask about family planning—I was planning for Richie to be my last. I had two miscarriages since him—one and two years ago—and the doctors told me that I definitely shouldn't have any more children because my blood pressure gets so high. I discussed the problem with our priest, who then spoke to my husband about the rhythm method, but I guess he didn't get the right instructions. Since then, my girlfriends tell me that's a silly method anyway.

Nurse: So you and your husband are interested in limiting your family?

Mary: Not limiting my family! I don't want any more children. I don't have the foggiest idea what my husband thinks about this. I told him just yesterday that this was the end of kids for me, and he just looked and listened without a comment—and then just walked into the kitchen and got himself a beer. I can't talk to that man—that's the problem! When he has something on his mind, he sure lets me have it. But when I'm talkin', it's like I'm nagging or like it's not any of his concern.

Last time I tried discussing us not having anymore children about a year ago, he mocked me, saying, "Without little ones, what do you think you would do with your time, open up your own business?" He doesn't think much of women who work. Pat believes women belong in the home, tendin' to their own business of housework and the children and staying out of women's "gossip groups" or church or school activities. He doesn't mind me visiting my family or his, but sure doesn't want me hanging around the neighbors or outside the home very much.

Nurse: How long have you been married?

Mary: Well, we were married when I was 28 and he was 36. I guess that's been seven years. As you can see, babies started coming pretty quickly after that—one a year until now, including the two miscarriages. We both knew each other from the parish and our parents both live in the neighborhood. We both graduated from Catholic high schools in the neighborhood. After high school Pat went to work in his father's grocery store, was in the service for three years, and then when his older brother stopped working for his father, Pat got the job of being butcher in the store—been doing that for his father four years now. I worked as a sales clerk in a dime store after I graduated. I started seeing Pat three years after I finished high school, and we went together five-and-a-half years before he asked me to marry him. I was afraid I was going to be an old maid like some of my friends were. Sure was a lot easier being single though, but my family and friends were always hinting and pressuring me to "tie the noose around Patrick."

Nurse: Sounds like marriage has been hard on you. Is that right?

Mary: Yeah.

Nurse: Has it always been that way? What was it like in the beginning and after the children came?

Mary (looking at the nurse with tired, disappointed, overburdened expression on her face, and a look of both regret and sadness in her eyes): I think our marriage started out all wrong—not that it was so different from any of my friends' and cousin' or sisters' marriages— but it was just not like the marriages I read about in the papers and magazines and see on television. I was raised a strict Catholic, in an Irish school and parish. My grandparents came over from Ireland during the depression—not by choice, but by necessity. Pat's folks also are Irish, and his father came over here as a teenager and worked in construction until he could save enough to buy a small grocery store—the one he has now. I don't think either one of us were ever told about sex, except in negative terms, by our parents or priest. Even though I hear on TV that things are changing and that sex is all right, I can't help but feel that Pat and I both still see it as basically wrong, or at the very least embarrassing for me, and not very enjoyable. You asked how our marriage first was. Well, we never had sex before marriage, and after marriage our love life was awkward and unsatisfying to both of us, but to this day I can't talk to my husband about it, and he's never brought it up with me either. I often feel it's this "lack" that drives us apart.

Nurse: Do you ever talk to your sisters, mother, or friends about the problem?

Mary: Only my sister and one girlfriend, and they both have the same frustrations. My sister tells me it's just part of marriage and to put up with it.

In the beginning we used to go out to the movies or friends' homes together—and talk more. But, after the children came we drew further and further apart. Don't misunderstand me, we wanted the children and were happy to see them born, but somehow the demands in raising them caused problems between us. Now we don't talk much and seem to have little to say to each other, excepting about the children and money problems—we're always just barely making it through the month. Pat spends more and more time with the boys. You know, going to football, baseball, and basketball games or spending time at the tavern. And when he's home, he's really not home. I can't get him to do anything around the house. When I ask him to do something he looks at me as if I'm imposing on him and I'm making his life difficult. He refuses to face up to his responsibilities or to talk about our problems. When I try to talk about them, he'll say: "Don't bother me with that now. Can't you see that I'm tired. I'll do something about it tomorrow." And tomorrow never comes.

Nurse: Does he help with the children?

Mary: Only if he feels the urge! I really can't depend on him to help. Somehow I'm raising them. My sister helps me and sometimes my mother, but Patrick removes himself and really has never got to know any of them, except perhaps our youngest daughter, who he calls "his little darlin'."

The first visit also consisted of discussing the newborn, Daniel, and Mrs. Shea's physical health status. Ms. Bell planned to return in a week with information for her on clinic services for the baby and on family planning.

SECOND HOME VISIT

During the second home visit one week later, the nurse came at 3:30 P.M. when the children were home from school and the father would be there for part of visit (after he returned from work at 4:00 P.M.). After discussing Mary's and Daniel's health and giving Mary information on the well-baby clinic at the local health center, the nurse spoke briefly about family planning and asked Mary if she felt that this could be discussed with her husband. Mary agreed, although she did not seem sure about how her husband would react to a

woman talking to him about such an intimate subject. However, when Ms. Bell suggested that this might be a way to help both of them talk more directly about this delicate subject, she seemed to reconsider her previous hesitancy and said she thought it would be a good idea.

Before talking with the parents about family planning, Ms. Bell asked them for a brief health history of each of the children and was able to observe and elicit data related to parent–child relationships, parenting roles, and child rearing. She noted that Mary was very warm and cuddly with newborn Daniel. She held him close, handled him gently, and appeared relaxed and confident in his care and sensitive to his basic needs. Pat, in contrast, looked proudly at Daniel, but did not hold him, and according to Mary did not get involved in his physical care (nor did he with any of the other children when they were babies).

Both mother and father are warm, and Mary is physically quite affectionate with Richard, age three. She seemed quite indulgent with him, letting him "have his way" and giving him a lot of freedom to run around and play.

With the older children—Betty, four; Maureen, five; and Joseph, six—there was not the same permissiveness as observed with Richard. Mary said, "They are older and so need to be more responsible." All three older children were fairly quiet around the nurse. They spoke when spoken to, but otherwise talked quietly with each other or listened. Joseph is the mother's favorite, but both parents say he is too serious and has problems handling himself sometimes, becoming bossy and wanting to take over. Betty is the father's favorite, since she is petite, very sweet, and looks like Pat's mother.

The parents believe in children behaving and showing respect for their elders and carrying out their responsibilities, even if at these ages they are not much. The father spanks the children when they misbehave. He explained by saying, "None of these newfangled ideas about disciplining for us." It was noticed that children were asked to do several things—pick up the toys from the floor and help their mother. Both Maureen and Betty acted immediately, while Joseph ignored and then refused until his father yelled at him. No positive reinforcement followed when the children did obey. Maureen and Betty seemed pleased to have a new baby brother, while Richard is jealous of the baby and has been more demanding since the baby's arrival. The parents understand, though, that he feels displaced and jealous and that he needs more parental attention during this time. Joseph states he does not like the new baby. He rather unexpectedly explained his feelings by saying he did not like Daniel because the new baby made it hard for Mary and added, "Mama doesn't have enough money for food now." Mr. O'Shea looked shocked and sternly told Joseph that that was none of his business.

When asked about each of the children and what they were like, mother led the conversation and father started reading the paper, although he chimed in about Joseph and Betty. The descriptions follow in Table B.1.

The topic was then changed to family planning.

Nurse: Your wife mentioned that she did not want anymore children. How do you feel about that?

Pat: I was a little surprised she would bring this up with you, but since she did, I guess we can talk about it. I have

TABLE B.1
The O'Shea Parents' Descriptions of Their Children

	Mother's Description	Father's Description
Joseph, age 6½	He's a bright, independent child. Joseph is the leader of the children at home and school and likes to take over. I try to give him some responsibilities for caring for his sisters and brothers, but have to watch that he doesn't get too bossy. I'm able to talk to Joseph more than the other children. He's a sensitive child and listens to me. I know I'm a little protective of him, but that's just because we're so close to each other.	Joseph is always arguing and wanting his own way. My wife spoils him. He's going to grow up thinking he'll be the President by the time he's 35. He needs to be put in his place by my wife.
Maureen, age 5	Maureen is a helpful little girl who likes to help me. She is an easy child to raise. She's quiet, likes to play alone and doesn't cause any trouble. Maureen follows her brother Joseph all the time when they play together.	No comment.
Betty, age 4	Betty knows how to get people to like her. She's a "people pleaser"—can act cute and sweet when it is in her favor. She need special watching, however, as she can pull the wool over one's eyes very quickly with her sweet and cunning ways.	Father acts disgusted with his wife's statement and responds by saying: "That's not true. She is a sweet, affectionate little sweetheart. You're just jealous because we have a special relationship."
Richard, age 3	He's always into everything! Very active and inquisitive. I try to let him have a lot of freedom to run around in the house, otherwise he gets so bottled up that he shouts, screams, and makes the rest of us miserable.	No comment.

felt that my wife is taking things in her own hands—complaining all the time about her life and seeing her job as such a burden. My mother had seven children, and I never heard her complain. If the good Lord wants her to have more, then I think she'll just have to accept them and manage with what we have.

Nurse: Does that mean that religiously you're against any form of family planning?

Pat: Oh, I guess not, especially if Father O'Neal says it's okay, but I can't understand what all this unhappiness is all about. It seems that we're living on easy street compared to what my parents and hers had to go through. My wife listens to too much TV and hears too many tales from the neighbors and radio on what life is supposed to be like now.

Nurse: Yes, I understand that when you look back at your parents' life and your own, that it's apparent that you are, indeed, very fortunate. Bearing and raising children has never been an easy job. What do you think about that Mrs. O'Shea?

Mary: Pat ought to stay home one or two days—take over my jobs and see what raising kids is all about. You've never done that, Pat, and I bet you never will.

Pat: No, that's true. I'm not planning to stay home and find out either.

Nurse: What's the benefit of having more children if your wife feels it's so hard for her to manage now and further pregnancies are dangerous for her?

Pat: I didn't say I wanted anymore. I just said that she's pretty lucky and she doesn't know it. I suppose our family is big enough, but we can't depend on "Russian roulette," I mean the rhythm method, solving our problem.

Nurse: Do you understand the problem your wife has in having children now? I mean the hypertension during pregnancy which has grown worse with each succeeding pregnancy?

Pat: Not really. (Nurse explains the problem and how pregnancy makes problem worse.)

Ms. Bell then asks the spouses if they have discussed their problem or family planning methods with their priest and family doctor, and then suggest that they do this together, since neither priest nor doctor has been approached to discuss the problem in any depth. Nurse also explains fertility variations during woman's menstrual period and explains methods for detecting the safe and unsafe periods using the rhythm method.

THIRD HOME VISIT

As spouses relate to each other and the nurse, the nurse makes the following observations regarding Mr. O'Shea and the couple's relationship.

Mr. O'Shea seems easygoing, verbal, and quite a conversationalist—as long as he controls the flow. He likes to be the center of attention and loses interest if Mary is talking, in this case, jumping in to refocus attention on himself. He expresses an interest in getting some help for his wife from his mother, but feels that helping himself is "not his job." He says that Mary and his mother don't get along too well together, however, there being too much competition between the two of them. According to Mary, Pat's mother caused tremendous tension during their engagement and early years of marriage. She had bitter arguments with her husband about his mother, but as mother-in-law finally began to accept the reality of her son's marriage, their problems subsided.

In terms of the marital relationship, there was no expression of love or affection either physically or verbally. Their relationship was characterized by a lack of empathy or two-way communication between them. One received the impression that Mary was there to meet the needs of her husband, but that he had no similar responsibility to her. She was expected to serve him, care for the home and children, and manage with the limited funds he allotted to her weekly for groceries and other home and child expenses.

While the husband was present, Mary took little part in the discussions, except when asked direct questions. She acted very self-effacing and subservient in his presence, except when she voiced the opinion that he should spend two days with the children to see what it was really like.

Pat did communicate to the children that they should have respect for Mary—because she was their mother. However, in his own communications with her, he did not express very much respect. Most communications were in the form of commands, with few requests or room for feedback from wife. When Mary spoke to him, he seemed to tune her out. Most of the time he halfheartedly agreed that she was right and that he would follow through on such matters as on making appointments with the priest and the doctor, but would not do so.

Children and parents were quite talkative concerning the recent Thanksgiving holiday and other happy events. With pleasant subjects all of the family contributed verbally to family conversations, but unpleasant subjects or angry statements were cut off, such as Joseph's reaction to the new baby, or minimized, such as the mother's feelings of being burdened by too many children. It was also noted that children spoke directly to their mother, but only indirectly with their father. If they had a request, they would ask their mother to ask father for permission.

When asked what activities the family engaged in together, Mary reported that family visiting is the most popular and frequent activity. "Movies and eating out are beyond our reach. I like taking the kids to the park, but Patrick doesn't like coming. I go to Mass regularly and so does Pat. The kids go to Sunday School. We don't travel much—our close relatives live in town and we can't afford traveling much on Pat's salary. Pat's car isn't very dependable. Groceries, clothing, and the usual household items we buy at the shopping center. It's about a half-mile from here."

In terms of friendships, Mary states that she has old high school friends she still sees occasionally and that Pat sees his friends at sports events or the local tavern. But Pat and Mary have no couple friends with whom they engage in social activities.

Ms. Bell asked the couple how they liked the community. Both the parents related that this was the only community and neighborhood they had ever lived in and said, "We like it here. We know where everything is. All of the storekeepers and neighbors are old friends and acquaintances. Our only problem is that minorities are moving in close to here, and crime has risen quite a bit in the last several years." (Both are facts, although the relationship between them is less certain.)

The family, having lived in the community for many years, was familiar with the community agencies, health centers, and private doctors in town. Up until recently, they have used a nearby hospital for children's emergency care and a family doctor, a general practitioner, for all the health care that they needed, such as maternity and pediatric care. The parents do not go in for checkups (Pat never had as far as Mary knew), but Mary has had a physical with each pregnancy. Children are only seen when they are sick, with the exception of well-baby care at the health center when they were infants and for immunizations after infancy.

Two months ago, Pat received group medical insurance through his father's store (the father just arranged for it), so their choice of health care was expanded. The family doctor is an older physician whom the family has seen for years. His charges are very low, but Mary feels he is getting too old to keep up with all he needs to know. She used the county hospital to deliver Daniel, since they were not covered by medical insurance at that time and could not raise the money for a private hospital. Now they will have to pay the county back in small payments until their bill is taken care of.

Dental care for the family has been close to nonexistent. It is obtained at a private neighborhood dental clinic. The mother took Joseph in once when he complained of a toothache. One of his baby teeth had to be filled. The other children have not been seen. Pat and Mary go in when they have problems, and brush their teeth twice a day after meals. Mary is teaching Joseph to brush his teeth now, too.

When Ms. Bell did a nutritional survey of the family, she found that their diet consisted of a lot of starches; potatoes and breads primarily at every meal. Their diet was basically American, with certain Irish specialities made use of—stews and boiled dinners. The family made little use of fruit or fruit juices, except for bananas, apples, when in season, and canned peaches—and occasionally apple or orange juice. One vegetable, in addition to potatoes, was usually eaten with the evening meal and casseroles, stews, and processed food such as frozen dinners, pizza, and chicken pies were frequently served for dinner. Salads were infrequently eaten; soups were served about every other night, epecially in the colder months. The weights of the children were within normal limits, but both parents were 10 to 20 percent overweight (visually) for their frame and height. There were no food allergies among any of the family members, according to the mother.

Their diet for yesterday (excluding Daniel) was:

Breakfast   Cold cereal and whole milk
                 Toast—1 to 2 pieces for Joseph, Mary, and Pat
                 Coffee—2 cups (parents)

Snacks	Crackers for children (3 to 4 apiece) and milk
	Coffee—mother
Lunch	Soup (tomato)
	Dish of mashed potatoes and butter
	Canned peaches
	Milk
	(Husband and Joseph not home)
Snacks	None
Dinner	Stew with meat (½ lb.), carrots, potatoes, and celery
	White cake
	Milk—children
	Coffee—wife
	Beer—husband

Since having adequate money for food was mentioned as a monthly concern, Mary was asked whether she received food stamps. When she said she did not, information on the program was provided. The nurse also learned that the family had very little left over each month and that two years ago Pat borrowed $2,000 from his father to buy a used car (without Mary's knowledge) and still had not been able to pay his father back.

The family associates with several organizations in the community: the parish church and school primarily. The family can walk to both, since they are only five blocks away. The health department, the family doctor, and the family dental clinic are also visited. In addition, the taverns Pat frequents, the stores they shop in, and Pat's store (his father's grocery store) are all community places and people with whom friendly ties existed are visited daily or weekly. Mary makes all the contacts with church, school, dentist, and doctors. The family's relationships with church, teachers, doctor, health center, dentists, and emergency room seem to have been good. There is public transportation available when family needs it, but Mary drives Pat to work on days that she needs the car, since taking the children with her on the bus is not easy.

Stemming from Mary's extensive experience in raising children and taking them to doctors, she seems to have a good, basic understanding of how to handle common minor illness and injuries. She also is able to explain what to do when more serious injuries occur or symptoms appear. She uses over-the-counter medicines such as aspirin, Tylenol, first-aid medications, Sudafed, and milk of magnesia carefully and correctly and keeps medicines in a safe place out of the reach of the children.

Neither she or her husband watch their diet or weight or engage in regular exercise. Although she was never active (except doing housework), Pat was very active in sports until recently. For relaxation she watches TV and thinks her husband uses TV and socializing at the tavern as ways of relaxing.

Utilizing the form below, assess the O'Shea family. (Where information is not provided, leave blank or note that a lack of information exists.)

Two words of caution are called for before using the following guidelines in completing family assessments. First, not all areas included below will be germane in each of the families visited. The guidlines are comprehensive and allow depth when probing is necessary. However, the student should not feel that every subarea need be covered when the broad area of inquiry poses no problems to the family or concern to the health worker. Second, by virtue of the interdependence of the family system, one will find unavoidable redundancy. For the sake of efficiency, the assessor should try not to repeat data, but to refer back to sections where this information has been covered.

IDENTIFYING DATA

1. **Family Name**
2. **Address and Phone**
3. **Family Composition** (see Table C.1, p. 313)
4. **Type of Family Form**
5. **Cultural and Religious Orientation**
6. **Social Class Status**
7. **Social Class Mobility**
8. **Developmental History of Family** (optional)
9. **Family's Recreational or Leisure-Time Activities**

ENVIRONMENTAL DATA

10. **Home Characteristics**
11. **Characteristics of Neighborhood and Larger Community**
12. **Family's Geographic Mobility**
13. **Family's Associations and Transactions with Community**
14. **Family's Social Support Network**

FAMILY STRUCTURE

15. **Role Structure**
    Formal Role Structure
    Informal Role Structure
    Role Models (optional)
16. **Power Structure**
    Decision Making

TABLE C.1
Family Composition Form

Name (Last, First)	Sex	Relationship	Date/Place of Birth	Occupation	Education
1.					
2.					
3.					
4.					
5.					
6.					
7.					
8.					
9.					

Decision-Making Process
Bases for or Sources of Power
Variables Affecting Power
Overall Family Power

17. **Communication Patterns**
 Extent of Functional and Dysfunctional Communication (types of recurring patterns)
 Extent of Affective Messages and How Expressed
 Characteristics of Family Communication Network
 Areas of Closed Communication
 Familial and External Variables Affecting Communication

18. **Family Values:** Compare to American or family's influence group values and/or identify important family values and their importance (priority) in family.
 Are these values consciously or unconsciously held by the family?
 Presence of value conflicts in family.
 Effect of the above values and value conflicts on health status of family.

FAMILY FUNCTIONS

19. **Affective Function**
 Family's Need–Response Patterns
 Mutual Nurturance, Closeness, and Identification
 Separateness and Connectedness

20. **Socialization Function**
 Family Child-Rearing Practices
 Adaptability of Child-Rearing Practices for Family's Situation
 Who is (are) Socializing Agent(s) for Child(ren)?
 Value of Children in Family

21. **Health Care Function**
 Family's Definitions of Health/Illness and Their Level of Knowledge
 Family's Dietary Practices
 Adequacy of family diet (recommend 24-hour food history record).
 Function of mealtimes and attitudes toward food and mealtimes.
 Shopping (and its planning) practices.
 Person(s) responsible for planning, shopping, and preparation of meals.
 Sleeping and Resting Practices
 Exercise and Recreation Practices (not covered earlier)
 Family's Drug Habits
 Family's Self-Care Practices
 Family's Exposure to Environmental Hazards
 Medically Based Preventive Measures (physicals, eye and hearing tests, and immunizations)
 Dental Health Practices
 Family Medical History (both general and specific diseases—environmentally and genetically related)
 Health Services Received
 Perceptions Regarding Health Services
 Emergency Health Services
 Dental Health Services
 Source of Medical and Dental Payments
 Logistics of Receiving Care

22. **Family Coping Function**
 Short- and Long-Term Familial Stressors
 Family's Ability to Base Decisions on Objective Appraisal of Stress-Producing Situations
 Functional Coping Strategies Utilized (present/past)
 Dysfunctional Coping Strategies Utilized (present/past)

Assessment of the O'Shea Family

1. **Family Name:** O'Shea
2. **Address:** Maplewood district, New England city
3. **Family Composition:** See Table D.1 on page 315.
4. **Type of Family Form:** Nuclear
5. **Cultural and Religious Orientation:** The family is Irish-American and to a large extent unacculturated.[1-3] This conclusion derives from Mary's clearly stated ethnic and religious preferences; the fact that family's social network is from the same ethnic/religious group; family has resided in same ethnically homogeneous neighborhood for life; visits to extended family and church activities seem to be central activities for family; family roles and power structure are in keeping with traditional structures within Irish families; home decor lacking of much visual art and the presence of religious objects is indicative of culture and religious orientation; family stays primarily within ethnic neighborhood; family actively involved in Catholic religious practices and belief system: attend Mass regularly, consult priest on matters of importance, belief in family and children stressed.
6. **Social Class Status:** Father is sole breadwinner. Family sees income as marginal; nevertheless, it is steady. Based on the father's occupation, income (estimated only), and education of parents, family is part of working class.
7. **Social Class Mobility:** The parents of the O'Sheas were poor, and thus Pat feels he, Mary, and the children are more fortunate. In fact, however, the family's history does not indicate much, if any, upward mobility. Actually, with more children the standard of living within their own nuclear family has probably decreased.
8. **Developmental History of Family**
   Family's Present Developmental Stage: Family with school-aged children.
   Family's History: Parents both lived in same neighborhood and went to same church. Went together 5½ years before marriage. During engagement and early years of marriage, sex was an uncomfortable area and later awkward and unsatisfying, reported the wife. Wife feels this has created a lack of closeness between them. Both parents expected children and wanted them, with the exception of the last, which Mary did not want but now accepts warmly. Wife feels burden of so many children and that marital relationship has become distant.
   Parents' Families of Origin: Father's family: Father came over from Ireland as teenager. Worked for construction companies and saved his money until he could buy the grocery store he now has. Raised family in same neighborhood in a strict Catholic fashion. Mother's family:

TABLE D.1
O'Shea Family Composition

Name	Sex	Relationship	Age	Place of Birth	Occupation	Education
O'Shea, Patrick	M	Father	43 years	Maplewood district	Butcher	High school graduate
O'Shea, Mary	F	Mother	35	same	Housewife	High school graduate
O'Shea, Joseph	M	Son	6½	same	Student	In first grade
O'Shea, Maureen	F	Daughter	5	same	Student	In kindergarten
O'Shea, Betty	F	Daughter	4	same	—	—
O'Shea, Richard	M	Son	3	same	—	—
O'Shea, Daniel	M	Son	5-day-old infant	same	—	—

Her grandparents came over from Ireland during the depression for economic reasons. Raised as Catholic in same neighborhood as family now resides. Both Mary's and Pat's families were mentioned to be poor while they were growing up. No mention of what life with their respective families of origin was like.

9. **Family's Recreational Activities:** Whole family visits extended families together (their most frequent family activity). Parents and children (Joseph, Maureen, and Betty) go to Sunday school. Mother takes children to park to play. No travel, movies, or eating out because of finances and car's poor condition. Mary and Pat do not go out as couple by themselves or with friends.

10. **Home Characteristics:** Three-bedroom, older wooden house rented from cousin for $250 per month. Outside of house: fair condition, needs paint, loose stairs, and no outside lighting or railing present. Inside of house: minimally furnished. Living room has a color TV. Dining room has lace curtains and tablecloth, a wedding present from Mary's mother. Parents have own bedroom, presently shared with newborn who has a bassinet. The boys have one bedroom, while the girls share the other. Adequate sleeping arrangements in both. Minimal decorations: no pictures, plants, crafts seen, but several Catholic religious objects were noted. Kitchen contains small functioning refrigerator and stove. One bathroom with toilet and bathtub. Common towels used (dirty). Mary considers the house just adequate for their needs now, but becoming more crowded because of the new baby. Safety hazards: outside loose stairs, no railings or outside light.

11. **Characteristics of Neighborhood and Larger Community:** Neighborhood (Maplewood district) is residential and composed of Irish working-class families. Neighborhood is near industrial area and 5 miles from center of city of 300,000 located in New England. Family likes closeness and familiarity of neighborhood, though worried about influx of members of minority groups nearby and rise in crime in the past several years. Family uses nearby shopping center (half-mile away) for most of their shopping needs. Family's church and church school located five blocks away. Public transportation available, but Mary has access to husband's car when needed.

12. **Family's Geographic Mobility:** Family members have lived in the same community and neighborhood for all their lives.

13. **Family's Associations and Transactions with Community:** The family is known in parish church and school. Parents go to mass regularly and seem to have close trusting relationship with Father O'Neal. Women's group at church donated bassinet for new baby. Mother acts as liaison with school. Also relate to the family doctor (although Mary wants to change physicians), family dental clinic, and children's hospital emergency room. In addition to receiving community health nursing visits, mother has taken children to well-baby clinic and for immunizations at the local health department.

Family's Territorial Cluster and Complex: Family's territorial cluster appears to be church, school, shopping center, husband's store, and perhaps extended family's homes, who also live in same neighborhood. Territorial complex is constricted, and members seem to stay primarily within their neighborhood. Family not aware of food stamp program (which was explained to Mary).

14. **Family's Social Support Network**
Informal Systems
Family, especially parents on both sides and mother's sister, seem to be quite helpful. Pat's father employs son in his grocery store as butcher and loaned him $2,000 for the purchase of a car. Pat's mother helped with housework and children when Mary came home from hospital. (Although relations with wife were conflictual during early days of marriage, they are improved but still competitive according to Pat.) Mary's mother also helped with house and children after Mary returned from hospital and Mary's sister went shopping for her. In addition to her sister, Mary has neighbors she talks to sometimes about her problems. And Pat has his buddies

at the tavern that he relates to frequently (the degree of their support is unknown, however).

Formal Systems

Priest, doctor (?), community health nurse, teachers (?) have substantial ties with family.

FAMILY STRUCTURE

15. Role Structure

Formal Role Structure

Pat: Father and husband. He acts as sole provider for family, and is leader of family. Does not see his position as involving a companionship, recreational, or therapeutic role, however, and only occasionally does he help with the child-care role (when he feels like it). Marital roles enacted, although constricted, appear consistent with his expectations of marital roles.

Mary: Mother and wife. She acts as the homemaker (not shared), involving cooking, shopping, and cleaning home; enacts the child-care role (not shared to any real extent); the recreational role (taking children to park to play). No therapeutic role or companion role enacted in marriage. Sexual role inadequately performed. Wife has expressed disappointment that the therapeutic role is not present and that the sexual role is inadequate (distant communications, no enjoyment in sexual relationship). Wife appears to have some expectations of Pat which are more consistent with American middle-class ideals of marriage, although she seems also resigned to the fact that Pat's traditional expectations of both of their positions in the family are fairly stable and not likely to be changed. She enacts the roles needed to complement husband's role expectations of her, while at the same time trying to limit her family roles in future to some extent by having no more children. Mary definitely shows some role strain in trying to handle child care and all the other mother-wife roles by herself.

Joseph: Older son and brother to siblings.

Maureen: Older daughter and sister to siblings.

Betty: Younger daughter and sister to siblings.

Richard: Younger son and brother to siblings.

Daniel: Youngest (baby) son and brother to siblings.

Informal Role Structure

Pat: Leader; distant one (does not get involved in family life); irresponsible one (does wife see him in this way or is this the way she expects husbands to act?)

Mary: Subservient one; go-between role (between children and their father); martyr?

Joseph: Leader of the children, mother's favorite and perhaps confidant, since mother cannot confide in and share affectively with husband. Serious one.

Maureen: Cooperative, compliant one. Follower.

Betty: Sweet one. "People-pleaser" role. Mother perceives her to play cute, manipulative role, whereas father defends her sweetness as being genuine and not manipulative. Father's favorite. Mary is perhaps threatened by husband's affections toward Betty.

Richard: Active one (with explosive temper if exploration and freedom are restricted).

Daniel: No comments by parents.

Purpose of Informal Roles: Mother's and father's informal roles go along with culturally patterned formal roles associated with their formal positions. The roles of Joseph and Betty (the parents' favorites) are possibly due to the fact that the marital relationship is not adequate affectively, and so Joseph and Betty become displaced objects of affection for the mates.

Role Models: Not discussed.

16. Power Structure

Decision Making

Husband decides major purchases (car, for example).

Wife is delegated (or relegated) sole roles of housekeeper, child rearer, and allotted a certain portion of paycheck to cover home and family expenses.

Husband in charge of distribution of funds.

Husband in charge of calling priest and doctor to initiate appointment with them.

Decision-Making Process: Husband uses his formal position of dominance to influence family decisions. Process used is accommodation. He seemed to be compromising with wife, under pressure of community health nurse when he agreed to discuss family planning health problem with priest and doctor and attempt to come up with an effective plan to prevent further pregnancies; but since he has not followed through in making appointments, one can question his sincerity in this case. May use de facto process in these cases; by doing nothing he has made the decision.

Bases for or Sources of Power: Father-husband maintains legitimate power or authority, granted to him culturally by virtue of his position in family. Mother has referent power (position of mother is exalted in the Catholic Church), which is more salient in her relationships with her children than it is in her relationship with her husband. Both parents have reward and coercive power over children, and husband has reward/coercive power over his wife, although no description of his using this is evident.

Variables Affecting Family Power Characteristics: Wife's position as go-between in family communication network and as implementer of family decisions should give her increased power; there is no evidence that it is being exercised, however.

Interpersonal Resources: The wife's hesitancy and fear to speak out more often and confront husband reduces what power she does/could have.

Social class/cultural and life cycle factors: Marital expectations which are commonly found in working class predominate. These same marital and family role and power expectations are characteristic of traditional Irish family life. Life cycle of family reduces wife's power and increases husband's power, since wife is burdened with day-to-day household and child-care responsibilities and has no time or energy to exercise whatever influence/power she has.

Overall family power:

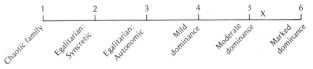

1	2	3	4	5	6
Chaotic family	Egalitarian: Syncretic	Egalitarian: Autonomic	Mild dominance	Moderate dominance	Marked dominance

Overall Family Power

Moderate dominance seen (father dominant), with some dissatisfaction of this situation expressed by wife.

17. **Communication Patterns**

Extent of Functional and Dysfunctional Communication (types of recurring patterns):

Dysfunctional communication used between husband and wife.

a. Husband gives commands and makes requests without leaving room for feedback.

b. Wife voices problems and husband minimizes them (does not validate or accept that her problems are real).

c. Wife voices concerns or asks husband's assistance, but he tunes her out, walks away, belittles her ("without children what would you do, open your own business"), or agrees with her and says he'll follow through, but does not (incongruency). Thus, Pat does not listen to Mary when she is communicating her needs to him.

d. Mary, in turn, does not express herself in some intimate areas due to cultural values and, possibly, fear of rejection. She probably does not directly express her needs in many areas.

e. Neither partner states needs and feelings clearly, except in case of Mary's expressed desire to curtail pregnancies.

f. Rules underlying communication patterns include the following: (1) don't question the status quo and tradition; (2) things are the way they are and complaining won't help or change things (powerless, fatalistic outlook); (3) closeness—husband doesn't want wife becoming exposed to any outside influences.

Extent of Affective Messages and How Expressed: Affective messages are not expressed openly (or privately according to Mary) between spouses. Mary is warm and affectively responsive to Daniel and Richard. She is also verbally warm and close to son Joseph. Father is verbally (and physically?) affectionate to daughter Betty. Pleasant emotions are more openly expressed, whereas negative emotions (anger, unpleasant events) are inhibited. Evidently, family rules exist which prohibit expression of these emotions.

Characteristics of Family Communication Network: Children make requests of father through mother. Little direct involvement and communication between father and children (except Betty–father relationship). Quality of communication between spouses poor. Limited in scope (mainly regarding children and money problems) and quality (see dysfunctional patterns). Interactions are distant and unsatisfying to wife.

Areas of Closed Communications: Between spouses: inner feelings and perceptions, especially sexual feelings and thoughts.

Familial and External Variables Affecting Communication: Cultural variables are important for this family. Men and women live in different worlds in traditional Irish culture. Roles and worlds are separate, and sexes never learn to communicate adequately with each other. Nor is expression of affection or warmth toward spouse seen as acceptable in public. Sex is riddled with guilt and ignorance, making it difficult for Irish couples to generate and retain close affective bonds. Socioeconomic stressors (marginal incomes and economic hardships) make family role enactment, housing, and fulfilling of family functions more onerous.

18. **Family's Values:** In comparing the O'Sheas' values with American and traditional Irish and Irish-American values, the O'Sheas' values are definitely much more in keeping with the traditional Irish values and the working-class values of today. Productivity and success are not primary values. Pat has worked for his father since graduation from high school, except for time he was in the Armed Services. Mary worked in dime store after graduation and until the first child was born. The work ethic and materialism do not seem central in family's life. The family does not value individualism, but the ethic of reciprocity (assisting one's extended family and church) is salient, as is the value of doing one's duty and playing expected family roles (conformity). Education is not highly valued, nor is progress, change, and mastery; conservatism and fatalistic thinking assume greater importance. No long-term plans were expressed, except Mary's ardent plans to prevent further pregnancies. Equality and individual freedom are not inferred to be important values either. The "doing orientation" does not fit this family. Time is not carefully allotted and used. Much time of Pat's is spent in recreational pursuits (spectator sports and social drinking with friends). Health care and practices are not of prime importance to family.

There appears to be a conflict in values, to some degree, between Mr. and Mrs. O'Shea. Mary obviously feels caught between the values of American society and those of traditional Irish culture which govern family roles, power relationships, and communication. She is trying—not very effectively—to assert herself with her husband, demonstrating the value of democracy-egalitarianism, rationality, and perhaps individualism and progress. Pat retains the old traditional values, as stated above. This directly affects the health status of the family, by creating strain in the marital relationship.

19. **Affective Function**

Need–Response Patterns

Pat: For the most part, he does not make any of his socio-emotional needs known to his wife or children; therefore, they are presumably not adequately met in family. (Perhaps his needs are met through work and socializing with buddies at sports events and tavern). He does, however, make his needs for affection and warmth known to daughter Betty, who responds in a sweet, affectionate manner toward him.

Mary: Expressed problem of not being able to talk to husband or feel emotionally close to him. He does not respond to her needs to communicate and does not empathize with her feelings regarding the responsibilities she assumes. Her son Joseph meets some of her socio-emotional needs, since she feels she can talk to him, whereas Pat is not available to meet her needs.

Joseph (age 6½): Has need to handle things, lead, and be assertive. His mother gives him this opportunity, Pat feels his son's behavior is inappropriate and feels he should be put in his place. The younger children follow him. Becomes rebellious or bossy when his needs to be assertive are frustrated.

Maureen (age 5): Expresses need to cooperate with and help her mother; emulates mother's behavior and roles. Mary gives her the opportunity to fulfill these needs.

Betty (age 4): Expresses need to please people and be liked. Mother sees this as a way to "get her way" (a form of manipulation). Father sees this need as genuine, and she is his favorite. He responds to Betty's sweetness, reinforcing her behavior and needs to please.

Richard (age 3): Richard has a need to explore and be autonomous. Mary realizes this and responds by letting him run around the house and explore. Also has need for extra attention because of arrival of new baby, which parents understand and are responding to.

Daniel (age 1 to 3 weeks): Needs to trust and have his basic physiological and affectional needs met. These are being fulfilled ably by the mother.

Mutual Nurturance, Closeness, and Identification: Adequate between mother and Joseph, Maureen, Richard, and Daniel.

Maybe attenuated between Mary and Betty, since Mary may feel threatened by her hsuband's favoritism and diversion of affections to Betty.

Adequate between father and Betty and father and Richard (?). Remainder of father's relationships with children are distant, and he is relatively uninvolved.

Inadequate between Mary and Pat. Mutual identification involving closeness and nurturance are weak, hence spousal bonds are weak also. She expresses need for greater closeness, whereas he does not express these needs.

Separateness and Connectedness: Not discussed here to any extent. It will become an issue with Joseph soon, since he is assertive, has leadership qualities and needs, and will increasingly wish to individuate. At present conformity and connectedness are valued much more highly than separateness.

20. **Socialization Function**

Family Child-rearing Practices: Observations limited. Pat advocated old-fashioned child rearing, not new-fangled methods. Believes in punishment, respect, and obedience. However, he has a minimal role in implementation, so that Mary may undermine some of his wishes regarding child rearing. From their behavior the children show they have been taught that "children should be seen but not heard" when adults are talking. Mary is very warm and physically affectionate, permissive, and tolerant when children are younger, but when they become pre-schoolers (age 4 up), she and Pat expect more self-restraint, self-discipline, respect, and obedience. Also could be seen that boys are allowed to be more assertive and aggressive than the girls of family (sex-linked socialization practices are evident).

Adaptibility of Child-rearing Practices for Family's Situation: They appear adaptive in that children are being raised to live in the world as the parents see and experience it. This involves the need to be respectful, obedient, and conformist, and for boys and girls to know their appropriate sex roles and behavior.

Who Is the Socializing Agent? Mother, almost exclusively. School (Catholic) teachers and priest, in addition to kin, are also socializing agents in children's lives and will become increasingly important as the children age.

Value of Children in Family: They were wanted and accepted. Children appear to be highly valued. Children are highly cherished in the Catholic religion and Irish-American families. Being a mother is the central role for Mary.

21. **Health Care Function**

Family's Definition of Health/Illness and Level of Knowledge: Preventive care for children (except for immunizations) is not given; mother did receive physicals with each pregnancy, hence her definition of health and illness is more enlightened than the husband's if his health-seeking behavior is indicative. Taking children and herself to receive medical care when they are not visually ill means that she acknowledges that health is more than just being able to function or a state of feeling well.

Wife is health leader and decides when children are ill and in need of medical services.

Mother has good basic understanding of how to handle common minor illnesses and injuries. She also knows what to do when more serious injuries occur or symptoms appear.

Family Dietary Practices: Adequacy of family diet: From data regarding the family the information was inserted into a food history record (Table D.2) to the extent possible.

Caloric Intake: Adequate, although husband and wife are a little overweight (children's weight is within normal limits). Data obtained via visual inspection only. Cultural food assessment: Stews and boiled dinners prepared. Extensive use of potatoes (the Irish staple); otherwise diet is basically American.

Typicality of 24-hour Diet: This report is typical. Mary said that their diet contains little fruit or fruit juices, except for bananas, apples (in season), and canned peaches— and occasionally apple or orange juice. One cooked vegetable besides potatoes is served at dinner each evening. Soups are eaten three to four times per week; salads are infrequently eaten.

Food Allergies: None noted.

Function of mealtimes and their attitudes toward food and mealtime: Not noted.

Shopping practices and person responsible: Mary goes to nearby shopping center. She has budgetary limitations and just barely gets by each month. She does not use food stamps but is interested in applying to obtain them.

Refrigerator and Stove: Functioning and adequate, though small. Wife is totally responsible for planning, shopping, and preparation of meals.

Sleeping and Rest Practices: Sleeping patterns not noted. Mary stated she used TV for relaxing and that Pat does same, in addition to going over to tavern to socialize and drink for the purposes of relaxation.

Exercise and Recreational Practices: Parents do not have regular exercise program for themselves. It is not mentioned as to whether they believe this is a necessity for health maintenance. Wife gets a moderate amount of

TABLE D.2
Family Food History Record

Meal	Food Served	Quantity	Individual Differences
Breakfast	Cold cereal	1 bowl	All family ate cereal
	Milk	½ cup for cereal	
	Toast, 1–2 pieces		Parents only
	Coffee	1 cup	Parents
	Milk	1 cup	Children
Snacks	Crackers	3–4 crackers	Children
	Milk	1 glass	
	Coffee	1 cup	Mother
Lunch	Tomato soup	1 bowl	Joseph, Maureen, and father not home.
	Mashed potatoes	½–1 cup	
	and butter	1 tbsp.	
	Canned peaches	½ cup	
	Milk	1 cup	
Snacks	None		
Dinner	Stew: containing		All ate stew, but children had smaller servings.
	meat	¼ cup	
	carrots	½ cup	
	potatoes	½ cup	
	celery	¼ cup	
	White cake	1 slice	All family
	Milk	1 cup	Children
	Coffee	1 cup	Wife
	Beer	1 cup	Husband
Snacks	None		

exercise doing housework and child-care activities. Husband used to be active in sports but is not presently. He stands at his job (as butcher).

Family's Drug Habits: Husband drinks alcohol (type and amount unknown); socializing at taverns is a frequent and central activity for him.

Both parents drink coffee (2 to 3 cups per day noted). Tobacco use not noted.

It is not mentioned whether use of tobacco or alcohol is considered a problem.

Family's use of prescription and over-the-counter drugs: Use of prescription drugs not noted.

Use of over-the-counter drugs directed by Mary. She uses cold medicines (Sudafed, etc.), gastrointestinal medicines (milk of magnesia, etc.), first-aid medications, and aspirin correctly and carefully. She also stores medicines in a safe cabinet away from children's reach.

Family's Self-Care Practices: See prior comments. Also administers medications carefully and correctly.

Environmental Exposure to Air and Noise Pollution: Not noted. Family lives close to industrial area, however, where a number of factories are located.

Use of common towels in bathroom may be potential source of spread of communicable disease. No other cleanliness problems noted.

Medically Based Preventive Measures: Children (except when infants) and adults do not have periodic physical examinations.

No information on recency or on vision/hearing examinations or immunization status of family members.

Dental Health Practices: Nutritional: breads and some desserts noted in diet. No candy noted.

Brushing teeth: Parents brush teeth two times a day after meals. Joseph is being taught to brush teeth. Other children have not started brushing teeth yet.

Use of flouride: Not mentioned.

Dental check-ups and cleanings: Not done.

Family Medical History: No information included.

Health Services Received: Receive pediatric and maternity services from family doctor. Last baby, Daniel, delivered at county hospital because family could not raise necessary funds for private hospital and did not have health insurance at the time. They are now covered by husband's employment, however. Receive well-baby care and immunizations through health department. Pat had never been seen by doctor for physical examinations to Mary's knowledge.

Perceptions/Feelings Regarding Health Care: Family physician (long-time family doctor) is liked, but since family has medical insurance now, Mary would like to switch doctors. Stayed with above physician because his rates were low; but he is old, and Mary is afraid he is not up-to-date in his practice.

No comments regarding health department services or dental services.

Emergency Health Services: Family uses children's hospital in community when emergency care is needed for children. No mention of where parents go or would go if emergency arose.

Dental Health Services: Family visits family dental clinic in neighborhood when dental problems arise. Joseph has had one cavity filled (baby tooth). Parents have been to dentist on a problem basis only. No regular checkups or cleanings. Chidren other than Joseph have not been seen by dentist.

Source of Payment: Family has had to assume total expense of medical and dental care up to now. Recently received group health insurance through Pat's father's business (the grocery store). No dental insurance mentioned. Provisions of health insurance not known.

Logistics of Receiving Care: No problems noted. Care has been accessible and mother has car for transportation.

22. **Family Coping Function**

Short-term Stressors

1. Recent addition to family (Daniel), causing need to reallocate resources and relationships in family.
2. Wife's potential to become pregnant again (lack of family planning).
3. Richard's sibling rivalry and acting-out behaviors, although this does not seem to be a serious stressor.
4. Role overload and strain experienced by mother due to the arrival of another baby and heavy household and child-care responsibilities.

Long-term Stressors

1. Economic: Marginally adequate income ("barely gets by every month") and two outstanding debts to pay off: car and hospital bills. With new baby and inflation, economic problems may increase.
2. Marital: Lack of communication between husband and wife.
3. Role strain of wife (role overload). Mary's role strain appears not to be recognized as burden by Pat and is minimized as a problem within their cultural/religous orientation.
4. Threat of future pregnancies (short- and long-term stressor).
5. Value conflicts between Irish-American subculture and American majority culture.

Strengths which Counterbalance Stressors: Family has several strong assets which counterbalance to a moderate extent the above family stressors:

1. Husband's steady job (stable provider).
2. Permanency of residence. Family knows neighborhood and community, familiar with resources. They like neighborhood's cohesiveness and are well integrated into neighborhood.
3. Social support system of family is strong. Extended family present and assistance available and utilized. Also, neighbors and friends were mentioned as helpful. Church and church school are important resources to family.
4. Health status of family members appears adequate to good with no obvious problems except Mary's hypertension during pregnancies mentioned.
5. Adequate housing and furnishings at present.
6. Adequate health care (except preventive), nutritional practices, and health resources (health services and insurance).

Family's Ability to Base Decisions on Objective Appraisal of Stress-Producing Situation: Role overload (role strain) experienced by Mary and her expressed need to prevent further pregnancies are the two stress-producing situations occurring during nurse's visits. Mrs. O'Shea seems to be able to appraise situations realistically, but Pat denies the significance of her concerns and strains. As a family they have not taken action yet, since Mr. O'Shea was supposed to call the priest and doctor for appointments but has neglected to do so. As a family, parents have not worked together to appraise problems objectively and solve them.

Functional Coping Strategies Utilized (Present and Past): The family uses their social support system of extended family and church primarily to assist them in time of need. Inner coping resources are not mentioned as means for dealing with stressors. The family is able to meet the usual stresses and strains of daily life, largely through the efforts of Mary, who is the central figure in the family.

Dysfunctional Coping Strategies Utilized (Past and Present): First, the family does not use its inner resources adequately to deal with stressors. There is no "pulling together," increased cohesiveness, or sharing of feelings and thoughts, during periods of greater demand. Pat goes his own way rather than pitching in as part of the family team. The more overt dysfunctional coping mechanism which can be identified is that of authoritarianism, coupled with an element of neglect. Interestingly enough, this pattern is an exaggeration of the traditional Irish or Irish-American pattern. The stance may be taken that Pat uses his position of dominance too extensively, however, since through his authoritarianism and neglect (his minimal involvement with family life) he stifles the growth and quality of their marital relationship, as well as reduces the quality of his relationship with his children (except with Betty). Mild dominance, where feelings and input are solicited and received from family members, especially the wife, is not detrimental, but the pattern observed in this case study affects the family unit, its subsystems, and the individual family members adversely (see Table D.3).

Other Family Nursing Diagnoses Generated from O'Shea Assessment

Father–child relationships weak (except for Betty).

Nutritional deficiencies: insufficient use of vegetables and fruits, especially ones containing vitamin C; lack of sufficient iron in diet.

Inadequate dental hygiene and care: brushing for Maureen and Betty; examinations for whole family.

Hygiene problem with use of common towels.

Lack of exercise program of the spouses.

Home safety hazards: no lighting or railings on outside steps. Stair boards loose.

Further Assessment Data Needed

Provisions within health insurance.

Family's knowledge regarding how to locate another family physician.

Family's knowledge of accessible emergency rooms for adults.

TABLE D.3
Family Nursing Care Plan and Further Assessment Needed

Family Nursing Diagnoses Including Major Variables	Signs and Symptoms (Behavioral Manifestations)	Further Assessment Data Needed	Goals*	Intervention	Evaluation
1. Weak Spousal Subsystem (marital roles inadequate)	No companion role present (couple does not do things together).	Do spouses wish to do leisure-time activities together?	**Short-term:** Spouses will be able to discuss their relationship and whether they feel they need to strengthen certain aspects of marriage.	**Modifying Behavior:** Encourage couple to discuss their communication difficulties—not listening to each other, etc.	To be completed after intervention. Would look at goals to determine to what degree these have been achieved.
Variables Cultural and religious values and norms regarding marital roles and adult roles for women and men.	Therapeutic role inadequate. Husband does not listen to wife's concerns. Lack of communication except for money and children problems.	Does husband feel there is a problem with communication?	**Long-term:** Spousal relationship (subsystem) will be strengthened, by enlarging number of roles involved in marital positions (companion, therapeutic, and perhaps sexual) and improving communications.	Assist wife in explaining to husband areas of concern in their relationship—facilitating communication of stressful areas.	
	Sexual roles unsatisfying to wife.	Does husband feel that sexual roles are problems and an area to improve? Would wife feel this is an area she would be too embarrassed to have discussed?		Ask questions which will help couple look at marital relationship and whether they are satisfied with it and help them problem solve to identify ways of enriching and strengthening relationship in a direction they feel comfortable with (such as engaging in social recreational activities together and sharing certain responsibilities).	
Life cycle of family: high demands being placed on both parents at this stage of family's life.	Mates do not "pull together" (become cohesive and reliant on own resources during periods of high demand of family).	Assess couple's, especially husband's, willingness and readiness to explore ways of strengthening marital relationship.		**Variables:** Suggest they discuss family/marriage with priest. See if couple can obtain new, enlightened information and guidance on family and marriage.	

TABLE D.3
Family Nursing Care Plan and Further Assessment Needed (cont.)

Family Nursing Diagnoses Including Major Variables	Signs and Symptoms (Behavioral Manifestations)	Further Assessment Data Needed	Goals*	Intervention	Evaluation
Socioeconomic position: marginal income, limited education, constricted world.				Socioeconomic: Refer to food stamp program.	To be completed after intervention. Would look at goals to determine to what degree these have been achieved.
2. Family Planning Problem	Further pregnancies harmful to mother's health.	How do priest and doctor feel about family planning for couple?	Short-term: Couple will be knowledgeable about the types of family planning methods available and acceptable to them (within their cultural/religious belief system).	Help couple explore feelings and thoughts regarding limiting family, effects of future children on family, risks to wife's health when pregnant, burden of more children economically and in terms of child rearing.	
Variables History of high fertility—pregnancies every year. Wife's hypertension during pregnancies.	Mother does not want more children—strain on herself, budget, housing, etc.	What is couple's relationship with priest and physician? Are they the most appropriate resources?	Couple will be able to explore their thoughts and feelings regarding having no more children and why.	Assist couple to problem solve in making and carrying out decision in this area (resources, who will follow up with contacting them, etc.)	
Cultural/religious influences on family planning.	Family planning methods inadequate (not a problem at present, but will be soon).		Long-term: Couple will successfully use family planning method(s) to prevent further pregnancies.	Refer family to religious and health resources (if needed) as part of problem-solving process.	
Weak spousal relationship (lack of spousal communication—Diagnosis 1).	Husband is not sufficiently empathetic with wife's concerns regarding having no more children.			Follow-through with spouses after they have met with priest and doctor, to discuss any questions, thoughts, or areas where further information is needed, making sure they have full knowledge about whatever family planning means advised is thoroughly understood.	

* These goals would need to be validated with family/spouses.

Eye/hearing examinations and immunization status of family members.
Family medical history.

Roles: role models of parents
Environmental exposure to pollutants from industrial area nearby.

REFERENCES

1. Connery DS: The Irish. New York, Simon & Schuster, 1968
2. Bestic A: The Importance of Being Irish. New York, Morrow, 1969
3. Shannon WV: The American Irish. New York, Macmillan, 1963

Index